Genoderms Made Ludicrously Easy
A Visual and Mnemonic Guide to Genodermatoses

Justin Finch, MD
and
Michael Payette, MD, MBA

JOURNAL OF DRUGS IN DERMATOLOGY

JDD
DRUGS • DEVICES • METHODS

The publishers of this guide will use reasonable efforts to include up-to-date and accurate information on this guide, but make no representations, warranties, or assurances as to the accuracy, currency, or completeness of the information provided. The publishers of this guide shall not be liable for any damages or injury resulting from your access to this guide, or from your reliance on any information provided in this guide. This guide is intended for U.S physicians only and is not in any means intended for use by the general public.

The author has worked to ensure that all information in this book is accurate as of the time of publication and consistent with standards of good practice in the general management community. As research and practice advance, however, standards may change. For this reason, it is recommended that readers evaluate the applicability of any recommendations in light of particular situations and changing standards.

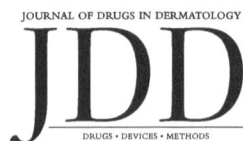

JOURNAL OF DRUGS IN DERMATOLOGY

JDD

DRUGS • DEVICES • METHODS

ISBN **978-0-9911919-8-7**

©2018 Published by *Journal of Drugs in Dermatology*
Written by Justin Finch, MD and Michael Payette, MD, MBA

Revised November, 2018
All images ©2012 Justin Finch

Foreword

We completed our dermatology residencies at the University of Connecticut School of Medicine in 2012. During our training together, we found the topic of genodermatoses to be particularly challenging–more like frustrating. Like the origin of many great ideas, however, the inspiration for this book was born at a bar over a couple of beers. Rather than try to actually memorize the seemingly endless list of genodermatoses and their myriad of associations, we began drawing funny cartoons. One cartoon turned into another…and then another. Soon we were creating lists of mnemonics for genoderms followed by more drawings, followed by searching for more genoderms. The original set of notes was only a couple dozen pages long, but it was a huge hit with our co-residents and faculty. After a few years of continuous updates, the idea to turn it into a book was born.

The title for the book, *Genoderms Made Ludicrously Easy*, was a combination of two experiences–medical school review books and the 1987 film, *Space Balls*. You may remember the *Ridiculously Easy* series of books to help medical students learn challenging topics and study for boards–maybe you even used them. And hopefully you have seen *Space Balls*, particularly the memorable discussion between Colonel Sandurz and Dark Helmet:

Col. Sandurz: "Prepare ship for light speed!"

Dark Helmet: "No, no, no, light speed is too slow!"

Col. Sandurz: "Light speed, too slow?!"

Dark Helmet: "Yes, we're gonna have to go right to…ludicrous speed!"

Col. Sandurz: "Ludicrous speed?! Sir, we've never gone that fast before. I don't know if the ship can take it."

Well, for anyone studying dermatology, light speed is too slow. You need ludicrous speed, especially when cramming for preposterous tests full of endless minutia. And for the subject of genodermatoses, the epitome of such topics, we created *Genoderms Made Ludicrously Easy*. We hope that you will find this book a complete reference for the majority of genodermatoses that have cutaneous symptoms, like we did. More importantly, we hope its light-hearted tone and memorable cartoons will help you learn and remember the important genoderms you'll need to know to be successful on the boards and even more so, to master dermatology.

Justin Finch, MD
Michael Payette, MD, MBA

Special thanks for contributions to the book include the following individuals:

Kristin Torre: for your meticulous attention to detail and text contributions

Fludiona Naka: for your work on obtaining patient consent

Amy Finch: for your cartoons and support

How to Use the Book

Genoderms Made Ludicrously Easy is designed to be a complete guide for the majority of genetic diseases that have cutaneous symptoms. It is organized into sections based on the primary phenotypic disorder of the genodermatoses (e.g. disorders of cornification, photosensitivity, malignant potential, etc.). Each syndrome discussed includes the name, common eponyms (if relevant), the inheritance pattern, the gene mutation, and the protein involved. Important clinical presentations, associations, lab abnormalities, and in some cases treatments are also included.

For many of the mnemonics, cartoons accompany the text, highlighting the salient features of the genoderm and serving as visual mnemonics to aid in the memorization of the disease. The visual mnemonics vary in degree of vulgarity, as we find that the more outrageous the mnemonic, the better it sticks in memory (think of how you learned the cranial nerves in medical school!).

There are also many clinical photos from our dermatology practice for which we are very grateful to have had the opportunity to meet these individuals, and for which we are even more grateful that they were willing to share their images for this book.

The book concludes with a series of tables and lists, which despite being quite ridiculous and preposterous, do serve as a succinct summary of the genodermatoses based on the primary phenotypic disorder. The two 17-page ludicrous tables at the very end serve as a quick reference for easy lookup. The first table is sorted alphabetically by genoderm name and the second is sorted alphabetically by gene.

This book is formatted for easy reference and maximum retention. The styles below will appear throughout the text to aid in your study. Each style has a specific purpose, and styles are formatted consistently throughout the book for at-a-glance recognition.

Dark Blue Shade – Genetic Diseases

- **Lamellar Ichthyosis**

Light Blue Shade – Non-Genetic Diseases

- Abs = Dermatitis Herpetiformis (along with Abs to gliadin, gliadin-TGase2 complexes, and TGase2)

Italicized – Gene Names

- e.g. defects in *TGM1* (Transglutaminase 1), *ABCA12, or CYP4F22* can all result in the phenotype Lamellar Ichthyosis

Blue Italicized - Genetic Diseases Without Prominent Dermatologic Manifestations

- *Muscular Dystrophy*
- *Meesmann Corneal Dystrophy*

Bold – High Yield (boards fodder)

- Mutated in several **ectodermal dysplasias**

Underlined – Disease Subtypes That Fall Within a Broader Category of Genetic Disease

- Leukocyte Adhesion Deficiency 1, Leukocyte Adhesion Deficiency 2, and Leukocyte Adhesion Deficiency 3

Common Abbreviations

- M.C. = most common
- Tx = treatment

Tips

Tip boxes offer relevant information and helpful pointers to the presented information. Tips are usually found alongside or directly under the related text.

> **Think "Plakoglobin is globally present" to remember that plakoglobin is the only protein present in both adherens *and* desmosomes.**

Mnemonic Boxes

All mnemonics are formatted similarly in these boxes, and can be easily identified on each page for easy scanning and quick study drills.

> ### *Refsum Syndrome*
>
> Picture a Referee holding salt/pepper shakers (salt and pepper retinitis pigmentosa), heart in a block on his shirt (heart block, arrhythmias), leaning on table (ataxia), X's over his ears (deafness), and an X over a head of broccoli (AR, PAHX encodes phytanoyl-CoA hydroxylase which is in peroxisomes = can't break down phytanic acid in veggies and fats). Also think "refereeing a fight" (phyte) to remember phytanoyl enzyme

Visual Mnemonic Boxes

The mnemonic cartoons add the potency of extra retention to help memorize the disease. Many are comical to visualize, because funny or peculiar things are harder to forget!

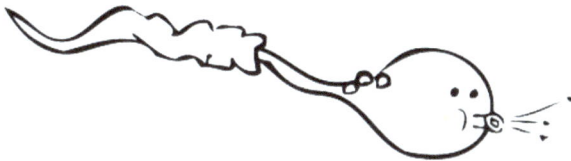

Mnemonic 4: Ichthyosis Bullosa of Siemens

Picture a molting sperm (siemen) with blisters, spitting "ktooey" (K2e)

Contents

1. Introduction to Genetics

Overview

- Human genome contains ~35,000 genes
- 46 chromosomes
  - 22 pairs of autosomes + 1 pair of sex chromosomes (XX in females and XY in males)
- Each chromosome is divided by centromere into short arm (p, petit) and long arm (q)
- Telomere = repetitions of **TTAGGG** sequences at the chromosome ends. Maintain chromosomal integrity
- Allelic Heterogeneity = when different disease phenotypes can result from defects in the same gene
  - e.g. mutations in *GJB2* gene that encodes connexin 26 can cause **KID**, **Vohwinkel**, or **Bart-Pumphrey Syndrome**
- Genetic Heterogeneity / Locus Heterogeneity = when defects in different genes can result in the same disease phenotype
  - e.g. defects in *TGM1* (Transglutaminase 1), *ABCA12, or CYP4F22* can all result in the phenotype **Lamellar Ichthyosis**

Mendelian Inheritance Patterns

- Autosomal Dominant (AD) inheritance
- Autosomal Recessive (AR) inheritance
- X-Linked Dominant (XLD) inheritance
  - (See mnemonic)
  - Frequently lethal in-utero to males, only manifesting in females
- X-Linked Recessive (XLR) inheritance
  - (See mnemonic)
  - Hallmarks of XLR inheritance:
    - Absence of male-to-male transmission
    - Female carriers asymptomatic

Non-Mendelian Inheritance Patterns

- Mosaicism
  - Two populations of different alleles
    - Examples: **Darier's**, Epidermal Nevi

X-Linked Dominant Genoderms

"My bad punk child goes oral and mends incontinent estrogen nodules"

My	MIDAS Syndrome
Bad	Bazex
Punk	X-linked Chondrodysplasia Punctata (Conradi-Hünermann)
Child	CHILD Syndrome
Goes	Goltz Syndrome
Oral	Oral-Facial-Digital Syndrome
And	Albright's
Mends	Mendes da Costa Syndrome (Macular-type Hereditary Bullous Dystrophy)
Incontinent	Incontinentia Pigmenti
Estrogen	Type III Hereditary Angioedema (estrogen-dependent)
Nodules	EDS with Periventricular Nodular Heterotopia

X-Linked Recessive Genoderms

"CHAD'S Kinky WIFE"

C	Cutis Laxa / Chronic Granulomatous Disease
H	Hunter's
A	Anhidrotic Ectodermal Dysplasia
D	Dyskeratosis Congenita
S	SCID
Kinky	Menkes Kinky Hair Syndrome
W	Wiskott-Aldrich / Woolf Syndrome (Albinism-Deafness)
I	Ichthyosis, X-linked / IFAP (and the nearly identical syndrome KFSD) / IPEX
F	Fabry's
E	Ehlers Danlos (Type V & IX)

Also:
Goeminne Syndrome
X-Linked Reticulate Pigmentary Disorder
Bruton's X-Linked Agammaglobulinemia
Properdin Deficiency

KFSD (Keratosis Follicularis Spinulosa Decalvans)

- Revertant Mosaicism = spontaneous correction of a pathologic mutation, like "natural gene therapy"
    - Examples: revertant mosaicism occurs in 35% of patients with non-Herlitz Junctional EB
- Type 2 Segmental Mosaicism = patient is heterozygous for a disease-causing mutation and loss of the remaining wild-type allele gives rise to affected skin
    - Examples: patients heterozygous for *GJB2* mutation (which causes KID Syndrome) get Blaschkoid porokeratotic eccrine ostial nevus
- X-Inactivation (Lyonization)
    - Examples: **Incontinentia Pigmenti**
- Genetic Imprinting
    - Epigenetic phenomena can influence expression of genes
    - Usually a result of DNA methylation
    - Examples
        - **Russell-Silver** and **Beckwith-Wiedemann** are both caused by epigenetic alterations of 11p15 - either *hypo*methylation (and thereby under-activation) in the case of Russell-Silver Syndrome, or *over*-methylation (and thus overactivation) in Beckwith-Wiedemann
        - **Prader-Willi** and **Angelman** are both due to the same deletion (15q), but phenotype differs depending on which parent the defective chromosome is inherited from
- Mitochondrial Inheritance
    - All embryonic mitochondria come from the egg (sperm have no mitochondria). Therefore, mitochondrial diseases are **inherited from mother only**
    - Hallmarks of mitochondrial inheritance: both men and women can be affected, but only women transmit the disease
    - Examples: **PPK with Deafness** is caused by a mutation in a mitochondrial serine tRNA (*MTTS1*). **Leigh Syndrome** (several genes involved in mitochondrial respiratory chain complexes)

Chromosomal Disorders

- Polyploidy = extra copy of all chromosomes
    - All forms are fatal in humans
- Aneuploidy = extra copy of a single chromosome
    - **Trisomy 21 (Down Syndrome)**, 18, or 13
    - **Klinefelter's Syndrome** (XXY sex chromosome aneuploidy)
    - Caused by nondisjunction of chromosomes during gametogenesis. Incidence of nondisjunction of chromosomes increases with maternal age
- Monosomy= single copy of a chromosome
    - **Turner Syndrome** (XO) is the only monosomy compatible with life
- There are only a few examples of chromosomal disorders in which derm findings are the predominant feature:
    - **Hypohidrotic Ectodermal Dysplasia** (X; autosome translocations)
    - **Ambras Syndrome** (chromosome inversion at 8q22)

Contiguous Gene Syndromes

- A deletion or mutation affecting a large portion of the genome may involve two contiguous genes, yielding a constellation of findings
- Examples
    - Steroid sulfatase [Xp22] **(X-Linked Ichthyosis)** + Arylsulfatase E gene [Xp22] **(XLR Chondrodysplasia Punctata)** + *KAL1* [Xp22] (Kallmann Syndrome)
    - *LMX1B* [9q34] **(Nail-Patella Syndrome)** + COL5A1 gene [9q33] (component of glomerular basement membrane) = Nail-Patella Syndrome plus glomerulonephritis
    - *TSC2* [16p13] **(Tuberous Sclerosis)** + PKD1 [16p13] = Tuberous Sclerosis with Polycystic Kidney Disease
    - 15q11 (Prader-Willi / Angelman) + P gene [15q12] **(Oculocutaneous Albinism Type 2)**

Prenatal Testing

- Chorionic villi sampling (week 10)
- Amniocentesis (week 12)
- Fetal biopsy (weeks 19-22) – 5% fetal death risk. Rarely performed in modern times

2. Disorders of Cornification

Keratinocyte Biology

Epidermis

- Cornified envelope = cross-linked proteins replace plasma membrane in terminally differentiated keratinocytes
  - Composed of **loricrin** (makes up 80% of cornified envelope), involucrin, small proline-rich proteins (SRPs), XP-5/late envelope proteins (LEPs), cystatin, envoplakin, periplakin, elafin, repetin, filaggrin, S100 proteins, keratins, desmosomal proteins
  - Proteins are cross-linked by ε-(γ-glutamyl) lysine isopeptide
  - **Catalyzed by transglutaminase enzymes**
    - TGase1 = **membrane bound** in keratinocytes
      - **Lamellar Ichthyosis**
      - **(Non-Bullous) Congenital Ichthyosiform Erythroderma**
    - TGase2 = aka "tissue transglutaminase" Tissue-bound in basal layer
    - TGase3 = "epidermal transglutaminase". Hair follicles and terminally differentiating keratinocytes
      - Abs = Dermatitis Herpetiformis (along with Abs to gliadin, gliadin-TGase2 complexes, and TGase2)
    - TGase5 = upper epidermis
      - **Acral Peeling Skin Syndrome**
- Epidermal stem cells – found in 2 locations
  - 1) Basal layer – constantly active
  - 2) Follicular bulge region – active only in response to skin injury
- Formation of cornified cell envelope (fig 2.1):
  - Basal Layer
    - Intracellular **calcium influx** in suprabasal epidermis triggers terminal differentiation of keratinocytes
      - Calcium concentration increases with increasing cell maturity (upper epidermis > basal layer)
  - Spinous Layer
    - Cornified envelope assembly begins with intracellular cross-linking of scaffold proteins envoplakin, periplakin, & involucrin by TGase1 and TGase5
  - Granular Layer
    - Keratohyalin granules (contain **profilaggrin** & **loricrin**)
      - Loricrin translocated to cell periphery and cross-linked to small proline-rich proteins (SRPs)
        - **Vohwinkel Syndrome, variant form**
        - **Progressive Symmetric Erythroderma**
    - Lamellar granules (Odland Bodies) (contain **lipids**)
      - ABCA12 transports lipids into lamellar granules
        - **Harlequin Ichthyosis**
        - **(Non-Bullous) Congenital Ichthyosiform Erythroderma**
  - Upper Granular Layer
    - ω-hydroxyceramides replace cell membrane and are cross-linked to scaffold proteins
    - Keratin, filaggrin, & involucrin complexes become cross-linked to the cornified envelope
    - Profilaggrin mutation = **Ichthyosis Vulgaris**
    - Filaggrin = mutated in 50% of Atopic Dermatitis

Keratin Intermediate Filaments

- Type I = acidic keratins, include K9-K28, K31-K40
- Type II = basic keratins, include K1-8, K71-86
- Other intermediate filaments:
  - Type III = vimentin, desmin, glial fibrillary acidic protein (GFAP), peripherin
  - Type IV = neurofilaments (low, med, & high molecular weights), α-internexin, syncoilin, nestin, synemin
  - Type V = laminins A/C, B1, B2
  - Others = filensin, phakinin

Initiation (spinous layer) → Reinforcement (granular layer) → Lipid-envelope formation (upper granular layer) → Desquamation (cornified layer)

Epidermolytic Ichthyosis (K1, K10)
Ichthyosis Hystrix of Curth–Macklin (K1)

Desmosome

Cornified Envelope

Acral Peeling Skin Syndrome (transglutaminase 5)

Lamellar Ichthyosis
Nonbullous Ichthyosiform Erythroderma (transglutaminase 1)

Ichthyosis Bullosa of Siemens (K2e)

Ichthyosis Vulgaris (filaggrin)

Protease Defects
Netherton Syndrome (serine protease inhibitor LEKT1)
Papillon-Lefevre Syndrome (cathepsin C)

Golgi

Lamellar Body

Defects of Lipid Metabolism
X-Linked Ichthyosis (steroid sulfatase)
Lamellar Ichthyosis (lipoxygenase-3)
Nonbullous Ichthyosiform Erythroderma (lipoxygenase-3)
Neutral Lipid Storage Disease (CGI-58/ABHD5)
Sjogren-Larsson Syndrome (fatty aldehyde dehydrogenase)
Refsum Disease (phytanoyl-CoA hydroxylase)
CHILD Syndrome (NSDHL)
Conradi-Hunermann-Happle Syndrome (emopamil-binding protein)

Loricrin Granule

Vohwinkel Syndrome
Progressive Symmetric Erythrokeratodermia (loricrin)

Harlequin Ichthyosis
Lamellar Ichthyosis
Nonbullous Ichthyosiform Erythroderma (ABCA12)

Legend:
ABCA12 lipid transporter
Small Proline-rich protein
Fatty Acids, Cholesterol, etc
Involucrin
Periplakin
Envoplakin
Cross-link
Filaggrin
Loricrin
Transglutaminase
Desmosome
Keratin 1, 2, 10

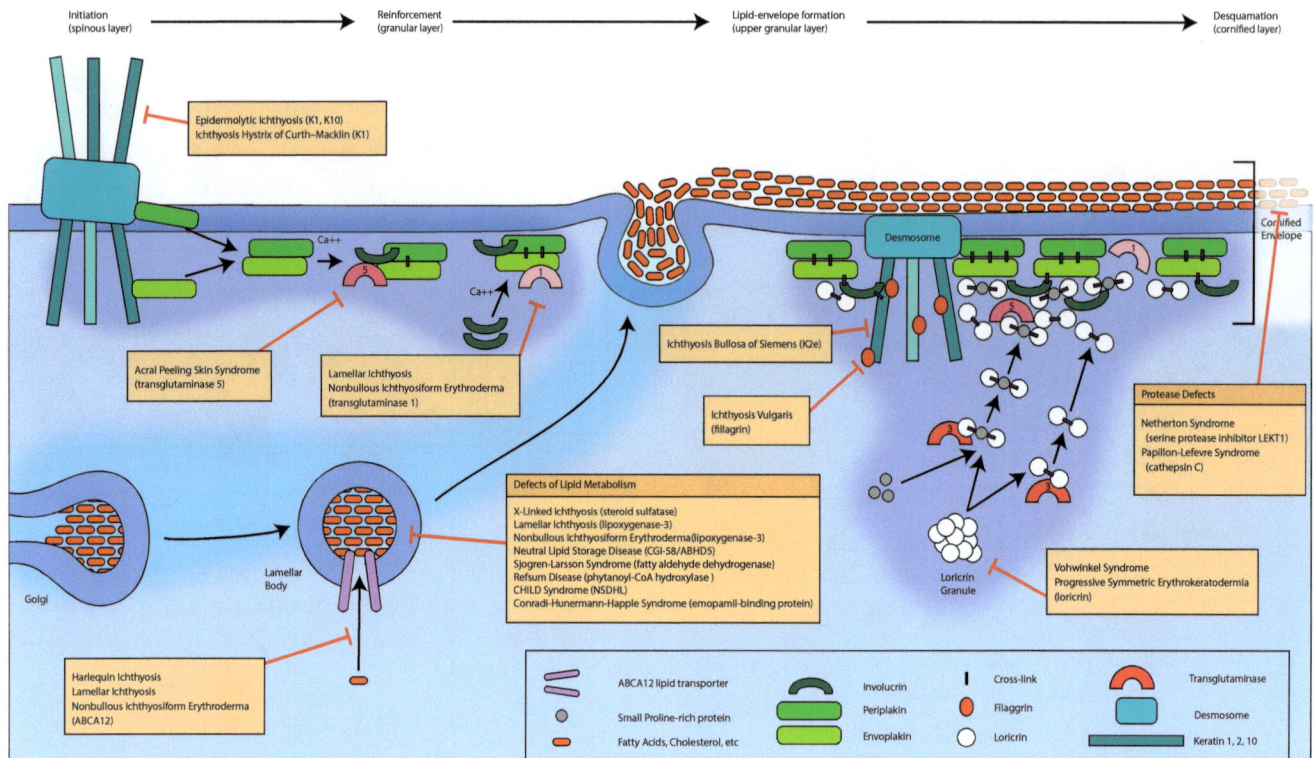

Figure 2.1: Formation of the Cornified Envelope

- Keratins form heteropolymer pairs of acidic + basic
- K1 is the only Type II keratin in palmoplantar skin
- K1/K9 mutations = **PPK**
  - **Vörner PPK** (aka epidermolytic PPK)
    - K9>K1
    - Histopath: EHK and keratin clumps
  - **Unna-Thost PPK** (aka non-epidermolytic PPK)
    - K1
    - Histopath: no EHK or keratin clumps

> **Think of the umlaut (¨) in Vörner as basophilic keratin clumps, to remember that Vörner gets EHK**

- Diseases with mutations in Type I or II keratins
  - K1/K10 = **Epidermolytic Hyperkeratosis** (aka Bullous congenital ichthyosiform erythroderma)
    - K1 = PPK
    - K10 = no PPK
    - **Keratin clumps in suprabasilar keratinocytes**

- Annular EHK variant (cyclic ichthyosis with EHK) = flares of polycyclic psoriasiform plaques with PPK
  - K4/K13 = **White Sponge Nevus of Cannon**
    - Benign, white plaques on oral mucosa, suprabasal cytolysis and keratin clumps
  - K5/K14 = **Epidermolysis Bullosa Simplex (EBS) (including Weber-Cockayne, Koebner, Dowling-Meara, EBS with mottled pigmentation)**
  - K6a/K16 = **Pachyonychia Congenita I (Jadassohn-Lewandowsky)**
  - K6b/K17 = **Pachyonychia Congenita II (Jackson-Lawlor)**
- Diseases with Type 1 mutations only:
  - K14 = disorders with reticulate hyperpigmentation
    - **Naegeli-Franceschetti-Jadassohn Syndrome**
    - **Dermatopathia Pigmentosa Reticularis**
  - K17 = **Steatocystoma Multiplex**
- Diseases with Type 2 mutations only:
  - K1 = **Ichthyosis Hystrix of Curth-Macklin**

- K2 = **Ichthyosis Bullosa of Siemens**
- K5 = **Dowling-Degos Disease (Reticulate Acropigmentation of Kitamura, Reticulate Pigment Anomaly of the Flexures)**
- K81, 83, 86 = **Monilethrix**. Also Dsg-4
- K85 = **Hair-nail type ectodermal dysplasia (pure type)**

Epidermal Differentiation

- Cytokeratin expression varies by level of epidermis
  - Basal layer (mitotically active) = K5 & K14 > K15
    - Palmoplantar epidermis only = K6b & K17
  - Spinous layer = K1 & K10
    - Upper spinous layer = K2
    - Palmoplantar epidermis only = K9, K6a & K16
- Also varies by anatomic site
  - Palms/soles, nail bed, hair follicles, sebaceous glands, & sweat glands = K6, K16, & K17
    - K6, K16, & K17 expression also induced by injury, UV radiation, wounding, & hyperproliferative states
  - Cornified mucosa = K12 & K76
  - Non-cornified mucosa = K4 & K13
  - Cornea = K3 & K12
    - *Meesmann corneal dystrophy*
  - Hepatocytes = K8 & K18
    - *Cryptogenic liver cirrhosis*

Keratinocyte Regulatory Pathways

- p63
  - Induces K14 expression, initiating maturation. Prevents onset of terminal differentiation
  - No p63 = no epidermal maturation, resulting in single-layer epithelium
  - Mutated in several **ectodermal dysplasias**
    - **AEC Syndrome** (Hay-Wells, Rapp-Hodgkin)
    - **EEC Syndrome**
- *ΔNp63α* (p63 isoform)
  - Controls formation of spinous layer by synergizing with Notch signaling to induce K1 expression
  - Induces cell cycle inhibitors and represses cell cycle progression genes

- Notch
  - Controls formation of spinous layer along with *ΔNp63α*
  - Promotes terminal differentiation via ↑ K1 expression and withdrawal from cell cycle
- Protein kinase C proteins
  - ↓ K1 & K10 expression
  - ↑ expression of granular layer markers (loricrin, filaggrin, Tgases)

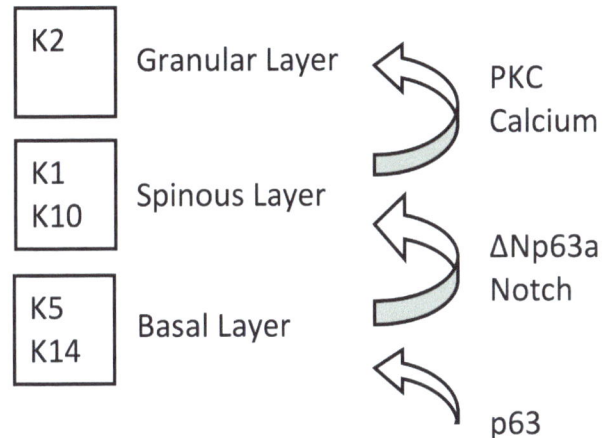

Figure 2.2: Keratinocyte Regulatory Pathways

Keratinocyte Adhesion

- Desmosomes
  - Slow but strong cell-cell adhesion
  - Provide attachment sites for **keratin** intermediate filaments
  - Cadherin Family
  - Desmosomes are very prevalent in both myocardium and skin, so mutations frequently manifest in both heart and skin problems
    - Core of desmosomes formed by desmogleins (Dsg) and desmocollins (Dsc), both of which are calcium-dependent cadherins
    - Dsg1
      - **Striate PPK**
      - Pemphigus Foliaceus
      - Bullous Impetigo
      - Staph Scalded Skin Syndrome
    - Dsg2 = **Arrhythmogenic right ventricular dysplasia/cardiomyopathy (ARVD/C)**
    - Dsg3 = Pemphigus Vulgaris
    - Dsg4

- – **Localized AR Hypotrichosis**
- – **AR Monilethrix**
  - Dsc1
    - – Subcorneal pustular dermatosis
    - – IgA pemphigus
  - Dsc2 = **ARVD/C**
  - Dsc3 = No known disease
- – Armadillo Family of desmosomal proteins:
  - Plakoglobin = **Naxos Disease** (<u>right</u> ventricular cardiomyopathy)
  - Plakophilin 1 = **Ectodermal Dysplasia/ Skin Fragility Syndrome**
  - Plakophilin 2 = **ARVD/C**
  - Plakophilin 3 = No known disease
  - Corneodesmosin = **Hypotrichosis Simplex of the Scalp**
  - Others: desmocalmin (keratocalmin), desmoyokin, & band 6 protein
- – Plakin Family
  - Desmoplakin I (250kDa) & II (210kDa)
    - – **Striate PPK**
    - – **Carvajal Syndrome** (<u>left</u> ventricular cardiomyopathy)
    - – **Skin Fragility/Woolly Hair Syndrome**
    - – **Lethal Acantholytic EB**
  - Also contain envoplakin (210kDa), periplakin (190 kDa), plectin (500kDa), *BPAg1* (230kDa)
  - β-catenin (plakin family, but not in desmosomes)
    - – If mutated: 1) pilomatricomas; 2) colorectal carcinoma
- Adherens Junctions
  - – Quick but weak cell-cell adhesion
  - – Provide attachment sites for **actin**
  - – Contain transmembrane E-, N-, & P-cadherin as well as cytoplasmic α-, β-, and γ-catenin (aka plakoglobin), vinculin, radixin
    - P-cadherin expressed in basal layer
    - E-cadherin expressed in interfollicular epidermis
  - – **Plakoglobin** is the only protein present in **both adherens *and* desmosomes**

> Think "Plako<u>glob</u>in is <u>glob</u>ally present" to remember that plakoglobin is the only protein present in both adherens *and* desmosomes.

- Tight Junctions
  - – Form skin barrier in granular layer
  - – Contain occludins and claudins
- Focal Contacts
  - – Attach keratinocytes to BMZ
  - – Contain integrins, vinculin
  - – Fras1, Frem1, and Frem2 newly discovered proteins that form a complex within the BMZ
  - – **Fraser Syndrome**
    - AR; *FRAS1* or *FREM2* mutation
    - Cutaneous syndactyly, cryptophthalmos, and renal defects, but no postnatal cutaneous bleeding
- Gap Junctions
  - – Allow for communication between cells
  - – Six connexins oligomerize to form a connexin hemichannel. Two connexons form a gap junction (fig 2.3)
  - – Connexin mutations are the MC cause of genetic deafness
  - – Connexin 26 (*GJB2*) = **Vohwinkel's Syndrome, KID Syndrome, PPK with Deafness, Bart-Pumphrey Syndrome**
  - – Connexin 30.3, 31 (*GJB4, GJB3*) = **Erythrokeratodermia Variabilis**
  - – Connexin 30 (*GJB6*) = **Hidrotic Ectodermal Dysplasia**
  - – Connexin 43 (*GJA1*) = **Oculo-Dental-Digital Dysplasia**
  - – Connexin 47 (*GJC2*) = some cases of **Milroy Disease** (but most have *FLT4* mutation)

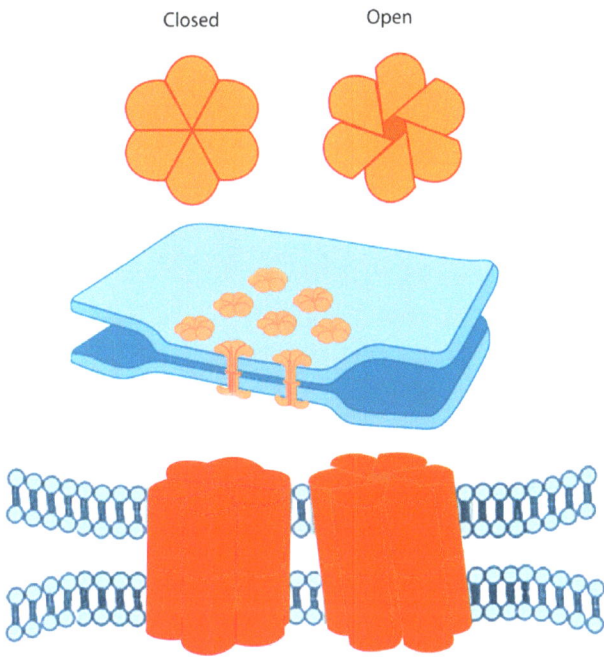

Closed   Open

Figure 2.3: Gap Junction

Table 2.1: Desmosome Defects

Dsc1	Subcorneal Pustular Dermatosis
Dsc2	Arrhythmogenic Right Ventricular Dysplasia/Cardiomyopathy (ARVD/C)
Dsc3	Hereditary Hypotrichosis and Recurrent Skin Vesicles
Dsg1	Striate PPK Pemphigus Foliaceus Bullous Impetigo & Staphylococcal Scalded Skin Syndrome
Dsg2	ARVD/C
Dsg3	Pemphigus Vulgaris
Dsg4	Localized AR Hypotrichosis AR Monilethrix
Desmoplakin	Striate PPK Carvajal Syndrome ARVD/C Skin Fragility/Woolly Hair Syndrome Lethal Acantholytic EB
Plakoglobin	Naxos Disease ARVD/C, SPPK
Plakophilin1	Ectodermal Dysplasia/Skin Fragility Syndrome
Plakophilin2	ARVD/C
Plakophilin3	--- (Hair abnormalities in mice)
Corneodesmosin	Hypotrichosis Simplex of the Scalp

Table 2.2: Keratin Defects

Type II (basic)	Type I (acidic)	Keratin Disorder
1	10	Epidermolytic Ichthyosis
1	10	Annular Epidermolytic ichthyosis (cyclic ichthyosis with EHK)
1		Ichthyosis Hystrix of Curth–Macklin
2		Ichthyosis Bullosa of Siemens
1	9,16	Epidermolytic PPK (Vörner)
1	16	Non-Epidermolytic PPK (Unna–Thost; focal)
4	13	White Sponge Nevus (of Cannon)
5	14	EBS, Dowling–Meara type
5	14	EBS, Koebner type
5	14	EBS, Weber–Cockayne type
5	14	EBS with Mottled Pigmentation
5		EBS with Migratory Circinate Erythema
	14	EBS, AR type
5		Dowling–Degos Disease
	14	Naegeli–Franceschetti–Jadassohn syndrome
	14	Dermatopathia Pigmentosa Reticularis
6a	16	Pachyonychia Congenita Type 1 (Jadassohn–Lewandowsky)
6b	17	Pachyonychia Congenita Type 2 (Jackson–Lawlor)
	17	Steatocystoma Multiplex
81,83,86		Monilethrix (autosomal dominant)
85		'Pure' Hair–Nail Type Ectodermal Dysplasia
3	12	Meesmann Corneal Dystrophy
	Loricrin	Vohwinkel Syndrome Progressive Symmetric Erythrokeratoderma
	Filaggrin	Ichthyosis Vulgaris Atopic Dermatitis

Table 2.3: Gap Junction Defects

Connexin 26 (*GJB2*)	**Vohwinkel's Syndrome** **Kid Syndrome** **Hid Syndrome** **Bart-Pumphrey** **Ppk with Deafness**
Connexin 30.3, 31 (*GJB4, GJB3*)	**Erythrokeratodermia Variabilis**
Connexin 30 (*GJB6*)	**Hidrotic Ectodermal Dysplasia**
Connexin 43 (*GJA1*)	**Oculo-Dental-Digital Dysplasia**
Connexin 47 (*GJC2*)	**Milroy Disease (Hereditary Lymphedema)**

PPK: palmoplantar keratoderma
EBS: Epidermolysis bullosa simplex

Ichthyosis

Ichthyosis Vulgaris

- AD; **profilaggrin** (*FLG*) mutation, with ↓ profilaggrin (and thus ↓ filaggrin, too)
- Scale on extensors and sparing flexures starting at puberty (fig 2.5), atopic diathesis, KP
- **Hyperlinear palms** (fig 2.4; differs from X-linked and Lamellar Ichthyoses)

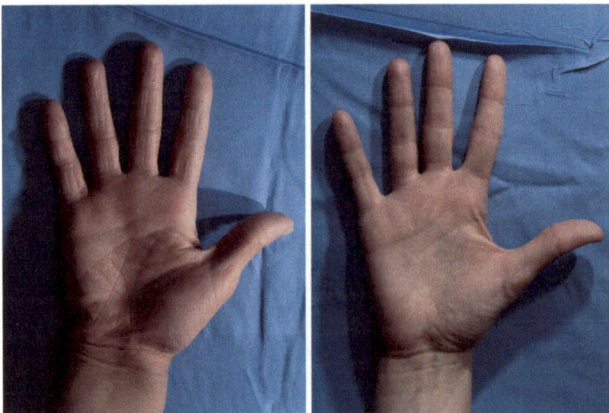

Figure 2.4: Hyperlinear Palms (left) of Ichthyosis Vulgaris Compared to Normal Hand (right)

- Path: **absent granular layer**. Poorly-formed keratohyalin granules on EM (filaggrin is the major component of granules)

X-Linked Ichthyosis

- **XLR**; *STS* gene, encoding **steroid sulfatase** (formerly arylsulfatase C)
- Brown scale sparing palms, soles, and flexures
- **Comma-shaped corneal opacities**, asymptomatic

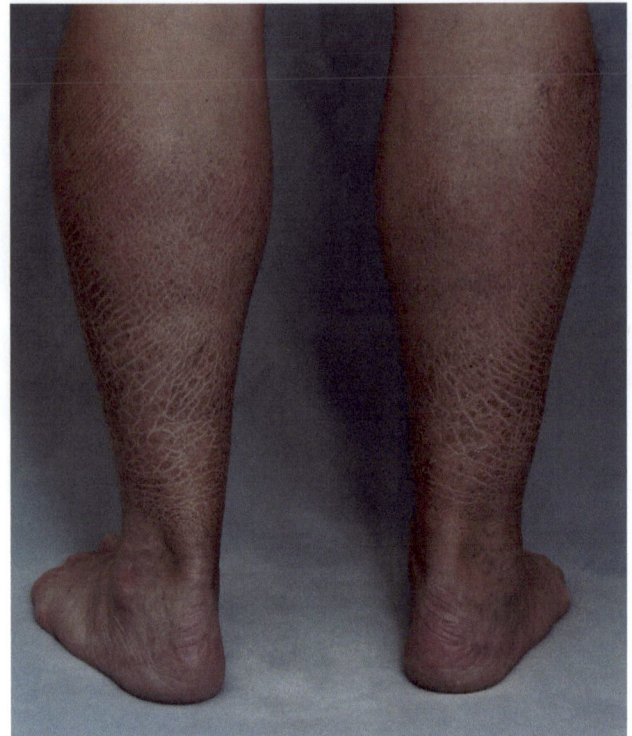

Figure 2.5: Ichthyosis Vulgaris

- **Failure of labor** progression (due to ↓ placental sulfatase and estrogen and ↑ DHEAS)
- **Cryptorchidism** (20%), ↑ risk testicular cancer
- Screen patients for *contiguous gene deletion syndrome* with Kallmann Syndrome and **XLR** Chondrodysplasia Punctata
  - Kallmann Syndrome (Hypogonadic Hypogonadism)
    - Ichthyosis + renal agenesis, anosmia, hypogonadism
    - *KAL1* gene encodes anosmin protein
  - **XLR** Chondrodysplasia Punctata
    - **XLR** mutation in **arylsulfatase E** gene
    - No skin findings

Table 2.4: Genoderms with Cryptorchidism

Noonan
Fabry's
X-Linked Ichthyosis
Rubinstein-Taybi
Goeminne
CMTC
Cornelia de Lange

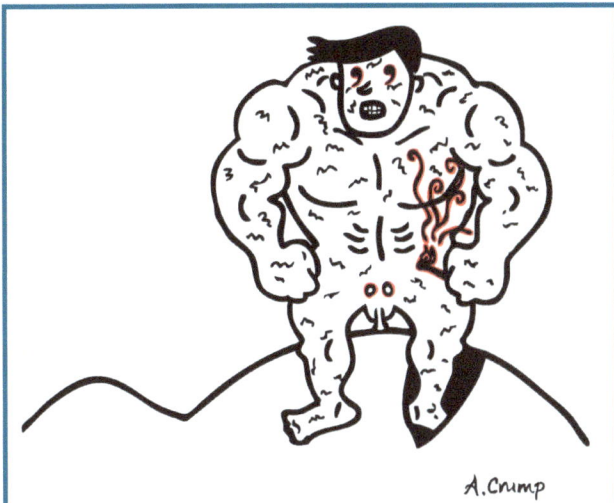

X-Linked Ichthyosis

Picture a scaly male body builder (steroids) with tiny, undescended testes, ichthyosis, and commas for eyes (comma-shaped corneal opacities), lighting a sulfurous match (arylsulfatase C mutation) climbing out of a C-section (prolonged labor)

- Arylsulfatase C deficiency
- C-section (Prolonged labor)
- Cryptorchidism
- Comma-shaped corneal opacities

Lamellar Ichthyosis

- AR
  - **TGM1** (Transglutaminase 1) most common
  - *ABCA12* (ATP binding cassette A12)
  - *CYP4F22*
- **Collodion baby** at birth, with subsequent large thick **plates of scale** especially on the flexures (fig 2.6), ectropion, and eclabium (more severe than **XLR** ichthyosis)
- Scarring alopecia, nail dystrophy, heat intolerance

Congenital AR Ichthyosis

- AR; ichthyin (*NIPAL4*) mutation
- Lamellar-like phenotype

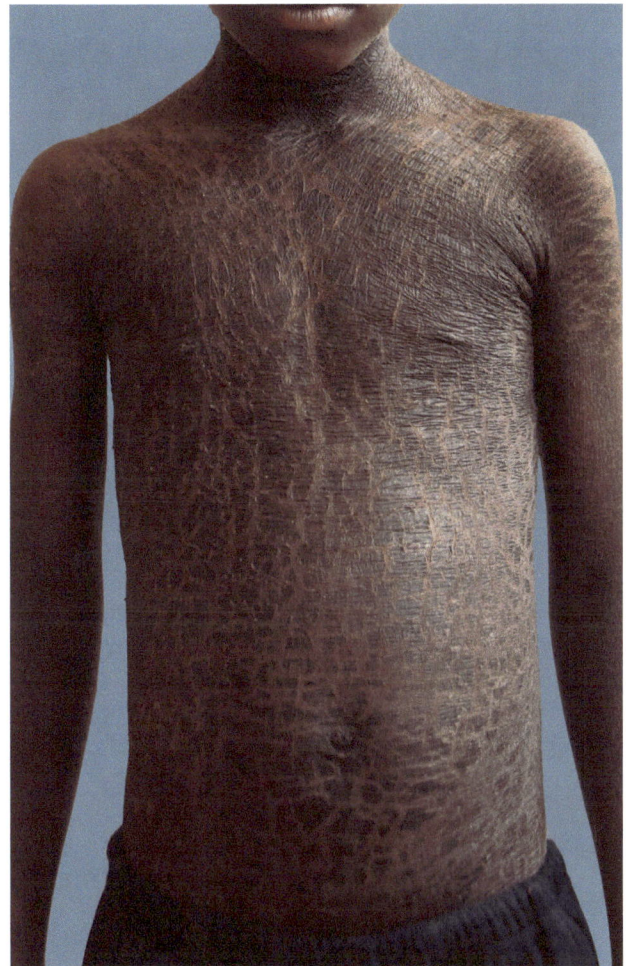

Figure 2.6: Child with Lamellar Ichthyosis

Epidermolytic Ichthyosis (Epidermolytic Hyperkeratosis [EHK], Bullous CIE)

- AD; **K1** & **K10** genes → deficient keratin filaments with **tonofilament clumping**
  - K1: PPK
  - K10: no PPK
- Bullae and erythroderma at birth (fig 2.7), generalized ichthyosis (**"corrugated cardboard"** scale) later in life (fig 2.8)
- Mosaic K1/K10 mutations manifest as large epidermal nevi ("ichthyosis hystrix")
  - Large epidermal nevi should be biopsied to look for EHK on pathology, because these patients may have a mosaic variant of Epidermolytic Ichthyosis. Therefore, they are at risk of having children with "full-blown" Epidermolytic Ichthyosis (if the gonads are involved)

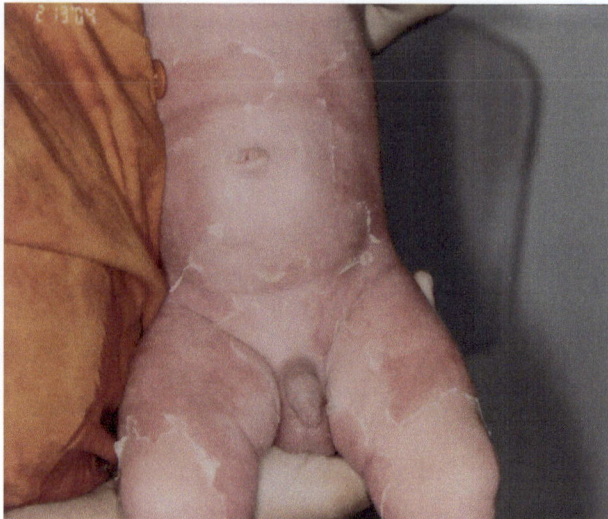

Figure 2.7: Bullae and Erythroderma at Birth in Epidermolytic Hyperkeratosis

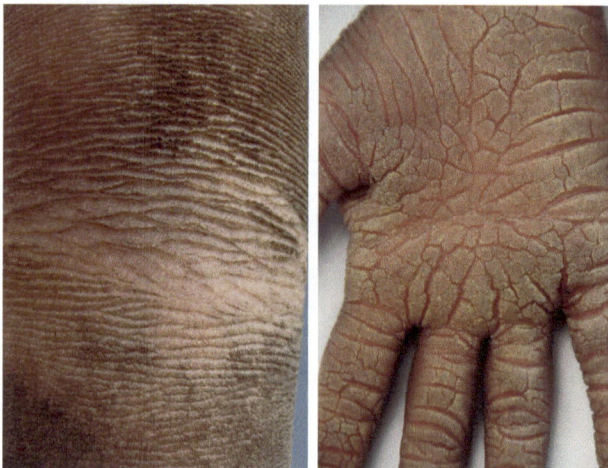

Figure 2.8: Corrugated Scale of Epidermolytic Ichthyosis

Ichthyosis Bullosa of Siemens

- AD; **K2e** gene
- Presents at birth with erythroderma and bullae
- Later, corrugated hyperkeratotic plaques on the flexures. No PPK
- Nearly identical to Epidermolytic Ichthyosis (above), except that **skin is unusually fragile**, with tendency to shed, called "**Mauserung**" (molting)

Ichthyosis Hystrix of Curth-Macklin

- AD; **K1** gene
- Clinically very similar to Epidermolytic Ichthyosis, but no skin fragility

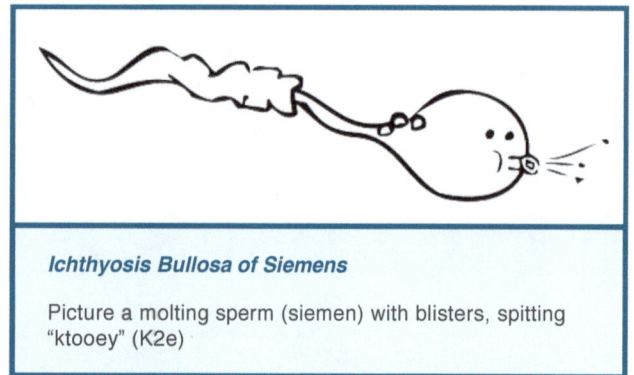

Ichthyosis Bullosa of Siemens

Picture a molting sperm (siemen) with blisters, spitting "ktooey" (K2e)

Congenital Ichthyosiform Erythroderma (Nonbullous CIE)

- AR
  - **TGM1** (Transglutaminase 1)
  - **ALOX 12B** (Arachidonate 12 lipoxygenase)
  - **ALOX E3** (Lipoxygenase 3)
  - Ichthyin
- **Collodion baby**, ectropion, eclabium at birth
- Generalized mild **erythroderma with fine white scale**
- Scarring alopecia, hypohidrosis with heat intolerance

Table 2.5: DDx of Collodion Baby		
Disease	Association with Collodion	% of Collodion Babies with This Disease
Self-Healing Collodion Baby	Always	6%
Congenital Ichthyosiform Erythroderma	Frequent	50%
Lamellar Ichthyosis	Frequent	11%
AD Lamellar Ichthyosis	Rare	
AD CIE	Rare	
Trichothiodystrophy	Rare	
Gaucher (infantile form)	Very Rare	
AEC and other Ectodermal Dysplasia	Very Rare	
Netherton	Very Rare	
Neutral Lipid Storage Disease	Very Rare	

Harlequin Ichthyosis

- AR/sporadic; **ABCA12** gene
- Massive hyperkeratotic plates w/ deep fissures encasing newborn ("harlequin fetus")

J. Finch & M. Payette

- Severe ectropion, eclabium
- Absent/deformed ears, nose, fingers, toes
- Erythroderma, most fatal
- Labs:
  - **No lamellar granules** (electron microscopy)
  - ↓ **calpain** (calcium-activated protein protease involved in calcium signaling and differentiation)
- DDx: collodion baby, Neu-Laxova Syndrome (severe IUGR, CNS malformations + harlequin phenotype. Gene unknown)

Sjögren-Larsson Syndrome

- AR; fatty aldehyde oxidoreductase/alcohol dehydrogenase deficiency. *FALDH* (*ALDH3A2*) gene
- Ichthyosis in infancy, mental retardation
- **Spastic tetraplegia**, epilepsy, "scissor" gait by age 2-3
- Glistening dot atypical **retinitis pigmentosa**
- Dental enamel dysplasia
- Very itchy from ↑ leukotriene B4 (treat with zileuton)

Refsum Syndrome

- AR; **phytanoyl coenzyme A hydroxylase** deficiency (*PAHX* gene, aka *PHYH*) or **peroxin 7** (*PEX7*)
- Neuro symptoms in childhood: cerebellar **ataxia,** peripheral **neuropathy, retinitis pigmentosa** (salt & pepper), and sensorineural **deafness**
- Ichthyosis in adulthood
- Heart block
- Tx: diet low in green vegetables, dairy, and ruminant fats

Chondrodysplasia Punctata

- Chondrodysplasia Punctata (CDP) is a heterogeneous group of disorders with limb defects, stippled epiphyses and sometimes ichthyosis. There is phenotypic overlap among this group
- Isolated CDP can also be caused by in-utero warfarin toxicity
- See also: Table 17.1: Genoderms with Bone/ Musculoskeletal Associations on p.117

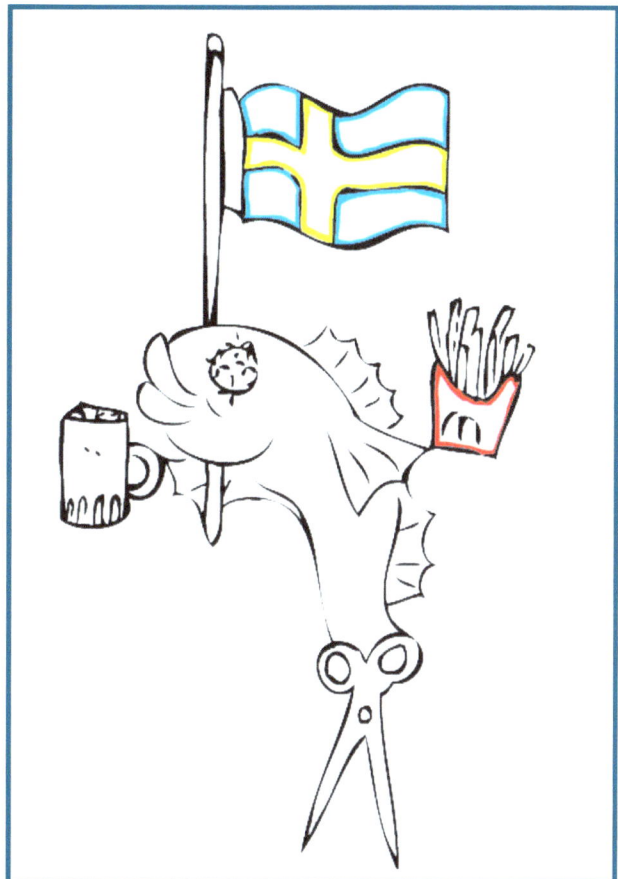

Sjögren-Larsson Syndrome

Picture a fish (ichthyosis) with scissor legs (scissor gait, tetraplegia), glistening dots in eyes, holding a Swedish flag (affects Scandinavians) and a beer and fatty french fries (fatty aldehyde alcohol dehydrogenase deficiency). Think of the umlaut (¨) in Sjögren as glistening dots

Refsum Syndrome

Picture a Referee holding salt/pepper shakers (salt & pepper retinitis pigmentosa), heart in a block on his shirt (heart block, arrhythmias), leaning on table (ataxia), X's over his ears (deafness), and an X over a head of broccoli (AR, PAHX encodes phytanoyl-CoA hydroxylase which is in peroxisomes = can't break down phytanic acid in veggies and fats). Also think "refereeing a fight" (phyte) to remember phytanoyl enzyme

Table 2.6: Chondrodysplasia Punctata Spectrum

CDP Subtype	Gene
Conradi-Hünermann (XLD CDP)	Emopamil-binding protein (EBP)
Rhizomelic CDP	Peroxin-7 (PEX-7)
XLR CDP	Arylsulfatase E (ARSE)
CHILD Syndrome	3β-hydroxysteroid-dehydrogenase (NSDHL)

Conradi-Hünermann Syndrome (XLD Chondrodysplasia Punctata)

- **XLD**; **emopamil-binding protein** (*EBP*) (formerly 3β-hydroxysteroid isomerase (3β-HIS)
- Rarely, AR peroxin 7 (*PEX7*) mutation
- Defective cholesterol biosynthesis
- Transient **blaschkoid ichthyosiform erythroderma** at birth, which resolves by age 1 with linear and **follicular atrophoderma**
- Cataracts, **stippled epiphyses**, limb asymmetry
- Increased risk in children born to **mothers with systemic lupus erythematosus**

Rhizomelic Chondrodysplasia Punctata

- AR; peroxin-7 (*PEX-7*) mutation
- Has features of Conradi-Hünermann and CHILD
- Stippled epiphyses + Rhizomelia (short proximal limbs)
- Deficient RBC plasminogen, Severe MR
- Skin: ichthyosis & alopecia in 25%
- Course: phytanic acid elevations after 6 months of age, X-ray changes within first year. Most die before age 2

CHILD Syndrome

- **XLD**; mutation in **NSDHL** gene (NADPH steroid dehydrogenase-like protein, aka **3β-hydroxysteroid-dehydrogenase**)
  - Rarely, emopamil-binding protein (*EBP*) mutation, similar to Conradi-Hünermann
- CHILD = **C**ongenital **H**emidysplasia with **I**chthyosiform erythroderma & **L**imb **D**efects
- **Unilateral ichthyosiform erythroderma**
- Ipsilateral alopecia, limb/visceral hypoplasia, and **stippled epiphyses**
- Organ hypoplasia/agenesis
- **Verruciform xanthomas**

Netherton Syndrome

- AR; *SPINK 5* → encodes **LEKT1** (serine protease inhibitor that decreases inflammation)
- Presents at birth with **erythroderma** and ichthyosis
- **Ichthyosis linearis circumflexa** (double-edged scale)
- **Trichorrhexis invaginata** (bamboo hair; esp lateral eyebrows)
- **Atopic** dermatitis, seborrheic dermatitis, anaphylactic food allergy, ↑↑ **IgE**, eosinophilia
- **Tacrolimus ointment contraindicated**

Netherton Syndrome

Think "BARE ASS Spank" to remember Netherton

B	Bamboo hair
A	Atopic Derm
R	Recessive
E	IgE
A	Anaphylactic food allergy
S	Seb derm
S	Serine Protease
Spank	= SPINK5

Erythrokeratodermia Variabilis (EKV)

- AD; connexin 31 & 30.3 mutations (*GJB3*, *GJB4* genes)
- Well-demarcated erythematous **migratory patches that change daily**, fixed hyperkeratotic plaques, PPK

KID Syndrome

- AD; **connexin 26** mutation (*GJB2*) (allelic with Vohwinkel & PPK with Deafness)
- **KID = K**eratitis-**I**chthyosis-**D**eafness
- Generalized mild hyperkeratosis, red keratotic plaques on face and extremities, **stippled PPK**, alopecia
- Congenital sensorineural deafness
- Progressive bilateral keratitis with secondary blindness (avoid systemic retinoids)
- ↑ **SCCs (skin, tongue),** ↑ infections
- **Porokeratotic Eccrine Ostial and Dermal Duct Nevus** (PEODDN) Note: patients heterozygous for *GJB2* mutation can get Blaschkoid PEODDN – Type II segmental mosaicism

J. Finch & M. Payette

- Senter Syndrome (Desmons Syndrome)
  - AR form of KID Syndrome, with liver problems
  - Glycogen storage defect leads to hepatomegaly, hepatic cirrhosis, growth failure and MR

Oculo-Dento-Digital Dysplasia (ODDD)

- AD; **connexin 43** mutation (*GJA1*)
- Oculo: microphthalmia, glaucoma
- Dento: underdeveloped teeth
- Digital: syndactyly of 4th & 5th fingers
- Abnormally small/thin nose

IFAP Syndrome (Ichthyosis Follicularis)

- **XLR**; *MBTPS2* gene → encodes zinc MMP
- **I**chthyosis **F**ollicularis with **A**trichia and **P**hotophobia
- Allelic with and phenotypic overlap with Keratosis Follicularis Spinulosa Decalvans (see p. 119)
- Congenital atrichia, KP, photophobia, MR, seizures, ichthyosis

Neutral Lipid Storage Disease (Chanarin-Dorfman Syndrome)

- AR; *CGI-58* (*ABHD5*) mutation
- Congenital generalized ichthyosis and erythroderma (presentation at birth is identical to nonbullous congenital ichthyosiform erythroderma)
- **Myopathy,** cataracts, sensorineural deafness
- **Vacuolated leukocytes** (fig 2.9)
- Prognosis dependent on course of liver disease

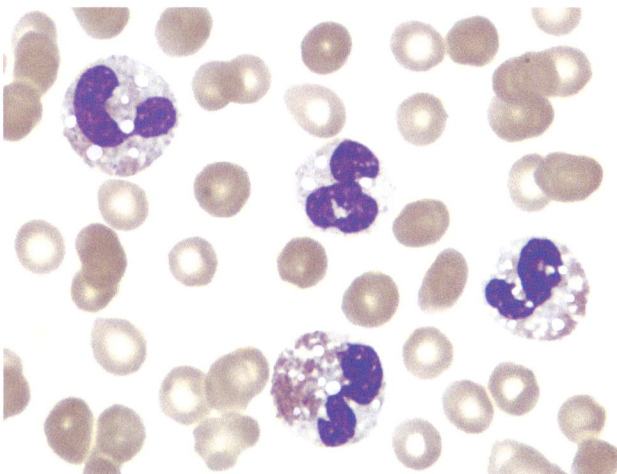

Figure 2.9: Vacuolated Leukocytes of Neutral Lipid Storage Disease

Darier's Disease (Keratosis Follicularis)

- AD; *ATP2A2* → encodes **calcium ATPase 2A2** (aka *SERCA2*)
- Presents in teens with
  - Hyperkeratotic papules in seborrheic areas (2.12)
  - Palmar keratoses and pits
- **Acrokeratosis Verruciformis of Hopf** – flat wart-like papules on dorsal hands (fig 2.11)
  - Patients with isolated Acrokeratosis Verruciformis of Hopf probably have a mosaic form of Darier's
- Red-white **longitudinal nail bands ("candy cane nails"),** v-shaped distal nail nicks (fig 2.10)
- **Cobblestoning** of oral and rectal mucosae
- Recurrent infections (*S. aureus*, HSV – eczema herpeticum)
- Worsened by lithium

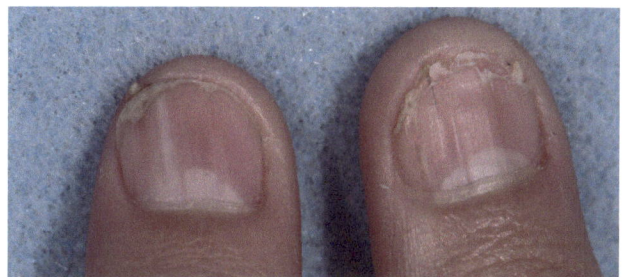

Figure 2.10: Darier's Disease - Nails

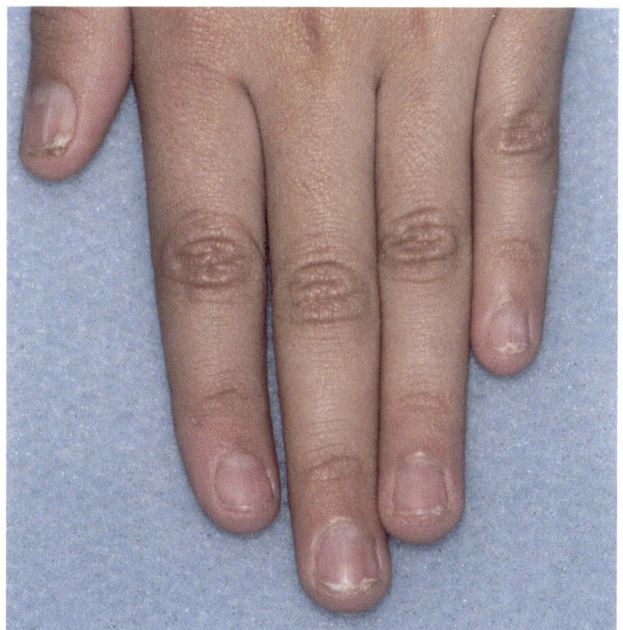

Figure 2.11: Darier's Disease – Acrokeratosis Verruciformis of Hopf

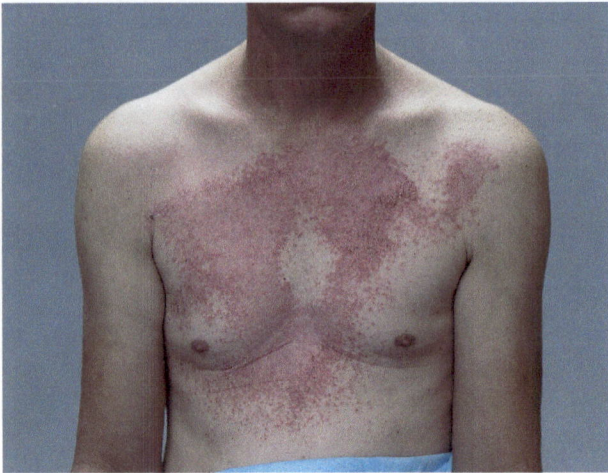

Figure 2.12: Darier's Disease
(image courtesy of Steven Brett Sloan, MD)

Hailey-Hailey Disease

- AD; *ATP2C1* → encodes **calcium ATPase 2C1** (aka hSPCA1)
- **Flexural** erosions and vesicles (fig 2.13)
- Longitudinal erythronychia
- Complete remissions and flares are common
- Path: acantholytic "dilapidated brick wall" appearance with dyskeratosis

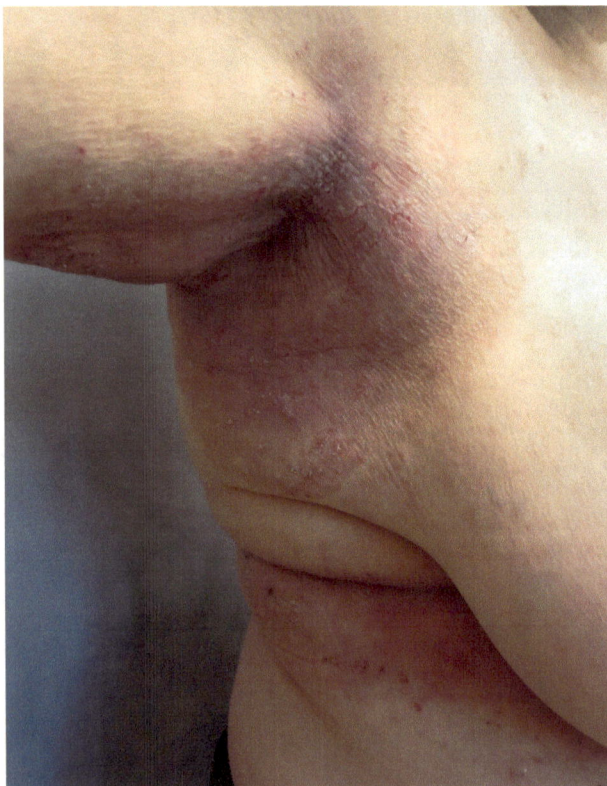

Figure 2.13: Erosions, Vesicles, and Scale Crust in Characteristic Flexural Areas of Hailey-Hailey

Poland Syndrome

- Ichthyosis + absent pec major muscle + ipsilateral syndactyly
- Gene unknown. Usually sporadic

> **Think of Halley's comet, which is visible only every 75 years – it's rare "to see one" (Hailey-Hailey = ATP2C1)**

Palmoplantar Keratodermas

Diffuse PPKs

- Vörner
- Unna-Thost
- Mutilating PPKs
  - Mal de Meleda
  - Olmsted
  - Vohwinkel
  - Vohwinkel variant
- PPK with transgrediens (top and bottom of hands/feet)
  - Mal de Meleda
  - Papillon-Lefèvre
  - Haim-Munk
  - Clouston (Hidrotic Ectodermal Dysplasia)
- Naxos
- Bart-Pumphrey
- Symmetric Progressive Erythrokeratoderma
- EBS, Dowling-Meara

Focal PPKs

- Richner-Hanhart
- Pachyonychia Congenita
- Howel-Evans
- EBS, Dowling-Meara
- EBS, Weber-Cockayne
- EBS, Koebner
- Kindler
- Dyskeratosis Congenita
- NFJ
- PPK with deafness
- Schöpf-Schulz-Passarge
- Punctate PPKs
  - Dermatopathia Pigmentosa Reticularis
  - Darier's
- Striate
  - Carvajal
  - Striate PPK (Brunauer-Fohs-Siemens)

Vörner PPK *(Epidermolytic PPK)*

- AD; **K9**>K1
- Diffuse symmetric, non-transgrediens PPK
- Clinically identical to Unna-Thost PPK
- Path: **EHK**

> **Think German Shepherd = K9 (Vörner is a German name)**
>
> **Think of the umlaut (¨) in Vörner as the histologic keratin clumps of epidermolysis, to remember that Vörner is epidermolytic**

Table 2.7: Lab Tests for Ichthyoses

Ichthyosis vulgaris	No laboratory tests needed. Skin biopsy if necessary
XLR Ichthyosis	Steroid sulfatase activity or level of cholesterol sulfate
Nonbullous CIE	No laboratory test indicated
Lamellar Ichthyosis	No laboratory test indicated
Epidermolytic Ichthyosis	Skin biopsy (epidermolytic hyperkeratosis)
Chondrodysplasia Punctata	No laboratory studies needed; X-ray (stippled epiphyses)
CHILD Syndrome	Usually no laboratory tests needed; radiographic studies (stippled epiphyses)
Trichothiodystrophy	Trichogram, with polarization (tigertail hair = pathognomonic)
KID Syndrome	Skin biopsy if necessary
Netherton Syndrome	Trichogram (bamboo hair)
Neutral Lipid Storage Disease	Peripheral blood smear (vacuoles); frozen skin biopsy
Refsum's Disease	Plasma phytanic acid levels
Sjögren-Larsson Syndrome	Fatty aldehyde oxidoreductase activity assay

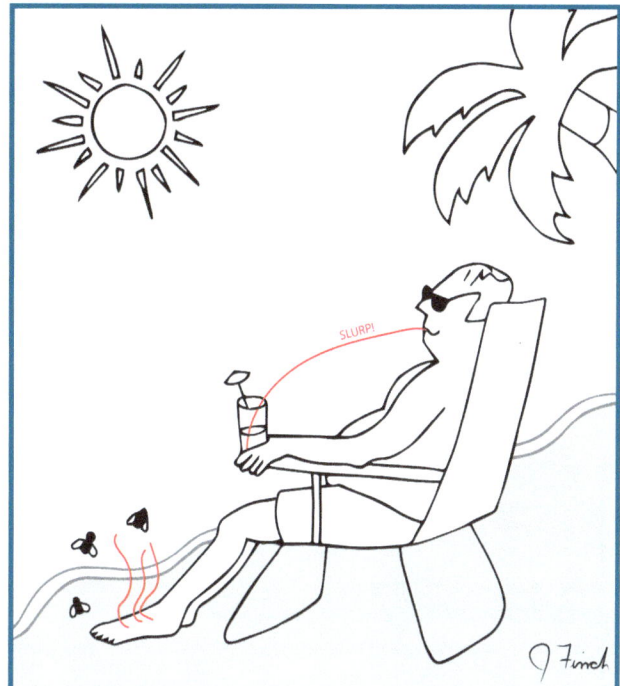

Mal de Meleda

Picture someone with smelly feet slurping a drink on a tropical island

Unna-Thost PPK
(Non-epidermolytic PPK)
- AD; **K1**
- Clinically identical to Vörner PPK
- Path: **no** EHK

KLICK Syndrome
(Keratosis linearis with ichthyosis congenita and sclerosing keratoderma)
- AR; *POMP* gene
- Ichthyosis at birth
- PPK with pseudoainhum and a sclerosing flexion deformity
- Linear hyperkeratosis w/o Koebner phenomenon

Mutilating PPKs

Mal de Meleda
(Keratosis extremitatum hereditaria transgrediens et progrediens)
- AR; *SLURP-1* (**s**ecreted **L**y-6/**u**Par **r**elated **p**rotein **1**) → cell signaling & adhesion protein
- Malodorous transgrediens PPK in **glove and stocking distribution**
- Hyperkeratotic plaques on elbows/knees
- Affects inhabitants of the island of Meleda, one of the Dalmatian islands in the Adriatic Sea

Olmsted Syndrome
- AD; *TRPV3* gene
- Mutilating PPK with prominent periorificial keratotic plaques
- Mal de Meleda can also have periorificial involvement, but less severe

Vohwinkel Syndrome, Classic
(Mutilating Keratoderma of Vohwinkel)
- AD; **connexin 26** (*GJB2* gene)
- Diffuse **honeycombed** PPK, **starfish**-shaped keratotic plaques over joints
- **Pseudo-ainhum** (constricting bands around digits, especially 5th toe) leading to auto-amputation of digits
- **Deafness**

Table 2.8: DDx - PPK Associated with Autoamputation

Vohwinkel Syndrome
Mal de Meleda
PPK of Sybert
Olmsted Syndrome
Acral Keratoderma
Pachyonychia Congenita

Vohwinkel, Variant

- AD; **loricrin** *(LOR)*
- Similar to classic Vohwinkel, but has ichthyosis and lacks deafness

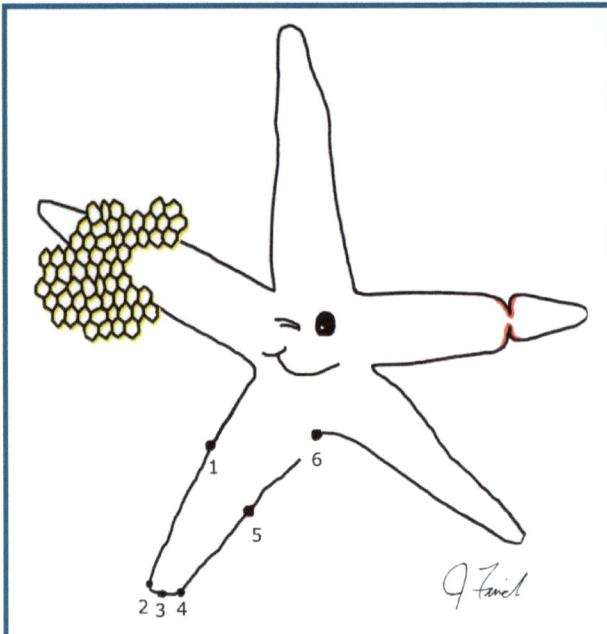

Vohwinkel Syndrome

Think "Winkle winkle little star" and picture a connect-the-dots (connexin mutation) starfish holding honeycomb, winking (vohWINKel) with an arm pinched off (pseudo-ainhum)

Progressive Symmetric Erythrokeratodermia

- AD; **loricrin** *(LOR)*
- Hyperkeratotic plaques and PPK

Papillon-Lefèvre Syndrome

- AR; *CTSC* gene → encodes **cathepsin C** (lysosomal protease involved in innate immunity & PMN function)
- Sharply demarcated, **transgrediens PPK** (stocking-glove) and hyperkeratoses over knees/elbows
- **Severe periodontitis** with tooth loss (attributed to PMN defect resulting in *Actinomyces* growth)
- Pyogenic infections
- Asymptomatic **dural calcifications of tentorium & choroid attachments**

Papillon-Lefèvre Syndrome

Picture a French Canadian hockey player with missing teeth (periodontitis), a calcified helmet (dural calcifications) and smelly, sweaty feet (malodorous PPK)

Haim-Munk Syndrome

- AR; **cathepsin C** (*CTSC*) (allelic with Papillon-Lefèvre)
- PPK + periodontitis + acro-osteolysis + onychogryphosis
- Compared to Papillon-Lefèvre:
  - No calcification of dura
  - No ↑ infections
  - Has arachnodactyly, acro-osteolysis, onychogryphosis

Naxos Syndrome

- AR; plakoglobin (*JUP*) mutation
- **Diffuse PPK + woolly hair + <u>right</u> ventricle** arrhythmogenic cardiomyopathy

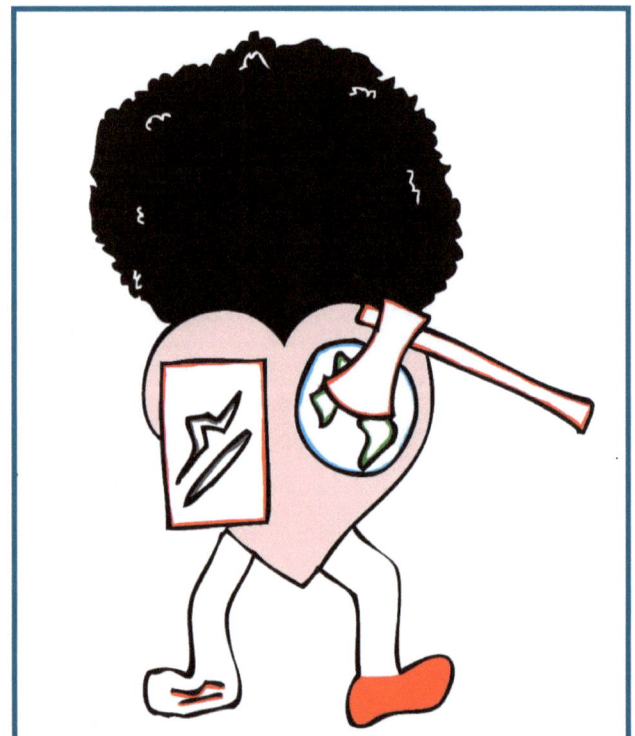

Carvajal and Naxos Syndromes

Picture a heart with woolly hair:
  On the right side is a globe and an axe (nAXos = plakoGLOBEin defect and R-sided heart problems, with diffuse PPK)
  On the left side is a carved plaque (CARVajal = desmoplakin, L-sided heart problems), with striate PPK

J. Finch & M. Payette

Striate PPK (Brunauer-Fohs-Siemens)

- AD; **desmoglein 1** (*DSG1*) and **desmoplakin** (*DSP*) or rarely keratin 1 (*KRT1*)
- PPK involving fingers and extending into streaks involving palms. No teeth/nail abnormalities

Howel-Evans Syndrome

- AD; *TOC* gene (**t**ylosis and es**o**phageal **c**ancer), aka *RHBDF2*, encoding a protein that **inhibits EGFR signaling**
- Focal, pressure-related, non-transgrediens PPK
- **Esophageal cancer**, oral leukoplakia

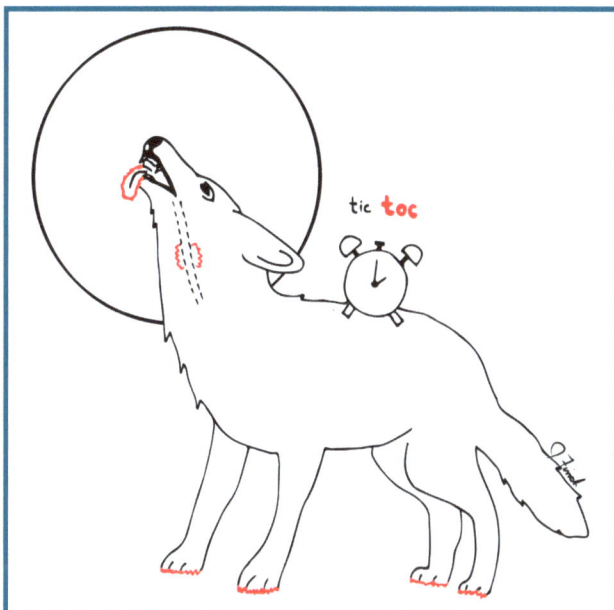

Howel-Evans Syndrome

Picture a coyote howling a raspy howl because he has esophageal cancer. He has a white tongue (oral leukoplakia) and PPK

Sclerotylosis (Huriez Syndrome)

- AD; *TYS* gene. Sclerosis of skin (esp sclerodactyly), nail hypoplasia, PPK
- 15% develop **SCC** of affected skin and ↑ risk of bowel cancer
- PPK with 46XX Sex Reversal
  - Same features as Huriez, plus hermaphroditism or 46XX phenotypic males, caused by AR *RSPO* mutation

PPK with Deafness

- Mitochondrial serine tRNA mutation (*MTTS1*)

Schöpf-Schulz-Passarge Syndrome

- AR; mutation in *WNT10A* (allelic with Odonto-onycho-dermal dysplasia)
- PPK, cystic eyelids, hypodontia, hypotrichosis, nail dystrophy, eccrine tumors (eccrine syringofibroadenoma)
- DDx: hidrotic ectodermal dysplasia. HED & SSPS are very similar, but SSPS gets eyelid hidrocystomas; HED does not

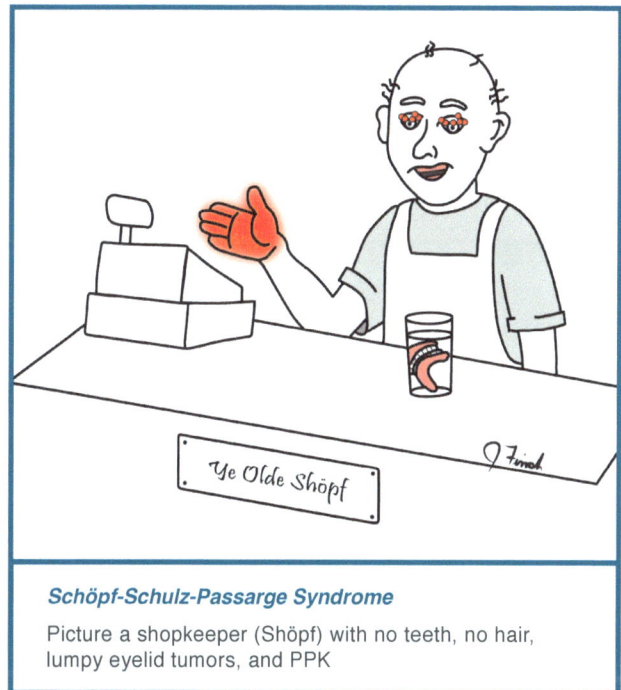

Schöpf-Schulz-Passarge Syndrome

Picture a shopkeeper (Shöpf) with no teeth, no hair, lumpy eyelid tumors, and PPK

Bart-Pumphrey Syndrome

- *GJB2* (connexin 26)
  - Allelic with PPK with deafness, Vohwinkel Syndrome (classic), KID
- PPK, knuckle pads, leukonychia and deafness
- Note: milder connexin 26 mutations are the #1 cause of nonsyndromic hearing impairment

Richner-Hanhart Syndrome (Tyrosinemia Type II)

- AR; *TAT* gene; deficient **hepatic tyrosine aminotransferase**
- Accumulation of tyrosine in all tissues
- **Eyes affected 1st** (pseudoherpetic keratitis, photophobia, ulceration, blindness)
- Focal, weight-bearing, non-transgrediens PPK
- Mental retardation
- Tx: low-tyrosine/phenylalanine diet
  - Nitisinone

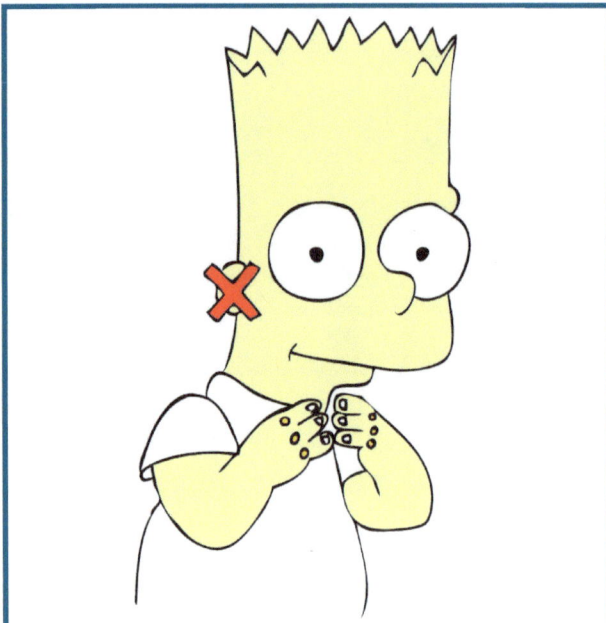

Bart-Pumphrey Syndrome

Picture a cartoon character with knuckle pads, white fingernails, deaf

Richner-Hanhart Syndrome

Richner-Hanhart = "Retard Hand Hurt"
Picture a retarded person standing in a large tire (tyrosine), with painful hands and dendrites on eyes

Epidermal Nevus Syndrome

- Numerous different findings
  - CNS findings of head/neck (MR, seizures, deafness, vascular malformations)
  - Skeletal findings (hemihypertrophy, limb deformity, vitamin D-resistant rickets)
  - Eye findings (lipodermoid tumors, corneal opacity, cortical blindness)
  - Neoplasms (syringocystadenoma papilliferum, Wilms' tumor, astrocytoma, rhabdomyosarcoma, salivary gland adenocarcinoma)
  - Lab abnormalities (low phosphate, low calcium)
- Mosaic mutations in *NRAS, HRAS, PIK3CA, and FGFR3* underlie most keratinocytic ENs
- Mosaic mutations in *RAS* (Usually *HRAS* or *KRAS*) underlie Epidermal Nevus Syndrome with rickets (Schimmelpenning Syndrome)

Table 2.9: Genoderms with Transgrediens PPK

Papillon-Lefèvre Syndrome
Mal de Meleda
Hidrotic Ectodermal Dysplasia (Clouston Syndrome)

Think "<u>T</u>ransgrediens = <u>T</u>op" to remember that transgrediens PPK involves the bottom *and* top of hands/feet. Non-transgrediens PPK involves only the bottom.

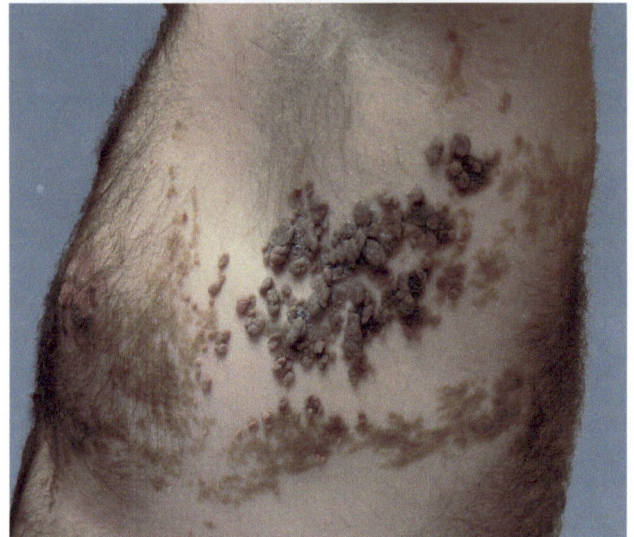

Figure 2.14: Extensive Keratinocytic Epidermal Nevus (nevus unis lateralis)

Specific Pathologic Analyses

- Decreased or absent lamellar granules
  - **Ichthyosis Vulgaris**
  - Acquired Ichthyosis
  - Netherton
  - Refsum
  - Trichothiodystrophy
  - Conradi-Hünermann
- Bamboo Hair
  - Netherton
- Tiger-Tail Hair (light areas = low sulfur content)
  - Trichothiodystrophy
- Parakeratosis & Hypergranulosis
  - Loricrin Keratoderma
- IHC staining
  - Ichthyosis vulgaris (filaggrin)
  - Netherton (*LEKT1*)
- Enzyme Assay (on frozen unfixed tissue)
  - TGase1 (*ARCI*)

3. Epidermolysis Bullosa & Other Bullous Diseases

Epidermolysis Bullosa

Overview

- Three major types: simplex, junctional, and dystrophic
- Clinical: in all types of EB, minor mechanical trauma leads to blisters, generally non-inflamed, and healing is with or without scarring/milia
- Nail dystrophy/alopecia can be present in all types (although less common in simplex)
- Leading cause of death in EB after adolescence = **SCC**, especially in RDEB

EB Simplex (EBS)

Overview

- All EBS has **AD** inheritance except for some rarer subtypes ("hemidesmosomal" and junctional EB are AR)
- Most are **K5** & **K14** mutations
- **Heals w/o scarring**, atrophy, or milia (vs JEB & DEB have scars)
- Most present at birth, except for Weber-Cockayne

Weber-Cockayne EBS (Localized EBS)

- MC form of EBS. **Affects hands/feet only**. Presents in childhood (not at birth)
- **Acral bullae** & focal PPK, oral erosions
- Often first manifests after prolonged walking/ running (e.g. military recruits during boot camp)

Dowling-Meara EBS

- **Herpetiform (grouped) blisters** at birth
- Generalized involvement (not limited to palms/ soles). **Most severe type of EBS**
- Progressive PPK occurs later. Dystrophic nails, minimal milia/scarring

Koebner EBS (Non-Dowling-Meara Generalized)

- At birth: **generalized blisters**, Focal PPK

EBS with Mottled Pigmentation

- K5 mutation (not K14)
- At birth: mottled **reticulate hyperpigmentation**, generalized blisters

- Note: Dowling-Degos (another K5 mutation) also has reticulate hyperpigmentation

EBS with Muscular Dystrophy

- **AR; plectin** mutation
- **Generalized blisters** at birth
- **Granulation tissue**/stenosis of respiratory tract
- Muscular dystrophy infancy-adulthood

EBS, Ogna Type

- AD; **plectin** mutation
- Very similar to Weber-Cockayne, but has easy bruising
- Presents at birth with **easy bruising, acral blisters, onychogryphosis**

Junctional EB

- All subtypes are **AR**, most are **laminin 332** defect
- **Enamel hypoplasia** is characteristic of all JEB types
- All types present at birth
- JEB is more severe than EBS. Blisters heal with scarring and milia

JEB-Herlitz

- AR; mutation in **laminin 332** (*LAMA3*, *LAMB3*, *LAMC2*)
- Generalized blisters (including face)
- **Exuberant granulation tissue** (perioral, axilla, neck, laryngeal)
- **Pitted teeth** (enamel hypoplasia)
- Note:
  - JEB-Herlitz shares laminin α3 (*LAMA3*) gene mutation with laryngo-onycho-cutaneous syndrome
  - Anti-Laminin 5 Abs cause antiepiligrin cicatricial pemphigoid

JEB non-Herlitz, Generalized (JEBnH-gen)

- AR; mutation in **laminin 332** or **Type XVII collagen**
- Similar to Herlitz, but no granulation tissue
- 35% exhibit revertant mosaicism, with areas of normal skin

JEB non-Herlitz, Localized (JEBnH-loc)

- AR; mutation in **Type XVII collagen**
- Localized blisters, abnormal teeth

JEB with Pyloric Atresia

- AR; mutation in α6β4 integrin (note: auto-antibodies to β4 integrin cause ocular cicatricial pemphigoid)
- Generalized blisters
- Dystrophic nails
- **Pyloric atresia**, **rudimentary ears**
- **Renal failure** due to urethral strictures & hydronephrosis

JEB Laryngo-Onycho-Cutaneous (Shabbir Syndrome, LOGIC Syndrome)

- AR; mutation in *LAMA3* (Laminin 5, subunit 3α)
- India
- LOGIC = **L**aryngeal and **O**cular **G**ranulation in **C**hildren from the **I**ndian subcontinent
- Mild blisters on face and neck
- Exuberant granulation tissue especially in conjunctiva and larynx, causing hoarseness
- Nail loss/erosions

Dystrophic EB

Overview

- All types of DEB are caused by AR or AD mutations in **Type VII collagen** (*COL7A1*)
- RDEB is secondary to a premature stop codon in collagen VII
- Note: **auto-antibodies to collagen VII cause EBA and Bullous SLE**
  - Recurrent denudation of small intestine → severe malabsorption

DDEB, Ggeneralized (DDEB-gen)

- At birth: generalized blisters, milia/atrophic scarring, albopapuloid lesions, oral blisters

Bart's Syndrome

- Variant of DDEB presenting with congenital aplasia cutis

EB Pruriginosa

- Prurigo nodularis-like lesions

RDEB, Severe Generalized (RDEB-sev gen) (Hallopeau-Siemens)

- At birth: generalized blisters, severe milia/scarring
- Dental caries, esophageal strictures
- **Tons of SCCs** (#1 cause of death, 80% incidence by age 45)
- **Renal failure** (both glomerulonephritis & hydronephrosis from strictures)
- Cardiomyopathy, osteoporosis
- **Mitten deformity** (pseudosyndactyly)

RDEB, Generalized Other (RDEB-O)

- At birth: less severe than RDEB-sev,gen

Table 3.1: Epidermolysis Bullosa Simplex		
Localized EBS (EBS-loc) (Weber-Cockayne)	K5, K14	AD
Generalized EBS (non-DM) (Koebner)	K5, K14	AD
Dowling-Meara generalized EBS (EBS-DM)	K5, K14	AD
EBS with muscular dystrophy (EBS-MD)	Plectin (PLEC1)	AR
EBS with Mottled Pigmentation (EBS-MP)	K5	AD
EBS, Ogna Type	Plectin	AD
Junctional EB		
JEB Herlitz (JEB-H)	Laminin 332 (laminin 5)	AR
JEB non-Herlitz, generalized (JEBnH-gen)	Laminin 332 (laminin 5) Type XVII collagen	AR
JEB non-Herlitz, localized (JEBnH-loc)	Type XVII collagen	AR
JEB with pyloric atresia (JEB-PA)	a6b4 integrin	AR
Dystrophic EB		
DDEB, generalized (DDEB-gen)	Type VII collagen	AD
Bart's Syndrome	Type VII collagen	AD
EB Pruriginosa	Type VII collagen	AD
RDEB, severe generalized (RDEB-sev gen) (Hallopeau-Siemens)	Type VII collagen (premature stop codon)	AR
RDEB, generalized other (RDEB-O)	Type VII collagen	AR
Transient bullous of the newborn	Type VII collagen	AD/AR

Transient Bullous Dermolysis of the Newborn

- Generalized moderate blisters at birth or in early infancy. Nail dystrophy. Blistering only for first 1-2 years of life, due to temporary delay in transport and deposition of collagen VII

EB Aquisita (EBA)

- Not a genoderm, but included for completeness
- **Anti-Collagen VII antibodies** result in blisters
- DIF shows linear IgG along the basement membrane

Non-EB Skin Fragility Syndromes

Table 3.2: Non-EB Skin Fragility Syndromes			
Disease	Inherit.	Protein	Gene
Ectodermal Dysplasia/ Skin Fragility Syndrome	AR	Plakophilin 1	PKP1
Kindler Syndrome	AR	Kindlin 1	KIND1 (C20orf42)
Lethal Acantholytic Epidermolysis Bullosa	AR	Desmoplakin	DSP
Skin Fragility/ Woolly Hair Syndrome	AR	Desmoplakin	DSP
Mendes da Costa Syndrome (Macular-Type Hereditary Bullous Dystrophy)	XLR	Unknown	Unknown
Nephropathy with pretibial epidermolysis bullosa and deafness	AR	Platelet-endothelial cell tetraspanin Antigen 3 (CD151)	CD151
Naegeli-Franceschetti-Jadassohn Syndrome	AD	Keratin 14	K14
Dyskeratosis Congenita	AD or AR	Telomerase complex components	ACD, CTC1, DKC1, NHP2, NOP10, PARN, RTEL1, TERC, TERT, TINF2, WRAP53

Kindler Syndrome

- Acral blisters, PPK and photosensitivity
- See p. 55 (Genoderms with Photosensitivity)

Mendes da Costa Syndrome (Macular-type Hereditary Bullous Dystrophy)

- **XLR**; gene unknown
- Bullae, absence of all hair, hyperpigmentation, depigmentation, acrocyanosis, dwarfism, microcephaly, mental inferiority, +/- nail dystrophy

Restrictive Dermopathy

- Uniformly fatal laminopathy due to mutation in **LMNA** (encodes **lamin A**) or **ZMPSTE24** (*FACE-1*, encodes endoprotease that processes lamin A)
  - Allelic with Progeria (Hutchinson-Gilford), Mandibuloacral Dysplasia, and Familial Partial Lipodystrophy
- Results in taut, shiny **translucent skin with prominent vessels** and **splits at flexural sites**
- Premature birth (mean 31 wks)

Acral Peeling Skin Syndrome

- AR; mutation in **transglutaminase 5** (*TGM5*)
- Periodic, painless, superficial (granular layer) skin peeling of dorsal hands and feet
- Path: split at level of stratum granulosum

Basan's Syndrome (Profuse Congenital Milia with Absent Dermatoglyphs)

- AD; *SMARCAD1* gene
- Profuse milia
- Absent dermatoglyphs, painful PPK, neonatal acral blisters and traumatic blisters in adulthood
- Palmoplantar hypohidrosis
- Single palmar crease (Simian crease)

Other Bullous Diseases of the Newborn

Hyper IgE Syndrome (Job Syndrome)

- Immunodeficiency disorder with papulopustular and vesicular eruption with crusting on the head and shoulders, as well as axillae and diaper area
- See p. 91 for full discussion

Vesiculopustular Eruption in Down Syndrome

- Extensive neonatal vesiculopustular eruption, **associated with congenital leukemoid reaction** (aka transient myeloproliferative disorder)
- 80% resolve spontaneously
- 20% early death
- 20% get Acute Megakaryocyte Leukemia (*GATA1* mutation)
- See p. 118 for full discussion of Down Syndrome

Epidermolytic Ichthyosis (EHK, Bullous CIE (Congenital Ichthyosiform Erythroderma)

- Generalized erosions and erythroderma at birth, followed by "corrugated cardboard" ichthyosis
- See p. 9 for full discussion

Incontinentia Pigmenti

- Blaschkoid lesions evolve through four distinct phases. Stages can occur in utero
    - 1) vesicular
    - 2) verrucous
    - 3) hyperpigmented
    - 4) hypopigmented/atrophic
- See p. 83 for full discussion

Naegeli-Franceschetti-Jadassohn Syndrome

- Bullae on feet in newborn period
- See p. 85 for full discussion

Dyskeratosis Congenita

- Frictional bullae, acrocyanosis, palmoplantar hyperhidrosis & PPK
- See p. 84 for full discussion

4. Biology of the Extracellular Matrix

Overview

- Functions of the ECM:
  - Structural
  - Cell adhesion and migration
  - Organization of cell shape and cytoskeleton
  - Cell division, differentiation/polarization and apoptosis
- Components of the ECM:
  - Collagens (28 types)
  - Elastin
  - Fibrillins (2 types)
  - LTBPs (4 types)
  - Fibulins (5 types)
  - Laminins (15 types)
  - Proteoglycans
  - Glycoproteins
  - Integrins
  - Modifying Enzymes

Collagen

- Comprises 75% of the dry weight of the dermis, 25% of the volume
- 43 genes → 43 proteins → 3 proteins combine to form trimers → **28 types of collagen**
- Each type has 3 polypeptide ("α") chains folded into a triple helix
- **Every 3rd amino acid is glycine**: Gly-X-Y
  - X = proline m.c.
  - Y = hydroxyproline m.c. (Hyp residues form hydrogen bonds, conferring stability)
- Collagen I has uninterrupted Gly-X-Y pattern, forming a very rigid rod (bone)
- Other collagens have non-collagenous interruptions in the Gly-X-Y pattern, creating flexible "joints" in the collagen rod
  - e.g. Col XVII has collagenous and non-collagenous domains
- Fibrils: always mixture of collagens and other
- All collagens are made by dermal fibroblasts, except these four:
  - VII, XVII = epidermal keratinocytes
  - VIII, XVIII = endothelial cells

- Biosynthesis (fig 4.1)
  - Synthesis of procollagen in the RER
  - Cleavage of signal peptides
    - Hydroxylation by prolyl hydroxylase and lysyl hydroxylase
      - Requires O_2, Fe^{2+}, α-ketoglutarate, **vitamin C** (vit C deficiency = Scurvy)
    - Prolyl hydroxylase converts Pro→Hyp
    - Lysyl hydroxylase converts Lys→Hyl
      - Mutated = **EDS, Kyphoscoliosis**
      - **Minoxidil** inhibits lysyl hydroxylase
    - Glycosylation of Hyl and Asp residues
    - Formation of procollagen triple helix when ~100 Hyp residues have accumulated. Procollagen is then transported extracellularly
  - N-and C-terminus cleavage
    - **Procollagen N-proteinase (*ADAMTS-2* gene, a zinc metalloproteinase) cleaves N-propeptide**
      - Mutated = **EDS Dermatosparaxis**
      - Note: the cleaved N-terminus of Procollagen III (PIIINP) is a surrogate marker for hepatic fibrosis in MTX therapy
    - **Procollagen C-proteinase (aka Bone Morphogenic Protein, *BMP-1* gene) cleaves C-propeptide**
  - Assembly into suprastructures
    - Once the propeptides are cleaved from each end, the mature collagen molecules assemble to form fibrils
  - Collagen fiber cross-linking
    - ***Lysyl oxidase*** (requires copper) crosslinks Lys and Hyl
      - Gene is on X chromosome
      - Mutated = **Cutis Laxa**
      - Inhibited in Lathyrism, caused by excessive ingestion of sweet peas (*Lathyrus sativus*), resulting in muscle weakness and atrophy
    - ***TGase2*** crosslinks collagen VII
- See Table 4.1 for diseases caused by collagen mutations

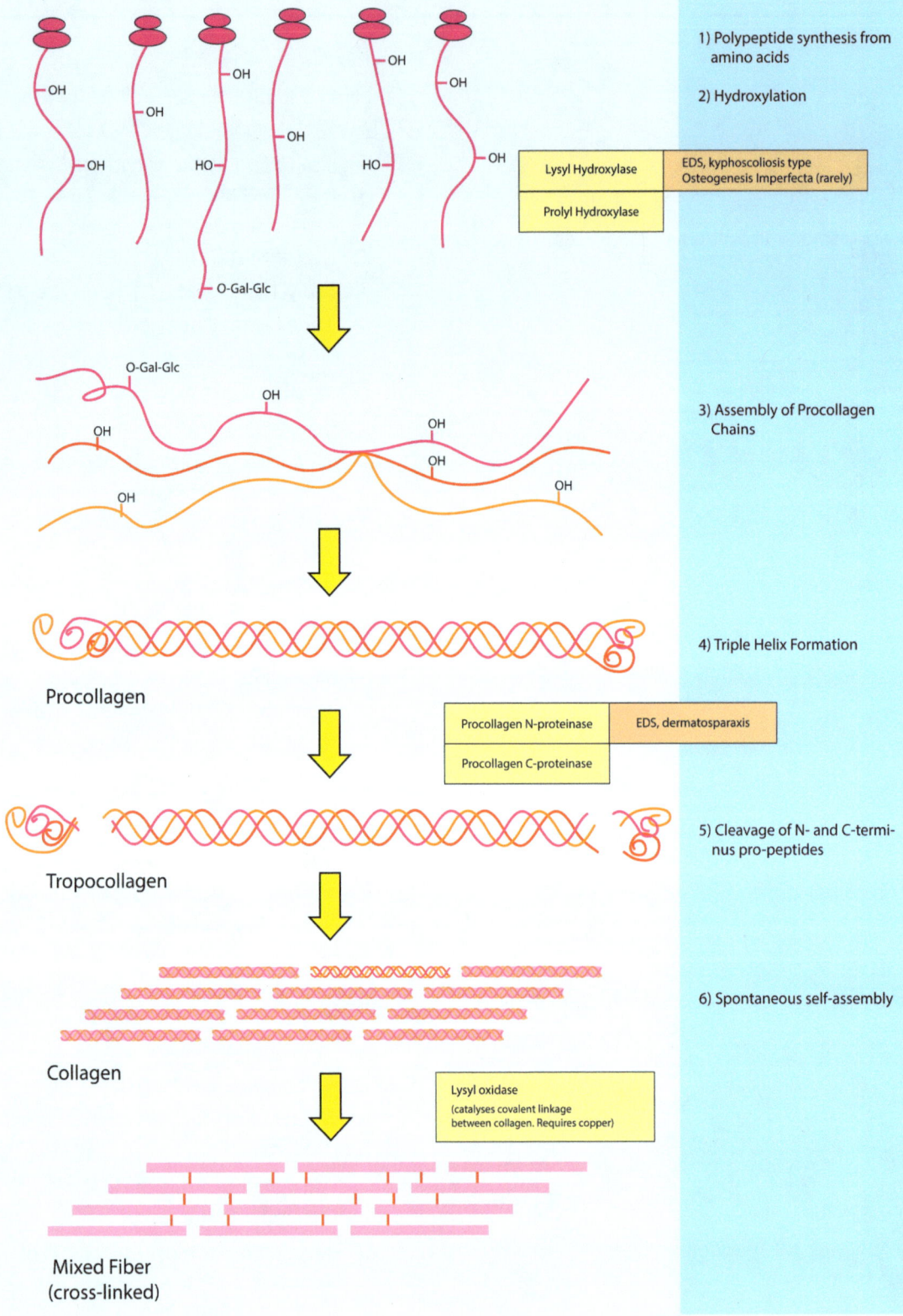

1) Polypeptide synthesis from amino acids

2) Hydroxylation

Lysyl Hydroxylase	EDS, kyphoscoliosis type Osteogenesis Imperfecta (rarely)
Prolyl Hydroxylase	

O-Gal-Glc

O-Gal-Glc

3) Assembly of Procollagen Chains

Procollagen

4) Triple Helix Formation

Procollagen N-proteinase	EDS, dermatosparaxis
Procollagen C-proteinase	

Tropocollagen

5) Cleavage of N- and C-terminus pro-peptides

6) Spontaneous self-assembly

Collagen

Lysyl oxidase
(catalyses covalent linkage between collagen. Requires copper)

Mixed Fiber
(cross-linked)

Figure 4.1: Collagen Biosynthesis

J. Finch & M. Payette

Table 4.1: Important Collagens

Collagen	Function	Disease
I	Major component of fibrils Skin, tendon, bone	**EDS Arthrochalasia** **EDS Cardiac Valvular** *Osteogenesis Imperfecta*
II	Cartilage, vitreous humor of eye	Relapsing Polychondritis, MAGIC
III	Form fibrils; **Wound repair; Fetal collagen**	**EDS Vascular**
IV	Basement membrane; Form tetramers	*Goodpasture's*
V	Skin	**EDS, Classic**
VI	Microfibrils	**Ullrich Scleroatonic Muscular Dystrophy**
VII	**Anchoring fibrils** Binds BM to dermal ECM	**Dystrophic EB** EBA, Bullous SLE
VIII	Strengthen vascular walls Form hexagonal networks beneath endothelial BMs	
XIII	Transmembrane collagen basal keratinocytes, focal contacts	
XVII (BPAG2)	Anchoring filaments Binds basal keratinocytes to BM	**Junctional EB** Bullous Pemphigoid Linear IgA Bullous Dermatosis
XVIII	Dermal side of vascular BM Cleaved C-terminus = **endostatin** (which inhibits angiogenesis)	

Elastin & Elastic Fibers

- *Elastin* = stretchable amorphous protein
  - Tropoelastin monomers (high in **desmosine and isodesmosine**) are crosslinked by *lysyl oxidase* (same enzyme that crosslinks collagen) to form elastin
  - Elastin (*ELN*) mutation = **Cutis Laxa (AD)**
  - 4% of the dry weight of skin is elastin
- Elastic fibers are composed 90% of elastin core, surrounded by microfibrils
  - Can be stretched 100% or more
  - *Oxytalan* = **vertical** microfibrillar elastic fibers
  - *Elaunin* = **horizontal** microfibrillar component plus some amorphous component
  - *Dermal elastic fibers* = microfibrillar component with a large amorphous component
- Elastic stains: Verhoeff-Van Gieson (elastic fibers black), Orcein, Resorcin-Fuchsin

> **Think:**
> oxyTALLan – fibers stand up TALL |||
> eLAYnin – fibers LAY flat ≡
> to remember that oxytalan is vertical and elaunin is horizontal

Microfibrils

- Connect to **perlecan** in the BM, extend through papillary dermis, then connect to horizontal elastic fibers (**elaunin**) in the reticular dermis
- *Fibrillins*: glycoproteins that contain EGF-repeats (epidermal growth factor) that bind calcium
  - *Fibrillin-1* = main component
    - Binds perlecan to microfibrils in the BM
    - Mutated = **Marfan Syndrome, Stiff Skin Syndrome**
    - AutoAb = Linear Morphea
  - *Fibrillin-2*
    - Guides elastogenesis
    - Mutated = **Congenital Contractural Arachnodactyly** (marfanoid body habitus with *crumpled ears*, but no ocular or cardiovascular defects)

> **Mnemonics for important collagens**
>
> I - b**ONE**
> II - car**TWO**lage
> III - "Wounded FBI"
>   **W**ounds
>   **F**etal collagen
>   **B**lood vessels
>   **I**ntestine

- *Microfibril-associated glycoproteins (MFAPs)*
- *Latent TGF-β binding proteins (LTBP)* – four types
  - **Repository for latent TGF-β**
  - TGF-β promotes tissue fibrosis
  - TGF-β is stored in an inactive form, bound to both LTBP & LAP (Latency Associated Peptide)
  - Thrombospondin 1 can bind to LAP, releasing active TGF-β
  - Loss-of-function mutations in LTBP4 cause **AR Cutis Laxa**
  - Activating mutations in TGF-β receptors 1 & 2 = **Loeys-Dietz Syndrome**
    - *Type I Loeys-Dietz* = aortic aneurysms, arterial tortuosity, craniofacial/skeletal defects, joint laxity, translucent skin
    - *Type II Loeys-Dietz* = bruising, atrophic scarring (~EDS type IV phenotype)
- *Fibulins*
  - Fibulins bind elastin
  - **Fibulin-4** mutation = **Cutis Laxa (AR)**
  - **Fibulin-5** mutation = **Cutis Laxa (AD & AR)**

Extrafibrillar Matrix

- Binds water, provides hydrated consistency
- Composed of proteoglycans, glycoproteins, hyaluronic acid, water
- **Glycosaminoglycans (GAGs, aka mucopolysaccharides):**
  - **Negatively charged** polysaccharides (carbohydrate) of repeating disaccharide units, with sulfated and acetylated sugars
  - Negative charge attracts Na+ ions, and Na+ subsequently **binds large amounts of water**
  - **Hyaluronic acid (HA)** = GAG + **protein-free** core
  - **Proteoglycan** = GAG + protein core
    - Four types of GAGs make proteoglycans:
      - Chondroitin sulfate (CS) – most prevalent GAG
      - Dermatan sulfate (DS)
      - Keratan sulfate (KS)
      - Heparan sulfate (HS) – similar to heparin

- **Proteoglycans of the skin**
  - *Versican* (GAGs = CS & DS)
    - Most important proteoglycan in dermis
    - Binds to a HA core, giving skin its tautness
    - Associated with elastic fiber system
    - Made by fibroblasts, smooth muscle cells, epithelial cells
    - Mutation (*VCAN* gene) = *Wagner Syndrome* (familial retinal detachment due to changes in vitreous humor)
  - *Perlecan* (GAGs = HS & CS)
    - Major HS proteoglycan of the **basement membrane**
    - Binds fibrillin-1 to BM
    - Mutation (*HSPG2* gene) = **Schwartz-Jampel Syndrome** (trichomegaly, characteristic facies, small muscle mass, congenital eyelid fusion)
  - *Decorin* (GAGs = CS & DS)
    - Binds collagen fibrils & TGF-β
    - Mutation (*DCN* gene) = *Congenital Corneal Dystrophy*
  - *Fibromodulin* (GAGs = KS)
    - Regulates formation of collagen-containing fibrils
  - *Lumican* (GAGs = KS)
  - *Keratocan* (GAGs = KS)
    - Mutation (*KERA*) = *Cornea Plana Congenita*
  - *Biglycan* (GAGs = CS & DS)
    - Cell surface proteoglycan, binds TGF-β
  - *Syndecans* (GAGs = HS & CS)
    - **1, 2,** & **4** are found in skin
    - Transmembrane HS proteoglycans on most cell types
    - Regulate coagulation cascades, lipase binding & activity, cell adhesion to ECM with cytoskeletal organization, and infection of cells with microorganisms

Laminins and Other Glycoproteins

- Laminins
  - Family of BM molecules (15 members)
    - 5 forms of α-chains: LAMA1, LAMA2, LAMA3, LAMA4, LAMA5
    - 4 forms of β-chains: LAMB1, LAMB2, LAMB3, LAMB4
    - 3 forms of λ-chains: LAMC1, LAMC2, LAMC3
  - Expressed in all tissue except bone & cartilage
  - Each molecule comprises αβγ trimers
  - Epithelial BM contains laminins 332, 331, & 511
  - Vascular BM contains laminins 411 & 511
  - **Laminin β1 mutation** (*LAMB1*) = **Cutis Laxa, Neonatal Marfanoid**
  - **Laminin 332** (*LAMA3, LAMB3, LAMC2*) mutation = **Junctional EB**
  - Laminin 221 mutation = *Muscular Dystrophy*
  - Laminin 521 mutation = *Nephrotic Syndrome*
- Other Glycoproteins
  - Fibronectin = cell adhesion & migration
  - Vitronectin = cell adhesion & migration
  - Thrombospondins = cell-cell & cell-matrix communication
  - Matrilins = matrix assembly & cell adhesion
  - Tenascins = regulation of cell function
    - Tenascin X deficiency =
      - **EDS, classic (AR form)**
      - **EDS, hypermobility**
  - Extracellular Matrix Protein 1 (*ECM-1*)
    - Mutation = **Lipoid Proteinosis**
    - Auto-antibody = LS&A

Integrins

- Integrins are cell receptors that mediate attachment to either the extracellular matrix or to other cells
- Binds laminin & Type IV collagen
- Capillary Morphogenesis Protein 2 (an integrin-like receptor encoded by *CMG 2* gene)
  - Mutated = **Juvenile Hyaline Fibromatosis** and **Infantile Systemic Hyalinosis**
- Mutation in β2 integrin or RASGRP2 (involved in integrin activation) = **Leukocyte Adhesion Deficiency**

- Mutation in α6 or β2 integrin = **JEB with Pyloric Atresia**
- Mutation in integrin α_M = ↑ risk for Systemic Lupus Erythematosus
- LFA1 (CD11a) = target of efalizumab - old psoriasis drug
- Integrin β3 (GPIIIa) = *Glanzmann Thrombasthenia* (platelet disorder that may present with bruising)
- GPIb (von Willebrand receptor) = *Bernard-Soulier Syndrome* (platelet disorder that may present with bruising)

Other Genetic ECM Diseases

- ABCC6 transporter: **Pseudoxanthoma Elasticum (PXE)**
- ATPase Cu^{2+} transporting α-polypeptide: **Occipital Horn Syndrome (Menkes)**
- Glucose transporter 10: **Arterial Tortuosity Syndrome**
- Galactosyl transferase-1: **EDS (progeroid)**
- Filamin A: **EDS (periventricular nodular heterotopia variant)**

Table 4.2: Elastic Fiber Defects

Disease	Defect	Clinical Manifestation	Associations	Biochemical Findings
Buschke-Ollendorff	AD; *LEMD3*	Dermatofibrosis lenticularis disseminata; ***osteopoikilosis***	Osteopoikilosis= long bones: coin-shaped opacities	↑**Desmosine** in skin
Cutis Laxa	AD; *ELN* (elastin) *FBLN4* (fibulin 4) *FBLN5* (fibulin 5)	Loose, sagging, inelastic skin, pulmonary emphysema, tortuosity of aorta, urinary and GI tract diverticula	Transient in baby associated w/maternal penicillamine dosage	↓**Desmosine and ↓ elastin mRNA levels**; ?inc elastase activity
Wrinkly Skin Syndrome ("Autosomal recessive cutis laxa")	AR; *ATP6V0A2* alpha-2 subunit of the V-type H+ ATPase	↓Elastic recoil of the skin; increased # of palmar & plantar creases		
Williams Syndrome	AD; Contiguous deletion up to 25 genes from 7q11, one of which is *ELN*	Velvety skin, dysmorphic facies	Autistic savant Supravalvular aortic stenosis	
Menkes Kinky Hair	*ATP7A*			↓Lysyl oxidase
Pseudoxanthoma Elasticum (PXE)	AR; *ABCC6* or sporadic (D-penicillamine)	Yellowish papules, coalescing into "Chicken skin" plaques, inelastic skin	Cardiovascular and ocular abnormalities	**Deposition of calcium apatite crystals**, excessive GAGs on elastic fibers
Marfan Syndrome	AD; *FBN1* Fibrillin 1	Skeletal, ocular, cardiovascular abnormalities, hyperextensible skin, striae distensae	Dissecting aorta (painless), M.C. skin lesion is striae (60%); spontaneous pneumothorax	
Congenital Contractural Arachnodactyly	AD; *FBN2* Fibrillin 2	Camptodactyly and joint contractures		
De Barsy Syndrome	AR	Cutis Laxa	Corneal clouding, mental retardation, dwarfism	↓Elastin mRNA levels
Anetoderma	Not inherited	Localized areas of atrophic, sac-like lesions		↓**Desmosine**

J. Finch & M. Payette

5. Disorders of Connective Tissue

See also Table 18.6: Connective Tissue Disorders (p. 127)

Ehlers-Danlos Syndrome

Overview

- Pathogenesis:
  - Defects in collagen family (28 distinct proteins)
    - Intracellular
      - S-S bonds at carboxyl ends → triple helix formation
    - Extracellular
      - Removal of propeptides and fibril assembly, stabilization by intermolecular cross-linking
  - 3 types of mutations
    - **Enzyme deficiency**
      - **Kyphoscoliosis, Dermatosparaxis**
    - **Dominant-negative effects** (loss of function mutation but **retains ability to di/trimerize**)
      - Splicing mutations resulting in **in-frame deletion of a single exon** or **missense mutations resulting in a glycine substitution in the collagenous domain**
      - **Classic (AD)**, **Vascular**, **Arthrochalasia**
    - **Haploinsufficiency**
      - 2 types
        - Loss of function mutations, often **premature termination codon** mutations resulting in **unstable mRNA and absence of corresponding peptide**
        - Missense mutations with **synthesis of polypeptides** that are **unable to be incorporated**
        - Reduced production (50% of normal)
      - **Classic (AD)**, **Vascular**

Presentation

- **Vascular** (IV) & **Kyphoscoliosis** (VI) **types do not have hyperelastic skin**
- All other types have velvety, hyperextensible skin and:
  - Easy bruising, poor wound healing, thin and atrophic appearing scars
  - Gaping **"fish mouth"** scars with minor trauma
  - **Molluscoid Pseudotumors** = soft fleshy nodules in areas of trauma (forearms, shins; fig 5.1)

- **Spheroids** = calcified subcutaneous nodules resulting from fat necrosis
- Histopathology
  - Generally non-diagnostic
  - Collagen fibrils appear "hieroglyphic" in cross-section in Dermatosparaxis type
- Treatment
  - No specific treatment
  - Prevention of trauma is most important
    - Shin guards, avoidance of contact sports
    - Prolonged use of sutures to avoid wound dehiscence

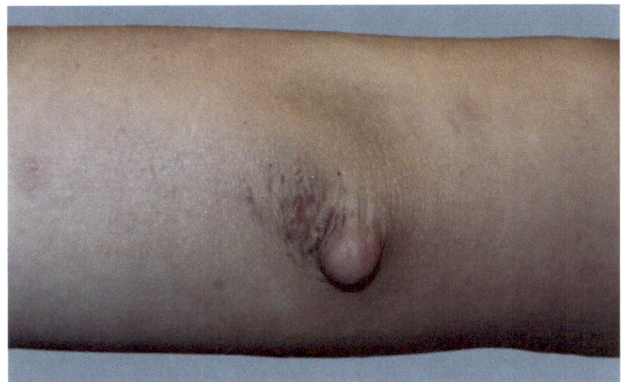

Figure 5.1: Molluscoid Pseudotumor (image courtesy of Hanspaul Makkar, MD)

EDS, Classical (I, II)

- Inheritance (AD, AR)
  - AD: **collagen V** (*COL5A1*, *COL5A2*)
  - AR: absence of tenascin-X leading to reduced collagen fibril density
- Clinical features:
  - Hypermobile joints, scoliosis
  - Hyperextensible skin
  - Mitral valve prolapse, dilated aortic root
  - Pes planus
  - Classical and Hypermobility types have absent lingual and labial frenula (Gorlin sign)
  - **AR tenascin-X cases get congenital adrenal hyperplasia**

EDS Hypermobility (III)

- AD; mutation in **tenascin-X** (*TNXB*)
- Clinical features
  - 90% female
  - Generalized joint hypermobility
  - Hyperextensible skin
  - Recurrent joint dislocations

EDS Vascular (IV)

- AD; mutation in **collagen III** α_1-chain (*COL3A1*)
  - Collagen III is present in arterial and intestinal walls. Less abundant in dermis but leads to small and variably sized dermal collagen fibrils
- Clinical features:
  - Thin, translucent skin, but <u>not</u> hyperelastic!
  - High risk for **arterial, intestinal, and uterine ruptures**
    - Often extensive bruising
    - Spontaneous arterial rupture highest in 3rd-4th decades
  - Characteristic facies: thin, pinched nose, thin lips, hollow cheeks, and prominent eyes
  - Vascular EDS is **the only type with premature death**
- Tx: celiprolol (β-blocker) ↓ risk of arterial rupture

> **Think "Wounded FBI" to remember that collagen III is present in healing wounds and EDS, vascular exhibits:**
>
> **F**etal Collagen (Col III) mutations, **F**etal (uterine) rupture, **B**lood vessel rupture, **I**ntestine rupture

EDS Kyphoscoliosis (VI)

- AR; mutation in *PLOD1*, encodes **lysyl hydroxylase** (normally converts lysine → hydroxylysine
  - Mutation results in ↓ hydroxylysine and altered collagen cross-linking
- Clinical features:
  - Skin is <u>not</u> hyperelastic!
  - Generalized joint laxity
  - Severe hypotonia at birth ("floppy baby") leads to delayed gross motor development
  - **Eye problems** are prominent, including glaucoma and scleral fragility → risk of globe rupture
  - Easy bruising
  - Progressive kyphoscoliosis, apparent at birth
- Labs: ↑ urine deoxypyridinoline: pyridinoline ratio
- Tx: ascorbic acid

> **EDS, Kyphoscoliosis**
>
> Picture a floppy baby with a crooked spine (kyphoscoliosis), exploded eyeballs, extensive bruising, but NO skin laxity. The baby has head lice (lysyl hydroxylase)

EDS Arthrochalasia (VIIA, VIIB)

- AD; mutation in **collagen I** (*COL1A1, COL1A2*) affecting α_1 and α_2-chains of type I collagen
- Clinical features
  - Severe generalized joint hypermobility with recurrent dislocations of large joints and **congenital bilateral hip dislocation**
  - Classic and kyphoscoliosis findings may be present

EDS Dermatosparaxis (VIIC)

- AR; mutation in **procollagen N-peptidase** (***ADAMTS2***), which cleaves amino-terminal propeptides from type 1 procollagen
  - Collagen fibrils are irregular and thin, and appear "hieroglyphic" in cross-section on EM
  - Type I collagen with intact N-propeptide (pN-collagen)
- Clinical features:
  - **Severe skin fragility and sagging, redundant skin** (like a hound dog)
  - May have soft, doughy skin with easy bruising, but normal wound healing
  - Premature rupture of membranes in pregnancy
  - Large umbilical or inguinal hernias
  - Delayed closure of fontanels, facies of puffy eyelids, micrognathia, blue sclera, may have gingival hyperplasia, abnormal dentition, and short limbs

Other Types of EDS

- <u>EDS cardiac valvular</u>:
  - AR; mutation in α_2-chain of Type I collagen (*COL1A2*)
  - Cardiac valve defects + classical findings

- EDS progeroid
  - AR; mutation in *B4GALT7* gene, encoding **galactosyltransferase-1** (xylosylprotein 4-β-galactosyltransferase), involved in the assembly of the **dermatan sulfate** chain
  - Progeroid facies, osteopenia, mental and growth retardation
- EDS periventricular nodular heterotopia variant
  - **XLD**; mutation in *FLNA* gene, encoding **filamin A** (actin-binding protein 280)
  - Aortic dilation, periventricular nodular heterotopias

Premature Aging Syndromes

Progeria (Hutchinson-Gilford)
- AD; **lamin A** mutation, a nuclear envelope protein
  - Allelic with:
    - Emery-Dreifuss muscular dystrophy
    - Familial partial lipodystrophy
    - Charcot-Marie-Tooth
    - Mandibuloacral dysplasia
- Sclerodermoid skin
- Prominent veins visible through thin skin
- Delayed eruption of permanent teeth (also seen in KID syndrome)
- Death in teens from atherosclerosis
- Tx: lonafarnib (farnesyltransferase inhibitor)

Werner Syndrome (Adult Progeria)
- AR; *RECQL2* mutation
- Does not present until 20's-30's (vs Progeria presents in infancy)
- **Bird-like facies** and high-pitched voice
- **Chronic leg ulcers**, especially at bony prominences
- **Sclerodermoid changes**
- Diabetes, premature atherosclerosis
- ↑ cancers, especially osteosarcoma & thyroid carcinoma

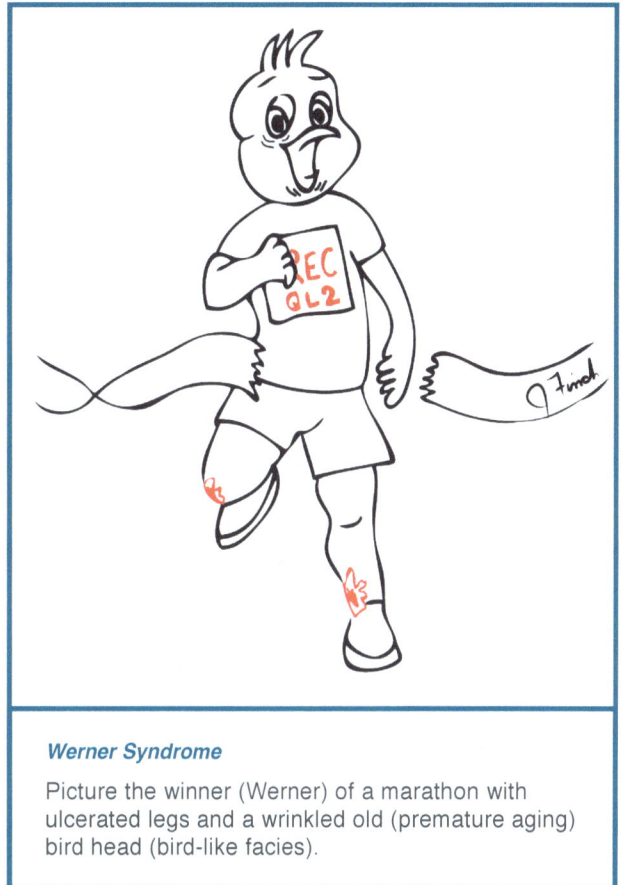

Werner Syndrome

Picture the winner (Werner) of a marathon with ulcerated legs and a wrinkled old (premature aging) bird head (bird-like facies).

Table 5.1: Leg Ulcers

Genoderms with leg ulcers	Drugs that cause leg ulcers
Werner	
Klinefelter	MTX
Homocystinuria	Hydroxyurea
Prolidase Deficiency	

Hallermann-Streiff Syndrome (Oculomandibulofacial Syndrome)
- Connexin 43 (*GJA1*) mutation
- Hypotrichosis, microphthalmia, congenital cataracts, beaked nose, micrognathia, short stature
- Natal teeth

Cockayne Syndrome
- See p. 56

Dyskeratosis Congenita
- See p. 84

Disorders with Lax Skin

Cutis Laxa

- Inheritance: AR, AD, **XLR**, or acquired
  - AD form: **elastin** (*ELN*) mutation. Rarely fubulin-5 (*FBLN5*)
  - AR form (m.c.): **Fibulin-4** (*FBLN4*) & **Fibulin-5** (*FBLN5*) mutation, a calcium-dependent, elastin-binding protein
    - Rarely *PYCR1, ATP6V0A2*
  - XLR form: *ATP7A*, a copper transporter
  - Acquired: following febrile illness, penicillamine
  - Cutis Laxa with Marfanoid Phenotype: Laminin β1 (*LAMB1*)
- Pathogenesis: elastic fibers are fragmented and diminished
  - Possibly abnormal copper metabolism (or copper chelation in the case of penicillamine), causing a reduction in lysyl oxidase activity, thereby decreasing desmosine crosslinks
- Clinical features:
  - Skin
    - Loose, baggy inelastic skin, giving 'bloodhound' look
    - Wound healing is normal
  - Extracutaneous (seen only in AR form)
    - Vocal cord laxity causing deep resonant voice, hoarse cry
    - Emphysema, leading to cor pulmonale
    - GI/GU-GI and urinary diverticula, umbilical and inguinal hernias

De Barsy Syndrome

- AR; *ALDH18A1*
- Severe Cutis Laxa, MR, growth retardation, dwarfism, corneal clouding

Wrinkly Skin Syndrome

- AR; *ATP6V0A2* (allelic with some forms of AR Cutis Laxa)
- ↓ elastic recoil of skin
- "Wrinkled" palms/soles (↑ palmar/plantar creases)
- Multiple musculoskeletal abnormalities

Costello Syndrome

- Cutis Laxa + nasolabial warts + rhabdomyosarcoma
- See p. 114 for full discussion

Ullrich Scleroatonic Muscular Dystrophy

- Collagen 6 mutation (*COL6A1, COL6A2, COL6A3*)
- Puffy skin, distal joint hypermobility (EDS-like), muscular dystrophy

Arterial Tortuosity Syndrome

- AR; mutation in glucose transporter 10 (**GLUT-10**, *SLC2A10*)
- Hyperextensible or lax skin, telangiectasias on cheeks
- Tortuous arteries

Loeys-Dietz Syndrome

- TGF-β receptors 1 and 2 (*TGFBR1, TGFBR2*)
- Translucent skin, bifid uvula, aortic aneurysms, arterial tortuosity, joint hypermobility, and craniofacial anomalies

Disorders with Aplasia Cutis

Goltz Syndrome (Focal Dermal Hypoplasia)

- **XLD**; mutation in *PORCN* gene (porcupine homologue), part of the Wnt pathway
- **Osteopathia striata** (80%)
- Syndactyly (**lobster hands**)
- Coloboma
- Soft yellow nodules (fat herniations) in Blaschko's lines
- Linear streaky atrophy with telangiectasias, aplasia cutis congenita (15%)

GOLTZ

Golden papules
Osteopathia striata
Lobster claw, Linear lesions
Teeth/hair/nail
ulcer**Z** and eye**Z**

Setleis Syndrome (Focal Facial Dermal Dysplasia)

- Most spontaneous. Some due to AR mutation in *TWIST2*
- Puerto Ricans; atrophic skin at the temples; eyebrows slant sharply upward and laterally; periorbital puffiness
- Low frontal hairline, pursed lips
- Double row of eyelashes (distichiasis)

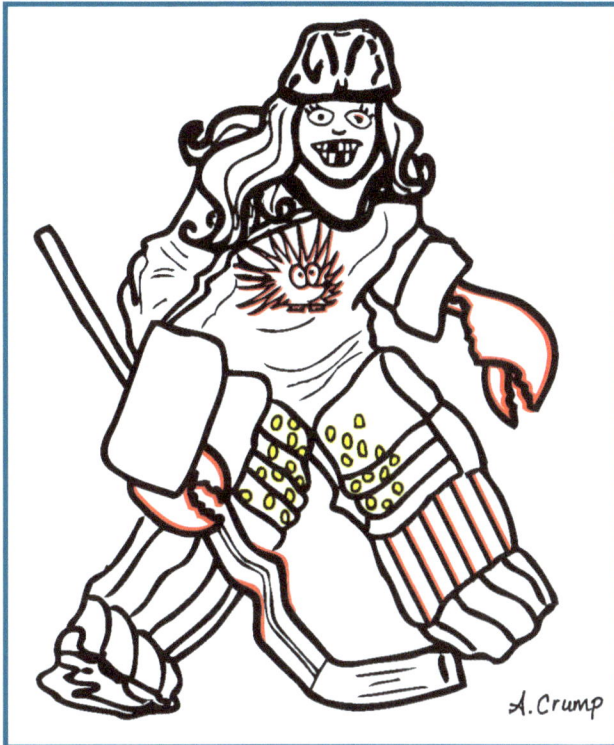

Goltz Syndrome

Picture a female hockey goalie (Goltz is XLD inheritance) with knocked out teeth (hypodontia), colobomas, a crooked stick (scoliosis) and lobster hands (syndactyly). The mascot on her jersey is a porcupine (PORCN gene) and her shin pads have vertical stripes (osteopathia striata)

Bart's Syndrome

- Form of Dominant Dystrophic EB (*COL7A1* gene) characterized by aplasia cutis congenita

Johanson-Blizzard Syndrome

- AR; *UBR1* mutation
- Aplasia cutis congenita w/ sparse hair, absent nasal alae, and pancreatic insufficiency

Adams-Oliver Syndrome

- AD; mutation in *ARHGAP31*, a GTPase
- AR; mutation in *DOCK6*
- Cutis marmorata telangiectatica congenita + aplasia cutis congenita + transverse limb defects (brachydactyly, syndactyly)
- Cryptorchidism, cardiac abnormalities

MIDAS Syndrome

- **XLD;** mutation in *HCCS* gene encoding Holocytochrome C Synthase
- **Mi**crophthalmia, **D**ermal **A**plasia, and **S**clerocornea

Miscellaneous Connective Tissue Disorders

Marfan Syndrome

- AD; mutation in **fibrillin-1** (*FBN1*)
- Clinical features:
  - Eye: **upward lens displacement** (ectopia lentis, 70%)
    - Myopia in ~100%
  - Cardiovascular: aortic aneurysm, mitral valve prolapse
    Skeletal: tall stature, arachnodactyly, pigeon chest, high arched palate, loose joints
    - Kyphoscoliosis, long extremities (fig 5.2)
  - Cutaneous: striae, elastosis perforans serpiginosa
- Tx: ECHO to monitor aortic root

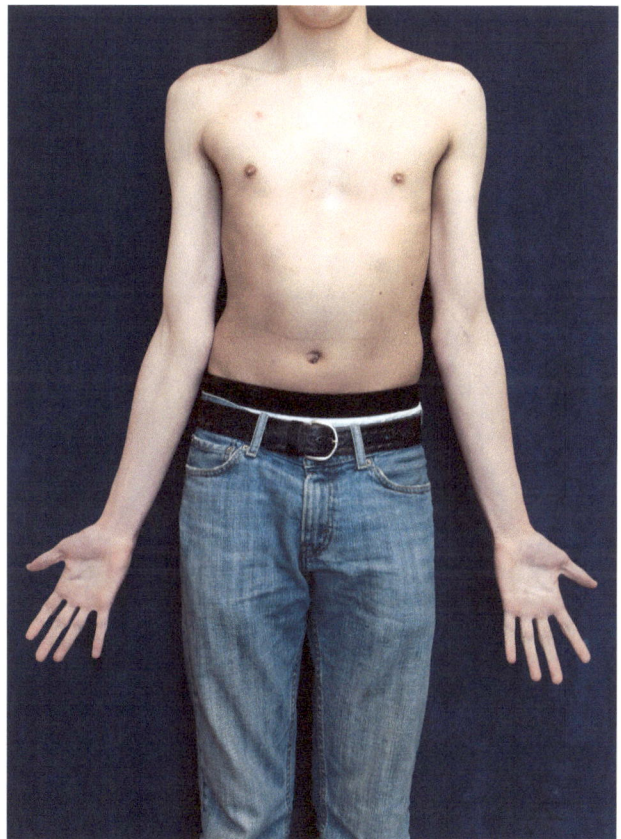

Figure 5.2: Marfan Syndrome

Table 5.2: Genoderms with Marfanoid Habitus
Marfan
MEN2B
Homocystinuria
Congenital Contractural Arachnodactyly
Cutis Laxa w/ marfanoid phenotype
Loeys-Dietz Syndrome
Klinefelter Syndrome

Stiff Skin Syndrome

- AD; mutation in *FBN* (fibrillin-1, same gene as Marfan)
- Congenital or develops in early childhood
- Rock-hard induration and thickening of skin and SubQ, especially on buttocks/thighs
- Spares inguinal folds, hands & feet
- Posture = hip/knee flexion and lordosis
- Stable or slowly progressive

Congenital Contractural Arachnodactyly

- AD; mutation in **fibrillin-2** (*FBN2*)
- Clinical features: similar to Marfan, but without cardiovascular and ocular problems
- "Crumpled" ears

Homocystinuria

- AR; mutation in **cystathionine β-synthase** (*CBS*), needed for methionine metabolism (specifically, conversion of homocysteine)
- Clinical features:
  - **Downward lens displacement** (vs upward in Marfan)
  - **Marfanoid** skeletal features, but no hyperextensibility (CBS involved in sulfur metabolism needed for collagen cross-linking)
  - Cutaneous: malar flush, thin hair, leg ulcers
  - **Thrombotic events**
  - MR
- Labs: ↑ urinary homocysteine and methionine
- Tx: some patients respond to **pyridoxine** (B$_6$), which is a cofactor for CBS. Avoid alfalfa and bean sprouts (which have lots of homocysteine)

Osteogenesis Imperfecta

- AD/AR; mutation in *COL1A1* or *COL1A2* (rarely, prolyl-3-hydroxylase)
- Clinical features: 8 types with varying presentation
  - Skin: thin skin with easy bruising and atrophic scars
  - Skeletal:
    - Skeletal deformities and fractures, "codfish vertebrae" (hollowing out by pressure of intervertebral discs)
    - Bimodal fracture peaks = prepubertal and late adulthood
    - Joint laxity, dislocation
  - Other: deafness by 3rd decade (due to otosclerosis), **blue sclera**, dentinogenesis imperfecta
- Death due to respiratory failure (from kyphoscoliosis)
- OI1: Collagen normal quality but insufficient quantity
  - Blue sclera, poor muscle tone, loose joints. **Heart valve problems**
- OI2: Collagen poor quality and quantity
  - **Death in first year** due to respiratory failure or hemorrhagic stroke
- OI3: Collagen sufficient quantity but poor quality
  - No blue sclera. Striking dentinogenesis imperfecta   ·
- OI4: Collagen sufficient quantity but poor quality
  - No blue sclera

Think "I Say A Good POEM" to remember diseases with blue sclera	
I	Incontinentia Pigmenti
Say	Steroids (one report, Prednisone)
A	Anetoderma
Good	Goltz Syndrome
P	PXE
O	Osteogenesis Imperfecta
E	EDS Type VI
M	Marfan's

J. Finch & M. Payette

Lipoid Proteinosis (Hyalinosis Cutis et Mucosae, Urbach-Wiethe Disease)

- AR; mutation in **ECM-1** gene, resulting in deposition of hyaline material
  - ECM-1 binds to **perlecan** and regulates basement membrane production
  - ↑ fibroblast production of collagen IV and laminin
- Clinical features:
  - First sign: **hoarse, weak cry**
  - Skin lesions by age 2
    - Skin stage 1: vesicles & crusts on face, mouth and extremities (trauma associated) →**ice pick scarring**
    - Skin stage 2: hyaline deposits in the dermis→ **thick, waxy, yellow skin**. Papules & plaques on axillae and face (**"string of pearls"** along eyelid margin). **Verrucous plaques on elbows and knees**
  - Other findings: thickened tongue, parotitis from Stenson's duct occlusion; absent incisor teeth, tooth loss
  - Seizures **(temporal and hippocampal comma-shaped calcifications)**
  - Slowly progressive, normal life span
- Path
  - Amorphous, laminated material (PAS+) around blood vessels and in connective tissues; "reduplication of BM" of blood vessels and sometimes DEJ containing Type II and IV collagens and laminin
  - Amorphous material contains non-collagen proteins, including neutral mucopolysaccharides & hyaluronic acid
- Ddx: EPP, amyloidosis, papular mucinosis, colloid milium, non-Langerhans histiocytosis, xanthoma
- Tx: scattered reports of penicillamine, oral retinoids, dimethyl sulfoxide

Table 5.3: Genoderms with Intracranial Calcifications

Lipoid Proteinosis	"Bean shaped" temporal (hippocampal)
Sturge-Weber	Tram track calcifications
Papillon-Lefèvre	Dural calcifications
Basal Cell Nevus Syndrome	Falx calcification
Tuberous Sclerosis	Paraventricular (basal ganglia)
Dyskeratosis Congenita	Basal ganglia
Cockayne Syndrome	Basal ganglia

Pseudoxanthoma Elasticum (PXE)

- AR/AD; or acquired
- Defect: inactivating mutations in *ABCC6*, or acquired (penicillamine)
- Pathogenesis: ABCC6 is an organic acid transporter expressed exclusively in liver and kidneys. Mutations result in accumulation of toxic metabolites that cause progressive calcification of elastin with fragmentation of elastic fibers
- Clinical features:
  - Cutaneous: yellow cobblestone plaques of "**chicken skin**" (average age 13), progressive, coalescing, may be total
    - Starts in lateral neck, then other flexural sites
    - Occasionally coexisting elastosis perforans serpiginosa
    - 2/3 have double chin
  - Ocular: **angioid streaks** in Bruch's membrane in 100%, macular degeneration, retinal hemorrhage
    - "Leopard spotting" = mottling of retinal pigment epithelium
  - Cardiovascular: due to calcification of elastic media
    - Gastric artery hemorrhage, claudication, HTN, MI, CVA, mitral valve prolapse, angina
  - Lungs not involved
- Management
  - Baseline CV and ophtho exams
  - Semi-annual ophtho exams
  - Avoid trauma, smoking
  - ↑ dietary Ca and Mg slows calcification

Buschke-Ollendorff Syndrome

- AD; *LEMD3* mutation (allelic with melorheostosis)
  - Encodes MAN1, which antagonizes SMAD
  - Loss of MAN1 leads to ↑TGF-β & BMP (bone morphogenesis protein)
- **Dermatofibrosis lenticularis disseminata**: widespread connective tissue nevi (elastomas) presenting as yellow papules, especially on the buttocks
- **Osteopoikilosis**: speckled epiphyses

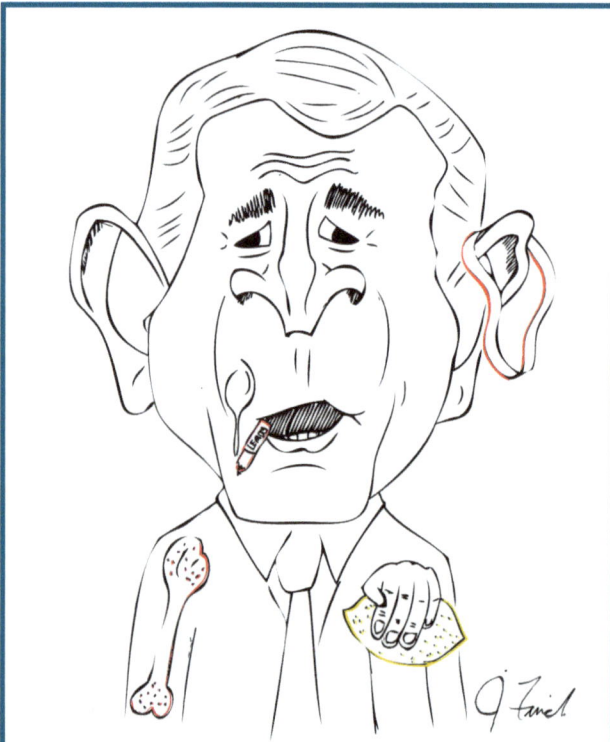

Buschke-Ollendorff Syndrome

Picture President George Bush with an elastic band around his ear, smoking a LEMD3 cigarette butt (elastomas on the buttocks). He is holding a lemon (LEMD3) and has osteopoikilosis

Melorheostosis

- Germline or somatic mutations in *LEMD3* gene
- Form of **linear scleroderma** with deep involvement of bone, affecting a single limb
- **"Dripping candle wax"** appearance of bone on X-ray
- Can be seen as an isolated finding or as part of Buschke-Ollendorff

Williams Syndrome

- AD; deletion of **elastin** gene, or possibly elastin gene downregulation by prenatal vitamin D exposure
- Clinical features:
  - Supravalvular aortic stenosis, HTN
  - Low IQ, attention deficit disorder
  - Dysmorphic facies
  - Gregarious personality
  - Infantile hypercalcemia

Genoderms with Dermal Hypertrophy

Pachydermoperiostosis (Hypertrophic Osteoarthropathy, Touraine-Solente-Golé Syndrome)

- AR; mutation in *HPGD* gene → ↑ PGE_2
- AR; mutation in *SLCO2A1* gene
- AD; gene unknown
- M:F = 7:1, with onset in late adolescence
- Clinical findings:
  - **Thickening of skin folds** and accentuation of creases on the face, scalp, **cutis verticis gyrata,** thickening of the eyelids, ears, lips, enlargement of the tongue
  - **Clubbing** of the fingers
  - **Periostosis of the long bones**
  - Elbows, knees, hands are enlarged and spindle-shaped
  - Hyperhidrosis, hyperkeratotic lesions of the palms and soles; stippled lines, resembling **"sand of the wind-blown desert"**
- AR variants have cleft palate & congenital heart defects
- Acquired forms: seen w/ chronic pulmonary, mediastinal, and cardiac diseases, chronic peripheral hypoxia; bronchogenic carcinoma (usually in men >40 w/ enlargement of forehead, hands, fingers)

Beare-Stevenson Cutis Gyrata Syndrome

- AD; mutation in *FGFR2* (allelic with Apert Syndrome)
- Furrowed skin on scalp (cutis verticis gyrata), forehead, preauricular, neck, trunk, palms and soles
- Acanthosis nigricans, craniosynostosis, prominent umbilical stump

Table 5.4: Genoderms with Dermal Hypertrophy	
Cutis Verticis Gyrata	**Beare-Stevenson**
	Pachydermoperiostosis
	Due to regressed lymphatic malformation
	– **Turner**
	– **Noonan**
	Acromegaly
	Infiltrative tumors
Knuckle Pads	**Bart-Pumphrey**
Keloids	**Rubinstein-Taybi**
	Goeminne
	Turner
	EDS-Vascular Type
Skin tags	**Cowden** (tags are actually sclerotic fibromas)
	Birt-Hogg-Dubé (tags are fibrofolliculomas)
	BCC Nevus Syndrome (tag-like BCCs, especially in children)
	Tuberous Sclerosis
Connective Tissue Nevus	**Cowden** (collagenomas)
	Tuberous Sclerosis (Shagreen patch = collagenoma)
	MEN-1 (collagenomas in 33%)
	Bushke-Ollendorff (dermatofibrosis lenticularis disseminata = widespread elastomas)
Angiofibroma	**Tuberous Sclerosis**
	Birt-Hogg-Dubé
	MEN-1
Desmoid Tumor (low grade fibrohistiocytic neoplasm)	15% of abdominal desmoids associated with Gardner or FAP

Juvenile Hyaline Fibromatosis & Infantile Systemic Hyalinosis (Murray-Puretic-Drescher Syndrome)

- JHF & ISH are allelic AR conditions caused by mutations in **capillary morphogenesis protein-2 (*CMG-2*)**
  - Encodes an **integrin-like** cell surface receptor that **binds laminin** and **Type IV collagen**, resulting in hyaline accumulation in the dermis
  - Mutations in **cytoplasmic domain** (in-frame mutations) → **JHF**
  - Mutations in **extracellular domain** (mostly truncating) → **ISH**
- Juvenile Hyaline Fibromatosis (JHF)
  - **Destructive keloid-like nodules on ears**. Also head/neck, anogenital, then hand
  - **Joint contractures**
  - Gingival hypertrophy
  - **Osteopenia**
- Infantile Systemic Hyalinosis (ISH)
  - More severe, with involvement of internal organs, IUGR
  - **Diffuse** thick, stiff skin
  - Papules are smaller (no nodules)
  - **Bluish plaques** over extensors. Joint contractures lead to frog-leg deformity
  - **Death by age 2** from recurrent pulmonary infections and diarrhea
- Treatment: physiotherapy, surgical release of joint contractures; systemic IFN-α2b for skin lesions, joint contractures and gingival hypertrophy
- Ddx
  - Winchester Syndrome: (AR; *MMP-2* mutation, short stature, coarse facies, corneal opacities, thickened, leathery lips, generalized osteolysis and progressive painful arthropathy
  - Nodulosis-Arthropathy-Osteolysis Syndrome: allelic with Winchester (AR; *MMP-2* mutation), shares clinical features (nodules, joint contractures, and osteopenia)

Familial Reactive Perforating Collagenosis

- AR; unknown gene
- Begins in infancy or childhood and appears clinically as recurrent koebnerizing umbilicated papules that resolve spontaneously in 6 to 8 weeks

Rubinstein-Taybi Syndrome

- AD; *CREBBP* mutation (CREB binding protein), 99% are sporadic
  - 3% are due to *EP300* gene mutation
- Key features:
  - Skin: mid-face vascular stain (50%); **spontaneous keloids**, **pilomatricomas**, **hypertrichosis** (lateral face, synophrys, trichomegaly)
  - Musculoskeletal: broad thumbs and halluces (broad terminal phalanges ± angle deformity)
  - Striking facies: large beaked nose; "grimacing" smile; high arched eyebrows, trichomegaly, microcephaly
  - Severe MR

Goeminne Syndrome

- **XLD** mutation of *TKCR* gene
- T Torticollis
- K **Keloids**
- C Cryptorchidism
- R Renal dysplasia

6. Metabolic Disorders

See also Table 18.12: Disorders of Metabolism (p. 134)

Sphingolipidoses

Overview

- Enzyme replacement therapy is available for Fabry and Gaucher

Fabry's Disease

- **XLR**; **α-galactosidase A deficiency** (*GLA*), resulting in **accumulation of globotriaosylceramide** (Gb3)
- Skin findings:
  - Accumulation of Gb3 in cutaneous endothelial cells weakens vessel wall and results in vascular ectasias (angiokeratomas)
  - **Angiokeratoma corporis diffusum** – starting around umbilicus & scrotum around age 5-10, extending to bathing trunk distribution
  - Anhidrosis
  - **Neuropathic pain**: chronic acral paresthesias in early childhood, plus severe crises of acral & GI pain
- Systemic findings:
  - Renal & heart failure, degenerative neuropathy, cerebral artery thrombosis
  - **Whorled corneal opacities (pathognomonic)**. Also present in 90% of female carriers
  - **"Maltese crosses"** = birefringent lipid inclusions in urine
- Path
  - "Mulberry cells" = lipid-filled epithelial cells
  - **Zebra bodies** on EM
- Fabry's often goes undiagnosed until ESRD or CV pathology develops in 20's. Affected men die in 30's from MI, CVA, or renal failure
- Female carriers: normal lifespan but 20% get angiokeratomas
- Tx: enzyme replacement

Fucosidosis

- **AR**; **α-L-fucosidase** (*FUCA1*) deficiency
- Accumulation of glycolipids, mucopolysaccharides, polysaccharides
- Skin changes similar to Fabry's, but without renal failure or CVA/CAD, and no cytoplasmic lipids

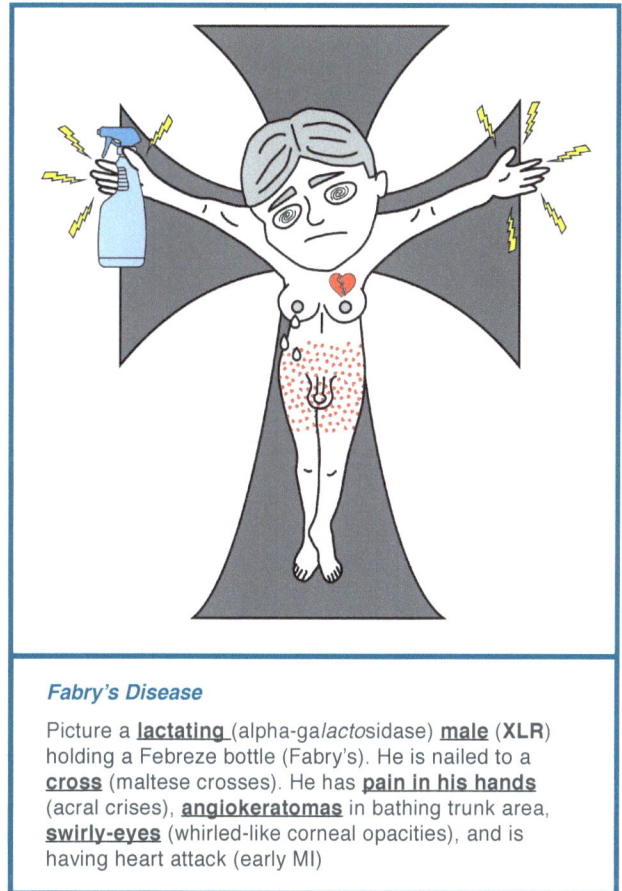

Fabry's Disease

Picture a **lactating** (alpha-ga*lacto*sidase) **male** (**XLR**) holding a Febreze bottle (Fabry's). He is nailed to a **cross** (maltese crosses). He has **pain in his hands** (acral crises), **angiokeratomas** in bathing trunk area, **swirly-eyes** (whirled-like corneal opacities), and is having heart attack (early MI)

3 Types

- Type I: patients die in a few years, only minimal skin changes (hyperhidrosis & thickened skin)
- Type II: is milder, mostly bony disease, no skin changes
- Type III: usually live until adolescence, diffuse angiokeratomas, purple nail bands, CNS involvement
- Tx: none

Gaucher's Disease

- **AR**; mutation in *GBA* gene, encoding β-glucocerebrosidase, resulting in **α-β-glucocerebrosidase deficiency**
- Hyperpigmentation
- Lipid-filled macrophages
- Tx: hematopoietic stem cell transplant, enzyme replacement

Niemann-Pick Disease

- AR; mutation in sphingomyelin phosphodiesterase-1 (*SMPD-1*) results in **accumulation of sphingomyelin**
- CNS issues, cherry red spots on fovea
- Yellow skin with **xanthomas** and waxy induration
- Also have foamy histiocytes on bone marrow biopsy

Bromhidrosis & Chromhidrosis

Table 6.1: Genoderms with Bromhidrosis and Chromhidrosis	
Apocrine Bromhidrosis	
Normal occurrence	Corynebacterium or micrococcus
Eccrine Bromhidrosis	
Keratinogenic	Plantar or intertriginous
Phenylketonuria	Stale, musty or 'mousy' odor
Maple Syrup Urine Disease	Sweet odor
Methionine adenosyl-transferase deficiency	Boiled cabbage odor
Methionine Malabsorption Syndrome (Oasthouse Syndrome)	Dried celery, yeast, or malt (An oasthouse is a place where hops are dried)
Trimethylaminuria	Fishy odor
Tyrosinemia Type 1	Cabbage or rancid butter odor
Dimethylglycine dehydrogenase deficiency	Fishy odor
Isovaleric acidemia	Sweaty feet odor
Apocrine Chromhidrosis	
Alkaptonuria	Black sweat
High lipofuscin content (normal variant)	Yellow, green, blue, or black, (depending on oxidation state) that fluoresce under Wood's
Eccrine Chromhidrosis	
Always extrinsic	e.g. clofazimine, rifampin

Trimethylaminuria

- *FMO3* mutation → ↓ **f**lavin-containing **m**on**o**oxygenase 3
- ↑ trimethylamine in sweat after eating fish or eggs (foods with choline, carnitine or lecithin)
- Fishy odor

Methionine Malabsorption Syndrome (Oasthouse Syndrome)

- Gene mutation unknown. Only a few cases described in 1960s
- Mental retardation, convulsions
- Urine and sweat have odor like an oasthouse (a building where hops are dried), akin to dried celery, yeast, or malt
- Odor is due to alpha-hydroxybutyric acid formed by bacterial action on the unabsorbed methionine

Disorders with Xanthomas and Lipid Abnormalities

Familial Chylomicronemia (Fredrickson Type I)

Lipoprotein Lipase Deficiency

- AR; *LPL* gene mutation
- Labs:
    - ↑ chylomicrons and ↑TGs (>1500)
    - ↓ LDL & HDL
- Skin: **eruptive xanthomas**
- Systemic findings:
    - **Presents in childhood with severe pancreatitis** (vs other lipoprotein disorders present as adult)
    - Hepatomegaly
    - Lipemia Retinalis
    - No ↑ risk CAD
- Tx: dietary modification

Apolipoprotein C2 Deficiency

- AR; *APO-C2* mutation
- Same phenotype as LPL Deficiency because APO-C2 is a cofactor for LPL

J. Finch & M. Payette

Familial Hypercholesterolemia (Type II)

Familial Hypercholesterolemia (Type IIa)

- *LDL-R* mutation
  - Rarely: *APO-A2, ITIH4, GHR, GSBS, EPHX2, ABCA1*
  - LDL receptor binds Apo-B100 on LDLs
  - Many Africans have accelerated LDL-R degradation rather than mutation
- M.C. **hyper-lipoproteinemia** (1:500 population are heterozygous)
- Derm findings:
  - M.C. **cause of tendinous xanthomas** (great majority of patients with tendinous xanthomas are heterozygous for *LDL-R* mutation)
    - **Heterozygotes only get tendinous xanthomas**
    - Homozygotes get all types (tendinous, eruptive, tuberous, plane)
- Labs: ↑ LDL, ↑ cholesterol
- Systemic findings
  - Arcus juvenilis (fig 6.1)
  - Atherosclerosis
- Tx:
  - Heterozygotes: statin
  - Homozygotes: liver transplant (get intact LDL-receptor from donor liver) or plasmapheresis

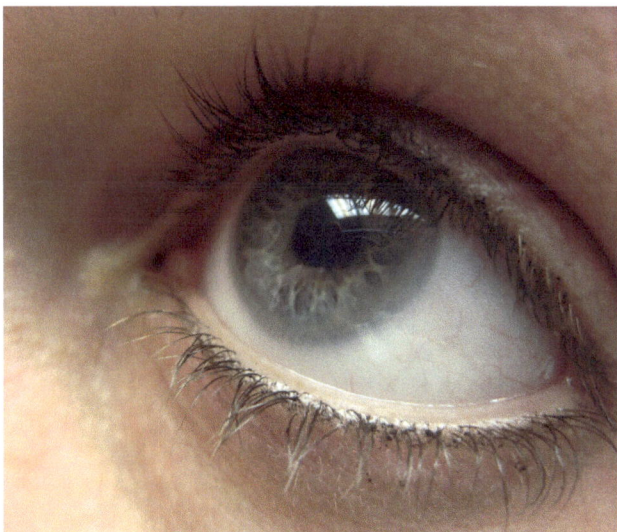

Figure 6.1: Arcus Juvenilis

Familial Defective APO-B100 (Type IIb)

- AR; *APO-B100* mutation
- Usually no xanthomas, but can have same phenotype as Familial Hypercholesterolemia because LDL receptor binds Apo-B100 on LDLs
  - **Plane xanthomas of finger webs** are characteristic (fig 6.2)

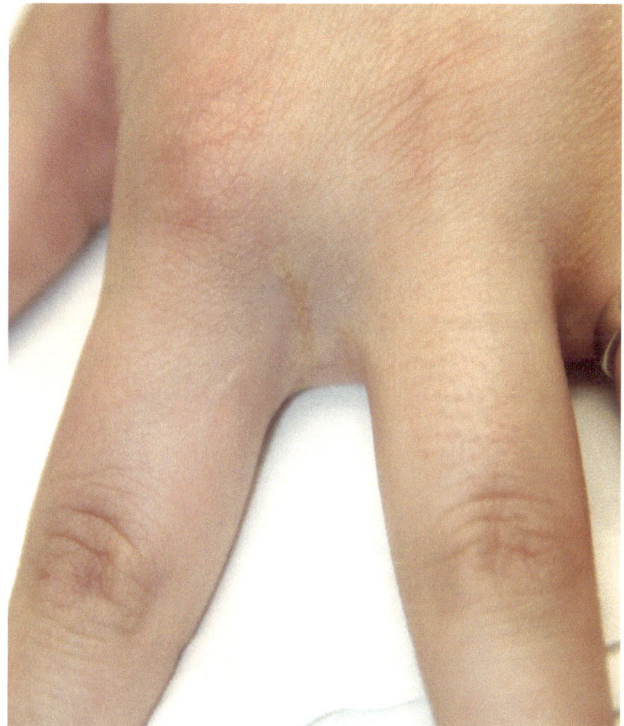

Figure 6.2: Plane Xanthomas of Finger Webs in APO-B100 Mutation

Defective Metabolism of Lipoprotein Remnants

Dysbetalipoproteinemia

- AR; mutation in *APO-E* gene
  - Patients only have Apo-E2, which is worse than E1 and E3
- Labs:
  - ↑ chylomicron remnants
  - ↑ cholesterol, ↑ TGs
  - **β-VLDL on electrophoresis**
- Skin findings:
  - Tuberoeruptive/tuberous xanthomas in 80%
  - Xanthoma striatum palmare: plane xanthomas of palmar creases in 66%
- Systemic findings:
  - Atherosclerosis
  - Diabetes, gout, obesity

Other Lipoprotein Disorders

Familial Hypertriglyceridemia
Familial HDL Deficiency

- AD; mutation in *APO-A1* gene or rarely *ABCA1* gene (allelic with Tangier Disease)
- AD; mutation in *LIPI,* lipase member I protein
- AD; mutation in *APO-A5*, Apolipoprotein A-V
- Skin findings are rare. Usually detected via routine lipid screening in adulthood

Xanthomas without Elevated Serum Lipids

Cerebrotendinous Xanthomatosis

- AR; mutation in *CYP27A1,* resulting in sterol-27-hydroxylase deficiency (a CYP450 enzyme in the bile acid synthetic pathway)
- Accumulation of **cholestanol** (intermediate in cholesterol metabolism) in virtually every tissue, particularly the Achilles tendon, brain and lungs
- **Tendinous xanthoma** = early finding, especially Achilles tendon
- Progressive neurologic dysfunction (cerebellar ataxia beginning after puberty), premature atherosclerosis, and cataracts

β-sitosterolemia (Phytosterolemia)

- AR; mutation in *ABC-G8* or *ABC-G5*, leading to **accumulation of plant sterols**
  - ABCG5 and ABCG8 heterodimerize to form efflux pumps that export free sterols from hepatocytes or enterocytes into the lumen
- Phenotype very similar to Familial Hypercholesterolemia (Type II)
  - Tendinous & tuberous xanthomas
  - Atherosclerosis
- Labs: ↑ cholesterol in childhood, but normalizes by adulthood
- Tx: dietary restriction

Tangier Disease

- AR; mutation in *ABC-A1* gene (cholesterol efflux regulator protein). Cells are unable to expel cholesterol into circulating HDLs
- **Tonsil xanthomas** (very large, yellow-orange tonsils)
- Enlarged liver, spleen and lymph nodes
- Hypocholesterolemia, and abnormal chylomicron remnants

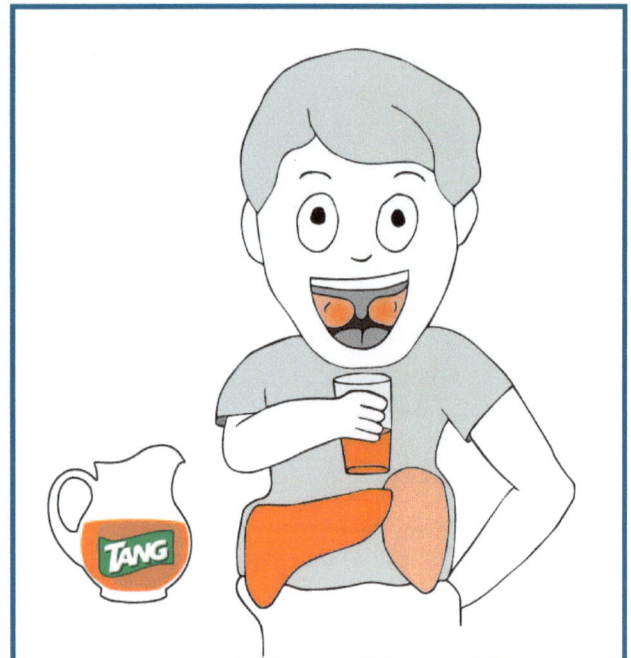

Tangier Disease

Picture a man drinking Tang (Tangier), which stains his tonsils and liver orange

Alagille-Watson Syndrome (Arteriohepatic Dysplasia)

- AD; deletion of *JAG1* gene in 5-7% of cases. 60% de novo mutations. Less commonly AD *NOTCH2* mutation
- **Direct hyperbilirubinemia** (caused by biliary hypoplasia) **+ congenital heart disease + triangle facies**
- Presents by age 3 months with liver failure
- Xanthomas

Alagille-Watson Syndrome

Picture an alligator (Alagille) with a triangle head (triangular facies), jaundice (hyperbilirubinemia) and xanthomas

J. Finch & M. Payette

Table 6.2: Hyperlipidemias (Fredrickson Types)

Fredrickson Type	Condition	Type of xanthoma
Type I	Familial Chylomicronemia (LPL)	Eruptive
Type II a	Familial Hypercholesterolemia (LDL-R)	Many types of xanthomas: tendinous, eruptive, tuberous, plane Heterozygotes: 15% by age 10 Homozygotes: 100% by age 6
Type II b	Familial Hypercholesterolemia (APO-B100)	Usually none, but can be similar to Type IIa
Type III	Familial Dysbetalipoproteinemia (APO-E)	Tuberoeruptive/tuberous xanthomas in 80% Xanthoma striatum palmare in 66% Can have any type
Type IV	Familial Hypertriglyceridemia	Rare, eruptive
Type V	Mixed Hyperlipidemia	Eruptive

Table 6.3: Genoderms with Xanthomas

Xanthoma Type	Genetic cause	Secondary cause

Eruptive xanthoma	Familial LPL Deficiency (Type I)
	APO-C2 Deficiency (Type I)
	Familial Hypertriglyceridemia (Type IV)
	Hyperchylomicronemia (Type V)
		Anything that causes increased triglycerides:
		  Obesity
		  Cholestasis
		  Diabetes
		  Drugs: retinoids, estrogen, protease inhibitors

Tendinous xanthoma	Familial Hypercholesterolemia (Type II) (great majority of patients with tendinous xanthomas are heterozygotes for Familial Hypercholesterolemia) Familial Dysbetalipoproteinemia (Type III) Familial Defective Apo-B Phytosterolemia Cerebrotendinous Xanthomatosis	
Tuberous xanthoma	Familial Hypercholesterolemia (Type II) Familial Dysbetalipoproteinemia (Type III) Familial Partial Lipodystrophy	Monoclonal gammopathies
Tonsil xanthomas	Tangier Disease	
Verruciform xanthoma	CHILD	
Xanthoma NOS	Niemann-Pick Alagille-Watson	

Atherosclerosis	Everything EXCEPT
	  Familial LPL Deficiency (Type I)
	  APO-C2 Deficiency (Type I)
	  Hyperchylomicronemia (Type V)	

Plane xanthomas		
Xanthoma striatum palmare	Familial Homozygous Hypercholesterolemia (Type II) Familial Dysbetalipoproteinemia (Type III)	Cholestasis
Xanthelasma	Familial Hypercholesterolemia (Type II) Familial Dysbetalipoproteinemia (Type III)	Monoclonal gammopathies
Diffuse plane Xanthomas		Monoclonal gammopathies, cholestasis

The Mucopolysaccharidoses

Hurler Syndrome (MPS I H)

- AR; mutation in α-L-iduronidase, resulting in **accumulation of dermatan sulfate and heparan sulfate**
- Clinical:
  - **Dermal melanocytosis** (anterior and posterior trunk)
  - "Gargoylism" (coarse facies), MR, cardiovascular involvement, hepatosplenomegaly, respiratory compromise, joint stiffness
  - Skeletal abnormalities, **dysostosis multiplex** (stiff joints)
  - Corneal clouding
- Heme: vacuolated lymphs

Hunter Syndrome (MPS II)

- **XLR**; mutation in iduronate 2-sulfatase, resulting in **accumulation of dermatan sulfate and heparan sulfate**
- Mild forms do not present until late childhood
- Clinical:
  - Distinctive **pebbly skin lesions**
  - MR, coarse facies, cardiovascular involvement, hepatosplenomegaly, joint stiffness
  - Dysostosis multiplex less severe than Hurler
  - No corneal clouding. Has retinal degeneration
- Heme: granulated lymphs

> **Hurler and Hunter Syndromes**
>
> Picture two cavemen (coarse "Gargoyle" facies) –
> One hurling a big rock (the Hurler) at a corncob shaped cloud (corneal clouding), with dermal melanocytosis
> One with a spear (the Hunter) on a cobblestone road (Pebbly cobblestone plaques)

Table 6.4: The Mucopolysaccharidoses

Type	Eponym	Enzyme
I-H	**Hurler (MPS I H)**	α-L-iduronidase
I-S	Schele	
II	**Hunter (MPS II)**	iduronate 2-sulfatase
III	Sanfilippo	
IV	Morquio A	
IV	Morquio B	
VI	Maroteaux-Lamy	
VII	Sly	

Low Yield

Lipodystrophy Syndromes

Congenital Generalized Lipodystrophy (Berardinelli-Seip Syndrome)

- AR; Type 1 = *AGPAT2* (TG & phospholipid synthesis); Type 2 = *BSCL2*
- **Generalized** loss of subcutaneous fat from birth, with **cadaveric facies, muscular appearing**, bone marrow and visceral fat deficiency
- **Metabolic Syndrome**: hepatosplenomegaly, insulin resistant DM, enlarged genitalia, acanthosis nigricans
- Death in 30s from hypertrophic cardiomyopathy or cirrhosis

Familial Partial Lipodystrophy

- AD
- FPLD Type 1 (Köbberling)
  - No compensatory fat accumulation on face/neck. Loss of fat on lower extremities
- FPLD Type 2 (Dunnigan)
  - Most common
  - *LMNA* gene encodes lamin A & lamin C → ↓ leptin, ↑ fasting insulin and C peptide
  - **Progressive symmetric** uniform loss of subcutaneous fat of extremities and trunk
  - ↑ compensatory fat in head and neck
- Accentuated subcutaneous veins, muscular appearance (fig 6.3)

J. Finch & M. Payette

- FPLD Type 3
  - *PPARG* gene encodes PPARγ → impaired adipogenesis
  - Similar to Type 2 but with more metabolic disturbances and less severe lipoatrophy
  - Metabolic disturbances: glucose intolerance/DM, CV disease, gynecologic abnormalities
  - Tuberous xanthomas, AN, hirsutism
- Mandibuloacral Dysplasia:
  - AR; *LMNA* or *ZMPSTE24* (Zn MMP to process prelamin A) mutation
  - Severe mandibuloacral dysplasia, premature aging, generalized lipodystrophy

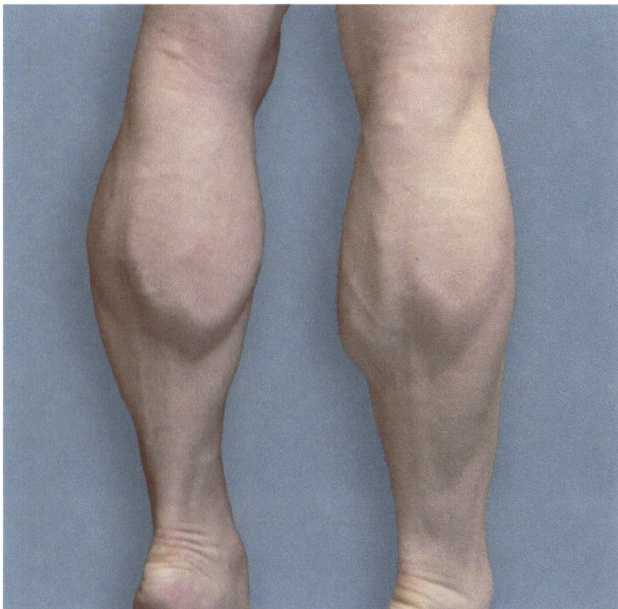

Figure 6.3: Familial Partial Lipodystrophy, Type 2, Demonstrating Very Muscular-appearing Calves in a Woman in Her 30s Due to Loss of Subcutaneous Fat

Leprechaunism (Donohue Syndrome)
- AR; mutation in **insulin receptor** (*INSR*)
- Generalized lipodystrophy, insulin resistance with paradoxical hypoglycemia, acanthosis nigricans, hirsutism
- Elfin facies, severe IUGR, large nipples/clitoris/penis, loose skin
- Death in infancy

SHORT Syndrome
- **S**hort stature, **H**yperextensible joints, **O**cular depression, **R**ieger anomaly/iridocorneal mesodermal dysgenesis, **T**eething delay

- Gene unknown
- Congenital lipoatrophy of the face, IUGR, delayed bone age, dysmorphic facies

AREDYLD Syndrome
- Congenital generalized lipoatrophic DM
- **A**cro**R**enal Field Defect, **E**ctodermal **Dy**splasia, And **L**ipoatrophic **D**iabetes
- Gene unknown

Poland Syndrome
- Rare congenital disorder with unilateral absence of breast/pectoralis major, ipsilateral symbrachydactyly, ichthyosis

Other Metabolic Diseases

Alkaptonuria (Ochronosis)
- AR mutation in **homogentisic acid oxidase** (*HGD*). Homogentisic acid (HA) accumulates, binds to collagen and inhibits lysyl hydroxylase
- Clinical
  - Presents in adulthood
  - Dark black pigmentation of cartilage, sweat, urine, ear wax, 3rd-5th decade
  - **Dark urine** when alkalinized (or after standing)
  - Severe arthropathy, especially knees (40s-50s)
  - Mitral & aortic valve calcification and regurgitation
  - Eye: dark spots on eye (**Osler's sign**)
- Path
  - Polymerized homogentisic acid causes collagen bundles to swell, forming "**banana bodies**"
  - Has a yellow-brown (ochre) color on H&E
- Tx: ascorbic acid (vitamin C), nitisinone (inhibits formation of HA)

> *Alkaptonuria (Ochronosis)*
>
> Picture a **homo**sexual guy (accumulation of **homo**gentisic acid) eating a banana, and wearing a baseball **CAP** (al**KAP**tonuria) with blue skin, joint pain, and black pee

Acrodermatitis Enteropathica
- AR; mutation in *SLC39A4* intestinal zinc transporter

- ↓↓ zinc
- Onset: 1-2 weeks after weaning from breast milk (breast milk has its own zinc binding factor)
- Clinical: diarrhea, dermatitis, and failure to thrive
  - **Periorificial and acral psoriasiform plaques** and erosions
  - Chronic form shows lichenified, psoriasiform plaques
  - **Alopecia** widespread
  - Nail changes: pustular paronychia, nail dystrophy
- Same phenotype can be caused by acquired severe zinc deficiency

Multiple Carboxylase Deficiency

- Periorificial dermatitis resembling zinc deficiency
- Alopecia, generalized eczema
- Prominent neuro findings (**seizures** by 6 months of age, hypotonia, ataxia)
- Lactic acidosis/ketosis, aciduria, hyperammonemia
- Neonatal form: AR; *HLCS*, holocarboxylase synthetase deficiency
  - Vomiting
- Juvenile form: AR; *BTD*, biotinidase deficiency
  - Optic atrophy and hearing loss
- Tx: biotin lifelong

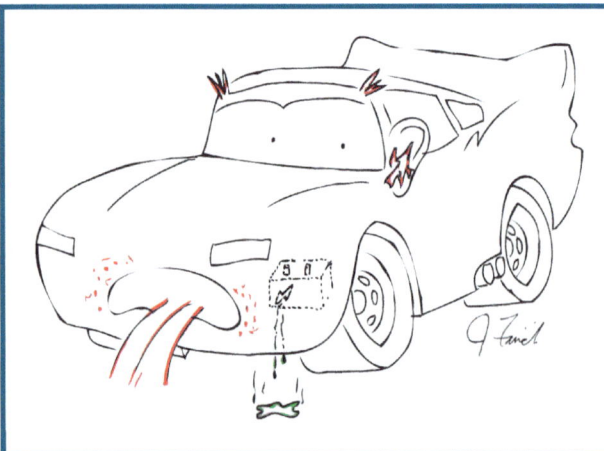

Multiple Carboxylase Deficiency

Picture a cartoon **CAR** (Multiple **CAR**boxylase deficiency) with hypotrichosis and periorificial dermatitis. He **can't see or hear, because of tinfoil in his ears** (bio**tin**idase deficiency causes optic atrophy & deafness) and that is **leaking acid through a hole and puking** (**holo**carboxylase deficiency causes vomiting and aciduria)

Phenylketonuria (PKU)

- AR; mutations in *PAH*, resulting in **phenylalanine hydroxylase deficiency**, leading to ↑ L-phenylalanine
- Rarely, mutation in *QDPR* (quinoid dihydropteridine or *PTS* (6-pyruvoyl-tetrahydropterin synthase) cause PKU
- Diffuse hypopigmentation of skin and hair (because L-phenylalanine inhibits the enzyme tyrosinase)
- Mousy-smelling urine

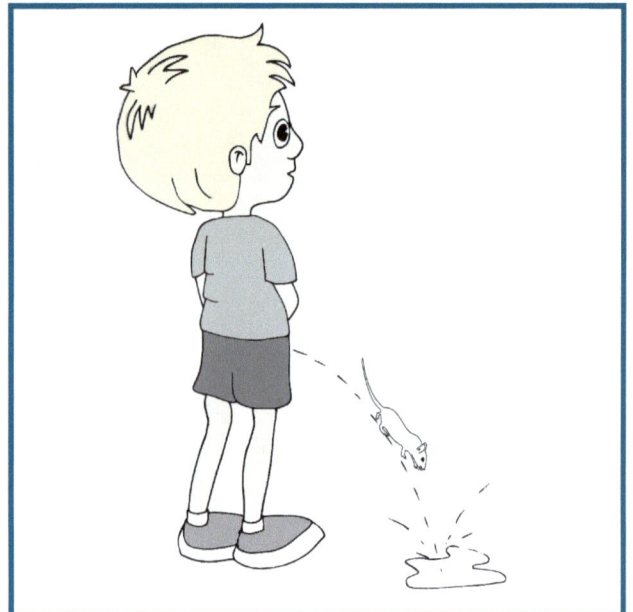

PhenylKIDonuria

Picture a hypopigmented **kid** peeing a **mouse** (mousy urine)

Wilson's Disease (Hepatolenticular Degeneration)

- AR; *ATP7B* mutation, a copper transporter, results in elevated copper
  - (Note: Menkes is a *ATP7A* mutation and gets low copper)
- Hyperpigmentation (pretibial), **blue lunulae** (fig 6.4)
- Ataxia, poor muscle coordination
- Hepatosplenomegaly, **cirrhosis**
- **Kayser-Fleischer Ring** (corneal limbus) occurs from copper deposition in Descemet's membrane of the cornea
- Tx: penicillamine, liver transplant

J. Finch & M. Payette

Table 6.5: Genoderms with Urine Findings

Argininosuccinic Aciduria	Hyperammonemia
Hartnup	Aminoaciduria
HEP, EP	Pink/red Fluorescing urine
AIP	Port wine urine
PCT	Pink fluorescing urine
Alkaptonuria	Brown urine
Fabry	Maltese cross in urine
Multiple carboxylase deficiency	Organic aciduria
PKU	Mousy urine → turns green with FeCl
Homocystinuria	↑ Homocysteine and methionine

> Think "copper is 'de cement' of Wilson's cornea" to remember that Wilson's gets copper deposition in Descemet's membrane of the eye

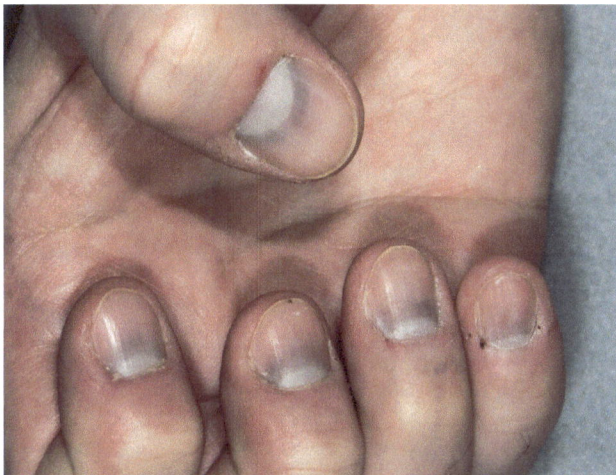

Figure 6.4: Wilson's Disease, Blue Lunulae

Argininosuccinic Aciduria

- AR; mutation in argininosuccinate lyase (*ASL*), resulting in ↑ **urea,** hyperammonemia
- Onset in first weeks of life
- MR, liver failure, seizures
- Brittle hair with **trichorrhexis nodosa** and red fluorescence

Hartnup Disease

- AR; mutation in *SLC6A19* gene
- Defect in BOAT1 neutral amino acid transporter
- Results in ↓ **tryptophan absorption** and **pellagra-like** syndrome (tryptophan is required for niacin production)
- Massive aminoaciduria with elevated tryptophan derivatives
- Clinical: photodistributed erythema (pellagra) and cerebellar ataxia

Hemochromatosis

- AR; mutation in *HFE* gene, or less commonly AR mutation in transferrin receptor (*TFR2*) or ferroportin (*SLC40A1*)
- ↑ iron absorption and deposition
- Tx: 1st line = phlebotomy

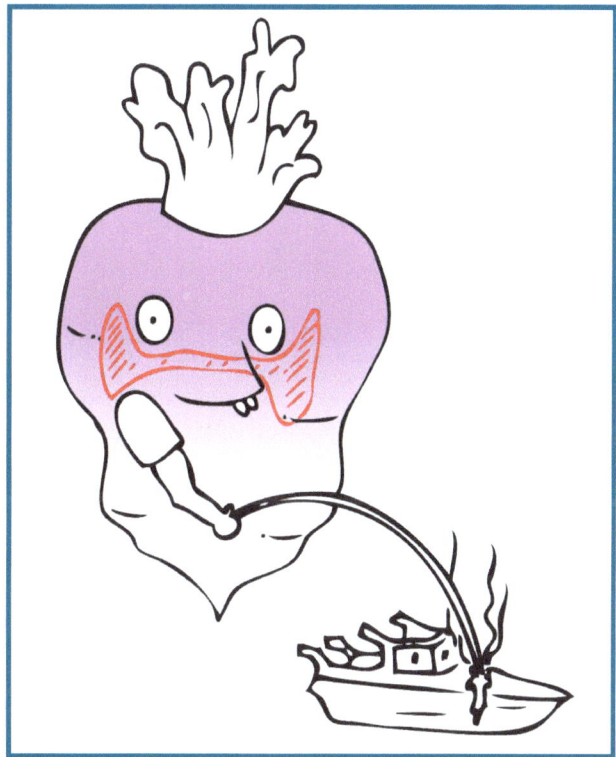

Hartnup Disease

Picture a turnip (Hartnup) with a scaly butterfly rash (photosensitivity) and acidic urine, peeing on a boat (BOAT1 transporter defect)

Lesch-Nyhan Syndrome

- XLR; HGPRT enzyme mutation (*HGPT*), involved in processing of uric acid
- Patients accumulate uric acid → **gout**, self-injurious behavior, MR
- Kelley-Seegmiller Syndrome = partial HGPRT enzyme deficiency. Develop gout only, no neuro symptoms

- Note: HGPRT is the same enzyme involved in **metabolism of azathioprine**

Tumoral Calcinosis

- Massive painful periarticular deposits of calcium phosphate
- Hyperphosphatemic TC
    - AR; mutation in *GALNT3*, encodes a glycosyl transferase
    - Less commonly *FGF23* or *KL*
- Normophosphatemic TC
    - AR; mutation in *SAMD9* (sterile alpha motif domain)

Homocystinuria

- See p. 34 (Connective Tissue Disorders) See p. 34 (Connective Tissue Disorders)

Porphyrias

- See p. 49 See p. 49

7. Porphyrias

Overview

- Every human cell makes heme for respiratory and redox reactions. Liver (CYPs) and RBCs (hemoglobin) make more heme than other tissues

- Porphyrias are inherited metabolic disorders in heme biosynthesis, leading to accumulation of hemoglobin precursors (porphyrins) in the skin

- There are 8 total enzymatic steps in heme biosynthesis

  - Inactivating defects in the first step do not cause a porphyria, rather, lead to X-Linked Sideroblastic Anemia (not a porphyria)

    - Rate-limiting step, occurs in the mitochondria

- Inactivating defects in the 7 remaining steps lead to 8 total porphyrias

  - 6 of the 8 porphyrias have skin symptoms

  - ALAD-Deficiency Porphyria & Acute Intermittent Porphyria are solely neurologic

  - PCT & Hepatoerythropoietic Porphyria share an enzyme, *Uroporphyrinogen Decarboxylase*

- The disorders consist of **acute** (with systemic symptoms, ★) & **non-acute** types

  - 2 acute porphyrias manifest skin symptoms; all 4 non-acute do

- Porphyrin absorption of radiation in the **Soret band (400-410 nm)** causes photosensitivity, blister formation & scarring

  - 400-410 is blue/violet visible light. Therefore, windows and UV sunscreens offer little protection.

> Note: ALA synthetase is the rate-limiting step in porphyrin/heme biosynthesis. Administration of exogenous ALA circumvents this rate-limiting step, leading ALA to be converted to protoporphyrin IX (PpIX). The addition of iron to PpIX by ferrochelatase would be the final step to create heme, but this step is tightly regulated by heme levels and iron availability, so it does not occur. Therefore, exogenous ALA administration (i.e. photodynamic therapy) results in a temporary iatrogenic Erythropoietic protoporphyria (EEP). Similarly, rare activating mutations in d-ALA Synthetase also overwhelm this first rate-limited step and cause EPP.

Use these 2 mnemonics to remember the order of porphyrias and what porphyrin accumulates in each disease

Porphyrias can go "Succ A PHUC and PP"	"Attempts at curing porphyria help vampires evolve"
Succinyl CoA	
delta-**A**LA	**A**LA-D
Porphobilinogen	**A**IP
Hydroxymethylbilane	**C**EP
Uroporphyrinogen III	**P**CT
Coproporphyrinogen III	**H**C
Protoporphyrinogen IX	**V**P
Protoporphyrin IX	**E**PP

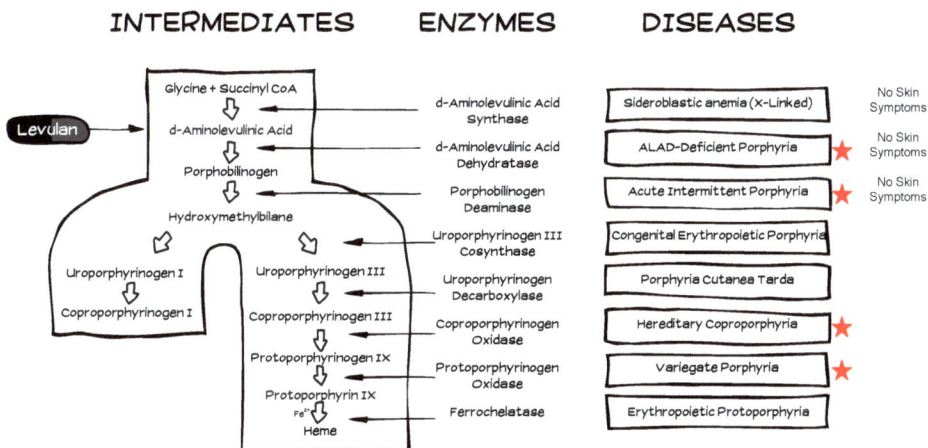

INTERMEDIATES   ENZYMES   DISEASES

Figure 7.1: Porphyrin Metabolism and Porphyrias

Acute Porphyrias

Overview

- **4 Types**
  - 2 w/o skin symptoms, (ALAD-D, AIP)
  - 2 with skin symptoms, (HC, VP)
- Symptoms associated with Acute Porphyric Attack
  - **Gastrointestinal & Metabolic:** colicky abdominal pain, nausea, vomiting, constipation, hyponatremia
  - **Neurologic:** paresthesias, weakness, muscle/back pain, seizures, encephalopathy, paralysis, anxiety, acute psychosis, coma
  - **Pulmonary:** hypertension, tachycardia, respiratory paralysis
- Attacks are infrequent. Peak in 3rd decade; rare before puberty. Recurrent attacks are rare; 90% of patients have only a single attack in their lifetime
- Diagnosis (during attacks)
  - All acute porphyrias have ↑urinary PBG and ALA
  - 1st line test for acute porphyrias: check urine for ↑ PBG. ALA is helpful but not essential. Urine porphyrins not helpful
  - Plasma fluorescence at 626 nm establishes VP diagnosis
  - AIP and ALAD have plasma fluorescence at 620 nm (not unique)

Acute Intermittent Porphyria (AIP)

- **Porphobilinogen deaminase** (3rd enzyme)
  - AD; *HMBS* gene
  - Porphobilinogen → Hydroxymethylbilane
    - M.C. acute porphyria
    - No skin manifestations
    - ↑ risk of liver cancer

ALA Dehydratase Deficiency Porphyria (Doss Porphyria)

- ALA dehydratase (2nd enzyme)
  - AR; *ALAD* gene
  - Accumulation of δ-ALA
  - δ-ALA → Porphobilinogen
  - Clinically identical to AIP, but extremely rare

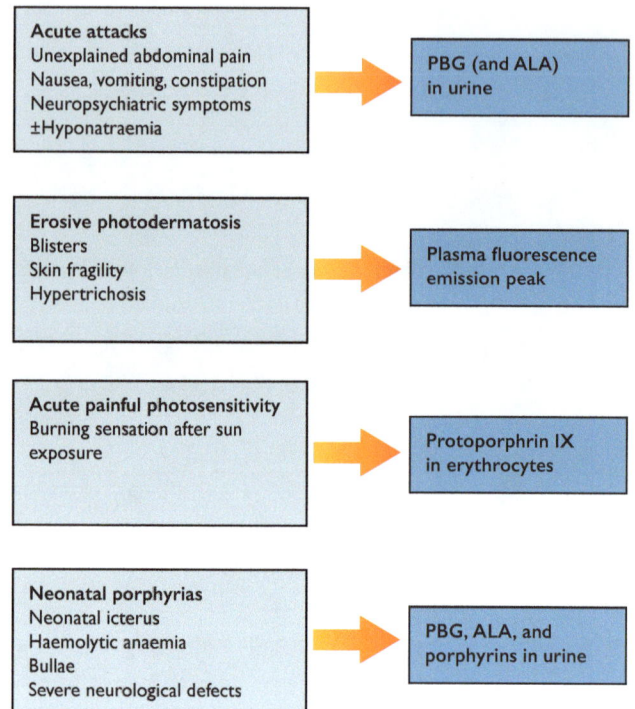

Acute attacks
Unexplained abdominal pain
Nausea, vomiting, constipation
Neuropsychiatric symptoms
±Hyponatraemia
→ **PBG (and ALA) in urine**

Erosive photodermatosis
Blisters
Skin fragility
Hypertrichosis
→ **Plasma fluorescence emission peak**

Acute painful photosensitivity
Burning sensation after sun exposure
→ **Protoporphrin IX in erythrocytes**

Neonatal porphyrias
Neonatal icterus
Haemolytic anaemia
Bullae
Severe neurological defects
→ **PBG, ALA, and porphyrins in urine**

Figure 7.2: Porphyria Diagnostic Clues

Porphyria Precipitants: "BEGS for Alcoholic Drinks"
Barbiturates
Estrogen (pregnancy), **E**rgot
Griseofulvin
Sulfonamides
Alcohol/**A**nticonvulsants
Dapsone

Variegate Porphyria (VP)

- **Protoporphyrinogen oxidase** (7th enzyme)
  - Accumulation of Protoporphyrinogen IX
  - AD; *PPOX* gene
  - Mitochondrial enzyme
  - Protoporphyrinogen IX → Protoporphyrin IX
- M.C. neurocutaneous porphyria, occurring in 1/300 Caucasian **South Africans**
- Clinical symptoms:
  - Skin findings identical to PCT (80%) + acute attacks identical to AIP (35%)
  - 60% of patients have only skin symptoms (i.e. no acute attacks)
- Labs
  - Blood: plasma fluorescence emission at **626 nm** is diagnostic
  - Stool: ↑ total stool porphyrins
    - **PROTO** > COPRO (opposite of HC)

J. Finch & M. Payette

- Treatment
  - Avoid triggers (see box)
  - Glucose infusion during attacks
  - No phlebotomy (can worsen symptoms)

Hereditary Coproporphyria (HC)

- **Coproporphyrin oxidase** (6th enzyme)
  - **Accumulation of Coproporphyrinogen III**
  - AD; *CPOX* gene
  - **Mitochondrial** enzyme
  - Coproporphyrinogen III → Protoporphyrin IX
- Neurocutaneous porphyria
- **Clinically identical to variegate porphyria**, but extremely rare (<50 reported cases)
- Labs
  - ↑ total stool porphyrins
  - **COPRO > PROTO (opposite of VP)**
- Note: **Coproporphyrin III** is synthesized by *Corynebacterium minutissimum*, producing the coral red fluorescence of **erythrasma**

Cutaneous Porphyrias

Porphyria Cutanea Tarda (PCT)

- **Uroporphyrinogen III decarboxylase** (5th enzyme)
  - **Accumulation of Uroporphyrinogen III**
  - Uroporphyrinogen III → Coproporphyrinogen III
- **Most common porphyria**
- M:F 4:1, manifests in adulthood
- Two types, depending on location of deficient enzyme
  - Type I (80%): **acquired** deficiency due to liver insult (m.c. type)
  - Type II (20%): **hereditary** deficiency due to AD mutation in *UROD* gene
- PCT, VP, and HC share the same chronic cutaneous photosensitivity
  - **Skin fragility**, vesicles/bullae, scarring w/ milia, **hypertrichosis**
  - Hyperpigmentation
  - **Sclerodermoid** changes
  - **↑ risk of hepatocellular carcinoma**
- Triggers:
  - Symptoms start when an additional liver insult decreases residual hepatic URO decarboxylase activity to <25% of normal
  - BEGS for Alcohol (see box)
  - Polychlorinated hydrocarbons, hemodialysis, iron overload, hemochromatosis, hepatitis C and HIV, dermatomyositis
- Labs:
  - Urine: ↑↑ **URO** > COPRO (8:1), hepta-carboxylated porphyrin
    - Urine is red/brown grossly, and **fluoresces coral red** under Wood's lamp (fig 7.3)

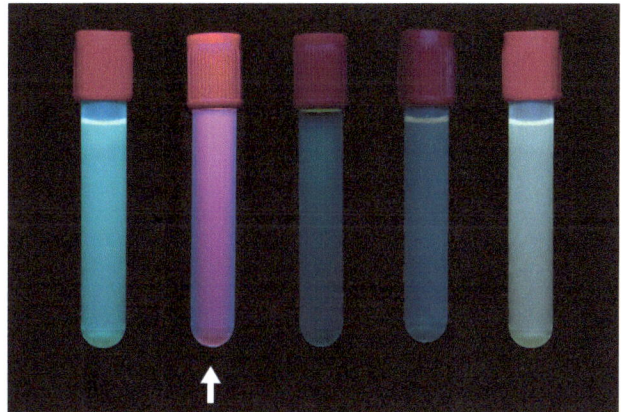

Figure 7.3: Urine Fuorescence in PCT Compared to Four Normal Controls

  - **Stool:** ↑ **isocoproporphyrin** (unique to PCT & HP)
  - Blood: ↑ iron, RBCs
  - Liver: fatty infiltration, hemosiderosis
- Path:
  - Subepidermal cell-poor (**pauci-inflammatory) blister**
  - **Festooning** of dermal papillae
- DDx: variegate porphyria
  - Distinguish by uroporphyrins in urine
    - URO: COPRO > 3:1 = PCT
    - URO: COPRO <1 = VP (and ↑ fecal ISOCOPRO)
- Treatment:
  - Photoprotection, sun avoidance
  - Avoid alcohol, iron, estrogens
  - 1st line: therapeutic **phlebotomy** 400-500 cc (1 unit) every 2 weeks for 3 to 6 months. Target is Hgb 10.0
  - 2nd line: low dose (weekly) hydroxychloroquine or chloroquine (binds and mobilizes porphyrins)
    - **Hydroxychloroquine can treat or worsen PCT**

Hepatoerythropoietic Porphyria (HEP, "Recessive PCT", "Homozygous PCT")

- **Uroporphyrinogen III decarboxylase** (5th enzyme)
  - **Accumulation of Uroporphyrinogen III**
  - Uroporphyrinogen III → Coproporphyrinogen III
- AR; complete absence of *UROD* gene
- Clinically, resembles CEP (but **no anemia**) with biochemical profile similar to PCT
- Presents in early childhood with dark diapers
- Clinical features:
  - Blistering, pruritus, hypertrichosis, hyperpigmentation
  - **Sclerodermoid skin changes,** nail damage
  - **Red fluorescence of teeth w/ Wood's lamp**
- Labs:
  - Urine: ↑ URO
  - Stool: ↑ **COPRO** (like PCT) & isocoproporphyrins
  - Blood: ↑ zinc-chelated PROTO
    - Also elevated in iron deficiency anemia & lead poisoning
- Treatment:
  - **PCT treatments (phlebotomy, antimalarials) are <u>not</u> effective**
  - Photoprotection (physical blockers), sun avoidance, change day-night rhythm, avoid trauma

Congenital Erythropoietic Porphyria (CEP, "Günther's Disease")

- **Uroporphyrinogen Cosynthase** (4th enzyme)
  - **Accumulation of Hydroxymethylbilane**
  - AR; *UROS* gene
  - Hydroxymethylbilane → Uroporphyrinogen III
- **Most severe porphyria**
- Clinical:
  - SEVERE photosensitivity and anemia that **manifests immediately after birth**
  - Extensive scarring with mutilation of cartilaginous structures
  - **Diapers stained red/brown** by urinary porphyrins
  - **Erythrodontia** and osteodystrophy due to porphyrin deposition in teeth and bones
  - **Hemolytic anemia** (from mild to as severe as hydrops fetalis)
  - Hepatosplenomegaly
- Labs:
  - Urine: ↑↑ URO: COPRO (20:1)
  - Stool: ↑ COPRO
  - RBCs: **stable fluorescence** under UVA (vs. transient in EPP)
- Treatment:
  - Photoprotection, strict sun avoidance, change day-night rhythm
  - Splenectomy to reduce hemolysis
  - Hematopoietic stem cell transplant
  - **Blood transfusions**
- Ddx: solar urticaria, PMLE, hydroa vacciniforme, EBA, bullous drug, pseudoporphyria, dystrophic EB (mitten deformity)

Erythropoietic Protoporphyria (EPP)

- **Ferrochelatase** (8th enzyme)
  - **Accumulation of Protoporphyrin IX**
  - AD; *FECH* gene
  - Protoporphyrin IX → Heme
- Clinical:
  - May be no abnormal cutaneous signs, but patients experience burning, stinging and pruritus (especially nose, cheeks, lips, dorsal hands) **minutes after sun exposure** (ddx: solar urticaria)
  - Begins in **early childhood**
  - Erythema → edema → petechiae → wax-like scarring
  - Characteristic linear scars (e.g. at angles of mouth)
  - Liver
    - Cholestasis from accumulation of protoporphyrin in bile canaliculi
    - 10-20% have ↑ LFTs
    - **2% cholestatic liver failure**
    - Porphyrin gallstones
- Labs:
  - **Check RBC porphyrins** (↑ free protoporphyrin in RBCs makes the diagnosis. Also elevated in plasma, feces, liver but unreliable test)
  - **Urine is normal** because protoporphyrin is highly lipophilic

- **RBCs: transient fluorescence** under UVA light (vs stable in CEP), emission at **634 nm**
- Path - EPP is the only porphyria with distinctive path features
  - Eosinophilic deposits around vessels that are highlighted by PAS stain
- DDx: solar urticaria
- Treatment:
  - Photoprotection, strict sun avoidance
  - **β-carotene improves sun tolerance** (except contraindicated in smokers)
  - **Afamelanotide (α-MSH analog)** improves sun tolerance
  - Cholestyramine to reduce enterohepatic recirculation of porphyrins

> Think "EPP = empty pee pee" to remember that there are no urinary porphyrins in EPP

Porphyria Work-up

- Plasma fluorescence is the best initial test for cutaneous porphyrias, differentiating between PCT and VP

- AIP, CEP, PCT and HCP all have plasma fluorescence at 619nm
- Only VP (626 nm) and EPP (634 nm) have unique fluorescence
- Check CBC
  - Hemolytic anemia = CEP
  - Erythrocytosis = PCT
- Check plasma erythrocyte protoporphyrin level (wrap tube in foil)
  - If elevated = erythropoietic protoporphyria
  - If normal = consider med-induced, solar urticaria, hydroa vacciniforme
- 24-hour urine in $NaCO_3$ buffered container
  - Check ratio of URO to COPRO in urine
  - PCT = 8:1
  - VP ≈ 1:1 (COPRO >URO)
- 24-hour stool
  - ISOCOPRO: PCT
  - PROTO: VP, EPP
  - COPRO: CEP, HEP, ECP, HCP

Table 7.1: Comparison of Porphyrias with Skin Manifestations						
Porphyria	Age at Onset	Clinical	Deficient Enzyme (gene)	Accumulated Porphyrin	Inh	Labs
Porphyria Cutanea Tarda (PCT)	3rd – 4th decade	Pruritus, blistering, milia, hypertrichosis Chronic = sclerodermoid	Uroporphyrinogen III decarboxylase (UROD)	Uroporphyrinogen III	AD	Urine: ↑ URO (URO:COPRO 8:1) (vs VP) Stool: ISOCOPRO
Hepatoerythropoietic Porphyria (HEP, "Recessive PCT")	Infancy	Most severe, identical to CEP	Uroporphyrinogen III decarboxylase (UROD)	Uroporphyrinogen III	AR	
Congenital Erythropoietic Porphyria (CEP, Günther's)	Infancy	Most severe type Erythrodontia, extensive scarring	Uroporphyrinogen Cosynthase (UROS)	Hydroxymethylbilane	AR	Urine: URO
Variegate Porphyria (VP)	After puberty if acute attack (35%) 4th decade if no attack (65%)	Neurocutaneous PCT-like skin + AIP-like neuro	Protoporphyrinogen oxidase (PPOX)	Protoporphyrinogen IX	AD	Stool: PROTO Plasma: 626 nm
Hereditary Coproporphyria (HC)	Identical to VP	Identical to VP	Coproporphyrin oxidase (CPOX)	Coproporphyrinogen III	AD	Stool: COPRO
Erythropoietic Protoporphyria (EPP)	Early childhood	Stinging within minutes of sun exposure Blisters	Ferrochelatase (FECH)	Protoporphyrin IX	AD	Stool: PROTO ↑ RBC protoporphyrin Plasma: 634 nm

8. Genoderms with Photosensitivity

Genoderms with Chromosomal Instability

Bloom Syndrome

- AR; mutation in **BLM** (**RecQL3**); encodes **DNA helicase**
- Mutation causes ↑ **sister chromatid exchanges**, chromosomal breakage
- **Quadriradial configurations of chromosomes in lymphs and fibroblasts** is pathognomonic (fig 8.1)
- Clinical:
  - Photodistributed malar erythema and telangiectasias, bird-like facies
  - Growth delay, short stature, CALMs, male sterility
- ↑ **risk leukemia, lymphoma, GI adenocarcinoma**
- ↓ IgA & IgM, +/- IgG

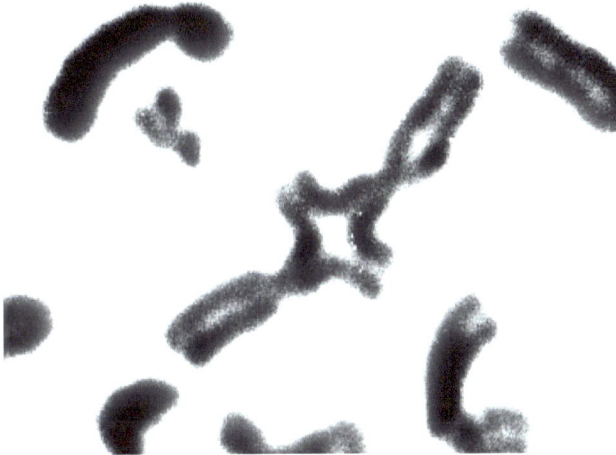

Figure 8.1: Quadriradial Configurations of Chromosomes. *(image courtesy of Bloom's Syndrome Registry Website http://weill.cornell.edu/bsr/)*

Rothmund-Thomson Syndrome (Poikiloderma Congenitale)

- AR; mutation in **RecQL4**; encodes **DNA helicase**
- Photodistributed erythema, edema, vesicles on face that progresses to poikiloderma
- **Absent radius, hypoplastic thumbs** (Fanconi's also has missing thumbs), osteosarcoma
- Cataracts, dental dysplasia

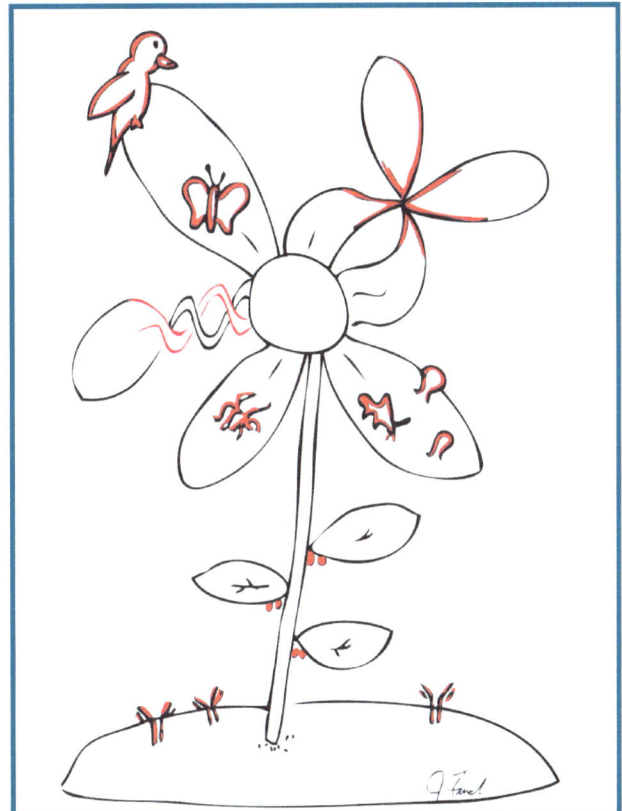

Bloom Syndrome

Picture flower <u>bloom</u> with three leaves on the stem (*RecQL3*) and a DNA helix petal (DNA helicase mutation), crossing leaves (sister chromatid exchange). Sitting on one petal are a bird (bird-like facies) and a butterfly (butterfly rash). The flower has telangiectasias and polyps (GI adenocarcinoma). Under the leaves are tiny balls (hypogonadism). Immunoglobulins are below the flower (low immunoglobulins)

Think Rothmund-ThomTHUMB (hypoplastic thumbs)

R	A**R**, No **R**adius
O	**O**steosarcoma, cataracts
T	**T**elangiectasias
H	**H**ypogonadism, **H**ypo-Thumbs, **H**ypo-Growth
M	**M**usculoskeletal (Short)
A	**A**lopecia, **A**cral Keratosis
N	**N**ail Dystrophy, **N**ormal Intelligence, **N**ormal life span

Table 8.1: Helicase Family Mutations	
Werner	RecQL2
Bloom	RecQL3
Rothmund-Thomson	RecQL4
XP (D)	ERCC2
XP (B)	ERCC3

Kindler Syndrome

- AR; mutation in *KIND1* gene; encodes kindlin-1 protein which links actin cytoskeleton to extracellular matrix
- Acral blisters, photosensitivity
- Diffuse poikiloderma
- Punctate PPK
- Periodontal disease

Sister Chromatid Exchange
"When Baby Chromatids Die Frequently"

Werner
Bloom
Cockayne
Dyskeratosis Congenita
Fanconi Syndrome
(also Trichothiodystrophy, XPB, XPD, Arsenic poisoning)

Genoderms with Defective DNA Repair

Xeroderma Pigmentosa (XP)

- Pathogenesis:
  - DNA Damage Binding Protein (A, E)
  - Endonuclease (C, F, G)
  - DNA helicase (B, D)
  - XP variant is the only one with intact nucleotide excision repair (it is the DNA polymerase-η that is screwed up)
- **Action spectrum 290-340 nm** (mostly UVB)
- Clinical:
  - Solar lentigines by age 2, NMSC by age 8
  - Ocular abnormalities in 40%
    - Photophobia, keratitis, corneal opacification, vascularization, loss of eyelashes, ectropion
  - 100,000x risk of tongue cancer, 6,000x risk of melanoma

- **Neurologic abnormalities** in 20-30%, **M.C. in XPA & XPD**
  - No neuro symptoms in XP variant
  - De Sanctis-Cacchione Syndrome
    - Describes a severe phenotype of XP + microcephaly, mental/growth/sexual retardation, deafness, ataxia, quadriparesis
    - Constellation of findings can occur in several forms of XP, but m.c. with XPA or ERCC6 mutations (allelic with Cockayne B)
  - 10-20x risk internal malignancies (brain, lung, mouth, GI, kidney, hematopoietic)
- Tx: photoprotection, Ca/Vit D, retinoids, imiquimod, bacterial DNA repair enzyme T4 endonuclease V

Trichothiodystrophy

- See p. 67 for full discussion
- AR; *XPB* and *XPD* genes (*ERCC3* & *ERCC2*)
- Unlike XP, is not associated with skin cancers, and pigmentary change is uncommon
- Clinical—**PIBI(D)S**
  - **P**hotosensitivity (in 50%, mostly with XPD mutations), **I**chthyosis, **B**rittle Hair, **I**ntellectual Impairment, **D**ecreased Fertility, **S**hort stature
  - Hair is brittle due to ↓ sulfur content

Cockayne Syndrome

- Action spectrum: UVB (cyclobutane pyrimidine dimers), UVA (8-oxoguanine)
- 2 types, both AR
  - CS-A = ***ERCC8*** mutation (more common)
  - CS-B = ***ERCC6*** mutation
- Photosensitive erythema without pigment changes
- Cachectic dwarfism, "Mickey Mouse" ears
- Extracutaneous features
  - Sensorineural deafness
  - "Salt-and-pepper" retinitis pigmentosa
  - Calcification of basal ganglia
  - No ↑ risk of internal malignancies
- *ERCC6* mutation causes both Cockayne Sx and De Sanctis-Cacchione Sx

Cerebro-Oculo-Facio-Skeletal Syndrome (COFS)

- Overlap with Cockayne

Table 8.2: Xeroderma Pigmentosum Subtypes

XP Subtype	Gene	Function of affected product	Features & Associations
XPA	DDB1	Affinity for DNA damage (? role in DNA repair assembly)	**De Sanctis-Cacchione** (neuro problems) Japan
XPB	ERCC3	3'-5' helicase; TFIIH subunit	also causes Trichothio-dystrophy
XPC	XPC	Recognizes DNA damage (global repair only)	No neuro abnormalities; **m.c. form in USA**
XPD	ERCC2	5'-3' helicase; TFIIH subunit	also causes Trichothio-dystrophy; COFS
XPE	DDB2	Affinity for DNA damage (? recognition)	Mild, no neurologic disease
XPF	ERCC4	5'-repair endonuclease	Mild, no neurologic disease
XPG	ERCC5	3'-repair endonuclease	Neurologic symptoms; XP/CS overlap syndrome
XP Variant	POLH	Polymerase η **responsible for intact NER**; Bypasses T-T dimers with correct insertion of two A residues (DNA polymerase-η)	No neurologic disease Accounts for 30% of all cases
Trichothio-dystrophy	ERCC3 ERCC2	TFIIH subunit	See below
Cockayne Syndrome A	ERCC8	Regulates recruitment of repair factors and chromatin remodelers upon stalling of RNA polymerase at DNA lesions (transcription-coupled repair only)	Ocular anomalies: retinitis pigmentosa (salt & pepper retina), cataracts before age 3, optic atrophy or disk pallor
Cockayne Syndrome B	ERCC6		

XP = xeroderma pigmentosum, TTD = trichothiodystrophy, CS = Cockayne Syndrome, ERCC = excision repair cross complementing gene, COFS = Cerebro-Oculo-Facio-Skeletal Syndrome

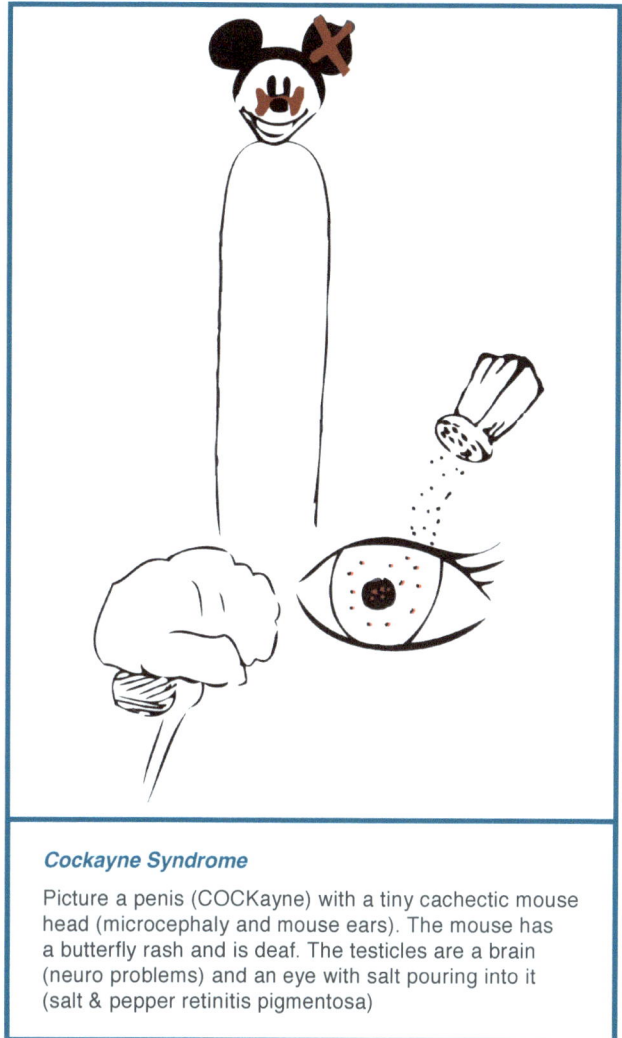

Cockayne Syndrome

Picture a penis (COCKayne) with a tiny cachectic mouse head (microcephaly and mouse ears). The mouse has a butterfly rash and is deaf. The testicles are a brain (neuro problems) and an eye with salt pouring into it (salt & pepper retinitis pigmentosa)

Other Genoderms with Photosensitivity

Smith-Lemli-Opitz Syndrome (Opitz Syndrome)

- AR; defect in cholesterol synthesis
- *DHCR7* encodes **7-dehydrocholesterol reductase**
- Photosensitivity, dysmorphic facies, mental retardation, microcephaly
- ↓ plasma cholesterol levels and ↑ cholesterol precursors, including 7DHC

Hartnup Disease

- See p. 47 for full discussion
- AR; mutation in *SLC6A19* gene, encoding BOAT1 neutral amino acid transporter
- Results in ↓ tryptophan absorption and pellagra-like syndrome (tryptophan is required for niacin production)

9. Vascular Disorders

Syndromes with Capillary Malformations

Table 9.1: Syndromes with Capillary Malformations
Sturge-Weber
Klippel-Trenaunay
Beckwith-Wiedemann
Von Hippel-Lindau
Macro/Micro-cephaly-Capillary Malformation Syndrome
CMTC
Phakomatosis Pigmentovascularis
Proteus

Sturge-Weber Syndrome (Encephalofacial Angiomatosis, Encephalotrigeminal Angiomatosis)

- Both sporadic port wine stains (PWS) and syndromic PWS caused by point mutations in **GNAQ** (*GNAQ* mutations also occur in blue nevi, nevus of Ota, and ocular melanoma)
- Sturge-Weber = PWS + leptomeningeal angiomatosis
- Occurs in 8% of patients with a PWS of V_1 dermatome
- Extracutaneous findings
  - Seizures (75%)
  - Glaucoma (60%)
  - Mental retardation (60%)
  - Hemiplegia (30%)
  - "Tram Track" calcifications of cerebral cortex
- ↑ risk of SWS with multi-dermatomal PWS, PWS involving both upper & lower eyelid, and bilateral PWS

Klippel-Trenaunay Syndrome (KT)

- KT = extensive PWS + venous varicosity + hypertrophy of bone and soft tissue
  - 95% involve lower limb
- **Parkes-Weber syndrome** = KT + AV malformation
- Venous varicosities present by age 12
- Hypertrophy is due to local hyperemia from increased arterial flow (fig 9.1)

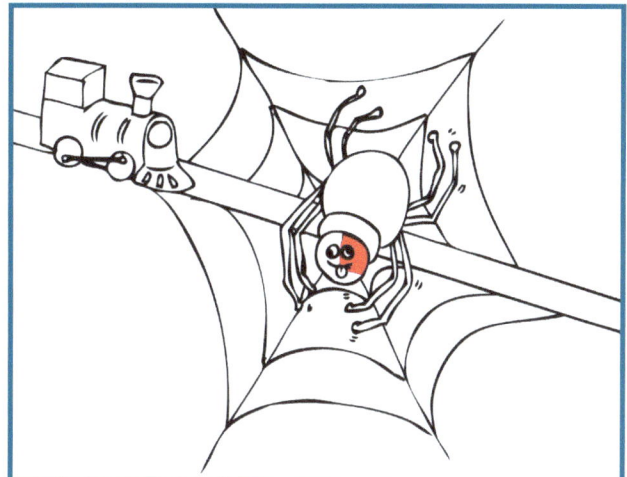

Sturge-Weber Syndrome

Picture a spider on a web (Sturge-Weber), with a facial port wine stain, having a seizure (m.c. CNS finding). There is a train driving across the web (tram-track calcifications in pia mater)

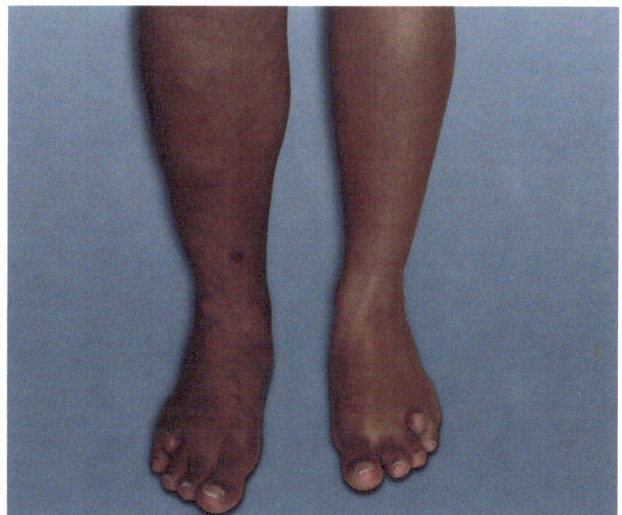

Figure 9.1: Klippel-Trenaunay Syndrome

Beckwith-Wiedemann Syndrome

- See p. 104 for full discussion
- *Epigenetic overgrowth syndrome caused by abnormalities of gene regulation of several genes on chromosome 11 (CDKN1C, H19, IGF2, and KCNQ1OT1 genes)*
- Organomegaly, **macroglossia**, **neonatal hypoglycemia**, omphalocele, **facial capillary malformation**
- Malignancies: **Wilms' tumor** (nephroblastoma) > hepatoblastoma > adrenocortical CA, rhabdomyosarcoma

Von Hippel-Lindau Syndrome

- AD; defect in tumor-suppressor gene *VHL*
- Key features:
  - Skin (<5%): **head and neck port wine stain**
  - Eyes: **retinal hemangioblastomas** with 2° visual impairment (blindness if untreated)
  - CNS: spinal cord hemangioblastomas (cerebellar > medullary) with 2° signs of ↑ intracranial pressure or spinal cord compression
  - Kidneys: **renal-cell carcinoma**; cysts
  - Endocrine: pheochromocytoma; pancreatic cysts; adrenal cancer
  - Heme: polycythemia due to ectopic erythropoietin (CNS hemangioblastoma or renal cell cancer)
- Death by age 40

> **Von Hippel-Lindau Syndrome**
>
> Picture a Hippo (Hippel) with red eyes (retinal hemangioblastomas), cerebellar & cord compression (ataxia, headache, spinal hemangioblastomas), endocrine tumors (pheo, pancreatic cysts, adrenal carcinoma), with red pee (hematuria).

*Macro*cephaly-Capillary Malformation Syndrome

- Reticulated PWS + macrocephaly
- *PIK3CA* mutation
  - PIK3CA mutations also cause CLOVE Syndrome (mosaic), keratinocytic epidermal nevus (somatic), and macrocystic lymphatic malformation (somatic)

*Micro*cephaly-Capillary Malformation Syndrome

- Multiple CMs, epilepsy, cortical atrophy, microcephaly, growth retardation
- AR inactivating mutation in *STAMBP* gene, resulting in upregulation of RAS and PI3K pathways

Syndromes with Telangiectasias

Table 9.2: Syndromes with Telangiectasias
Cutis marmorata telangiectatica congenita (CMTC)
Ataxia-Telangiectasia

Cutis Marmorata Telangiectatica Congenita (CMTC) (congenital generalized phlebectasia)

- Serpiginous bluish mottling resembling exaggerated cutis marmorata, trunk, extremities, face
  - Does not resolve with warming (vs cutis marmorata does)
- Associations: m.c. = ipsilateral limb hypoplasia (vs *hyper*plasia in PWS), coexisting PWS, microcephaly
- Adams-Oliver Syndrome: CMTC + aplasia cutis congenita + limb defects (brachydactyly, syndactyly) cryptorchidism/cardiac abnormalities. AD inheritance. (see p. 33)
- "CMTC with Macrocephaly"
  - Now referred to as "Macrocephaly-Capillary Malformation Syndrome" (above), because vascular lesion is actually a reticulated PWS (which improves with time), not CMTC (which doesn't improve)

Ataxia-Telangiectasia (Louis-Bar Syndrome)

- See page 97 (Disorders of Malignant Potential)

Syndromes with Hemangiomas

Table 9.3: Syndromes with Hemangiomas
Diffuse Neonatal Hemangiomatosis
PHACES Syndrome
SACRAL Syndrome (PELVIS Syndrome)
Bannayan-Riley-Ruvalcaba Syndrome

- Note: **infantile hemangiomas are GLUT-1(+) tumors** (vs vascular malformations which are GLUT-1 negative)

Diffuse Neonatal Hemangiomatosis

- Familial clustering noted, but causative gene unidentified
- Typically hundreds of hemangiomas (but may rarely have only a few lesions)
- May have internal organ involvement
  - GI hemangiomatosis (**liver** > bowel) has high risk of serious bleeding
  - GI hemangiomas **de-iodinate thyroid hormone**, causing severe hypothyroidism
  - AVMs result in CHF from shunting of blood

PHACES Syndrome

- Gene unidentified
- Segmental hemangioma of the face with associated anomalies, >90% female
  - **P**osterior Fossa defects (m.c. = Dandy-Walker, agenesis of CNS structures)
  - **H**emangiomas (extensive facial, plaque like, segmental)
    - V_1 segment has worst prognosis
  - **A**rterial abnormalities in nearly 100%. No venous malformations
    - M.C. location = neck
    - **Corkscrew arteries** nearly pathognomonic
    - Aneurysms, anomalous branches, stenosis
  - **C**ardiac abnormalities/**C**oarctation (PDA, VSD, ASD, etc). Aortic coarctation in 30%. Highest coarc association of any derm disorder
  - **E**ye (Horner's, retinal vascularity, microphthalmia, optic atrophy, cataracts, coloboma)
  - **S**ternal clefting/**S**upraumbilical abdominal raphe (ventral developmental defects)
- Tx:
  - ECHO to evaluate for coarctation
    - Coarctation is usually proximal, so UE/LE BPs not helpful
  - MRI/MRA at 6 months, or earlier if symptoms. Must include lower neck!
  - Ophtho consult

SACRAL Syndrome (PELVIS Syndrome)

- Large perineal hemangioma + anorectal, neurologic, renal or genitourinary defects
- SACRAL
  - **S**pinal dysraphism
  - **A**nogenital anomalies
  - **C**utaneous anomalies
  - **R**enal and urologic anomalies
  - **A**ngioma of **L**umbosacral localization
- PELVIS
  - **P**erineal hemangioma
  - **E**xternal genitalia malformations
  - **L**ipomyelomeningocele
  - **V**esicorenal abnormalities
  - **I**mperforate anus
  - **S**kin tag
- 50% of midline lumbosacral hemangiomas have underlying spinal anomaly
- Need MRI to diagnose. Ultrasound shown to be inadequate

Bannayan-Riley-Ruvalcaba Syndrome

- AD; *PTEN* mutation (allelic with Cowden)
- Lipomas + hemangiomas + macrocephaly
- Genital lentigines
- Shares features with Cowden's: warty papules that histologically are trichilemmoma

Syndromes with Venous Malformations

Table 9.4: Syndromes with Venous Malformations

Familial Cutaneous & Mucosal Venous Malformation (CMVM)

Maffucci Syndrome

Blue Rubber Bleb Nevus Syndrome (Bean Syndrome)

Familial Glomangiomatosis

Familial Cutaneous and Mucosal Venous Malformation

- AD; *TEK* → constitutive activation of **endothelial cell specific TIE-2/TEK tyrosine kinase receptor**
- Multiple lesions affecting skin, oral mucosa, & muscles
- **No visceral or intestinal VMs** (vs. Bean Syndrome)

Maffucci's Syndrome (Multiple Enchondromatosis)

- Somatic gene mutations in *IDH1* or *IDH2* gene, which encode isocitrate dehydrogenase 1 and isocitrate dehydrogenase 2, respectively
- Dyschondroplasia + venous malformations
- **Enchondromas** (benign cartilaginous tumors)
- Note: Ollier's Syndrome = Maffucci's w/o venous malformations
- 30% of patients develop associated **malignancy**: chondrosarcoma (20%), fibro-, angio-, adenosarcoma (pancreas), glioma, teratoma
- Finger/toe nodules in prepubertal years, then ossification defects with pathological fractures, usually extremity
- Neuro deficits from skull enchondromas encroaching on cerebrum

Blue Rubber Bleb Nevus Syndrome (Bean Syndrome)

- Compressible rubbery blue nodules
  - Compression leaves an empty, wrinkled sac that slowly refills (fig 9.2)
- Skin lesions up to 5 cm, solitary or hundreds, usually on trunk/arms or in nose/mouth
- GI blebs (especially small intestine) may bleed, causing chronic anemia
- Tx: excise symptomatic lesions; bowel resection if excessive bleeding

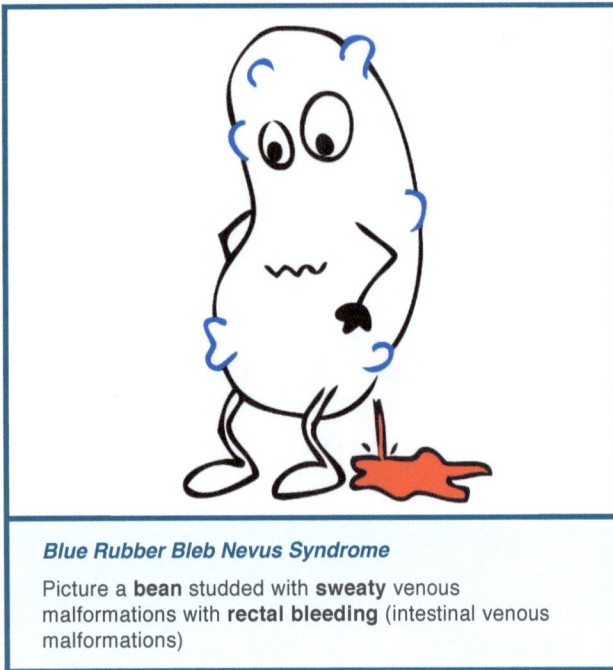

Blue Rubber Bleb Nevus Syndrome

Picture a **bean** studded with **sweaty** venous malformations with **rectal bleeding** (intestinal venous malformations)

Familial Glomangiomatosis (Glomuvenous Malformations)

- AD; mutation in *GLMN*, which encodes **glomulin** protein (role in vascular morphogenesis)
- Glomangiomas are **painful** tumors composed of glomus cells. Pain elicited with palpation or exposure to cold

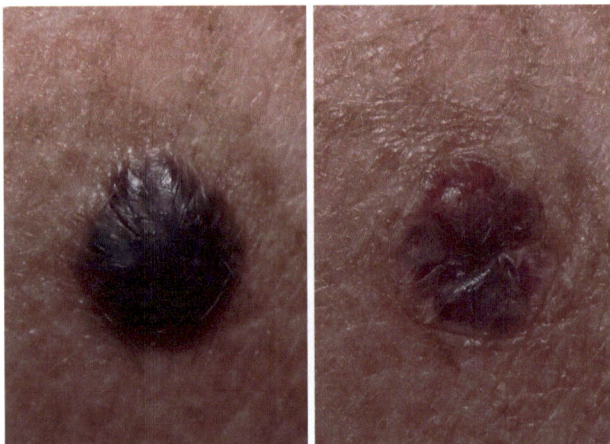

Figure 9.2: Blue Rubber Bleb Nevus. Compression With a Finger Tip Yields a Wrinkled Sac (Right) That Slowly Refills With Blood.

Syndromes with AVMs

Table 9.5: Syndromes with AVMs
Parkes Weber Syndrome
Hereditary Hemorrhagic Telangiectasia (HHT; Osler-Weber-Rendu Disease)
Capillary Malformation-AVM
Cobb Syndrome
Bonnet-Dechaume-Blanc Syndrome (Wyburn-Mason Syndrome)

Parkes-Weber Syndrome

- *RASA1* mutation
- Multiple AV fistulae + hypertrophy of affected limb
- Can look clinically identical to KT syndrome, but much more dangerous
  - KT = slow-flow capillary malformation (PWS)
  - PW = **fast-flow AVM**, may have a palpable "thrill", more pronounced hypertrophy
- Lytic bone lesions, high output cardiac failure

Hereditary Hemorrhagic Telangiectasia (Osler-Weber-Rendu)

- 2 subtypes, both AD mutations in TGF-β receptors that affect vessel wall integrity
  - HHT1: **endoglin** (*ENG*) (TGF-β binding protein found in endothelial cells)
  - HHT2: *ALK-1* (activin receptor-like kinase 1)
  - HHT with polyposis: *SMAD4*
    - ↑ risk of GI cancer
- 1st symptom = **recurrent epistaxis**; children age 8-10
- Mucocutaneous "telangiectasias" are actually small AVMs
  - Begin in 20s
  - Face, lips, tongue, hands (fig 9.3)

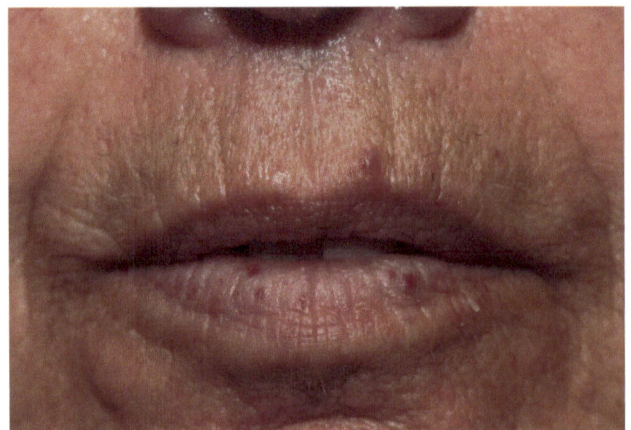

Figure 9.3: Arteriovenous Malformations in HHT

J. Finch & M. Payette

- Visceral hemorrhages later in life (especially GI & urinary → **iron deficient anemia**)
  - AVMs in other organs = hepatic (30%), pulmonary (30%), cerebral (10-20%)
  - **Pulmonary AVMs increased risk in HHT1** → risk of stroke from paradoxical emboli
  - **Hepatic AVMs increased risk in HHT2** → associated with fibrosis, cirrhosis, coagulopathies
- Tx: embolization of pulmonary AVMs

> Think "endLUNGin" to remember that endoglin mutations get lung AVMs
> Think of alk phos liver test to remember that ALK1 mutations get liver AVMs

Table 9.6: Genoderms that Present after Early Childhood

Hereditary Hemorrhagic Telangiectasia	Presents at puberty with nose bleeds > bloody stools. Telangiectasias not until $3^{rd} – 4^{th}$ decade
Meige Lymphedema (Hereditary Lymphedema II, Lymphedema Praecox)	Lymphedema presents around puberty
Ataxia-Telangiectasia	Ataxia age 3, telangiectasias age 6
Neurofibromatosis I	CALMs are early sign, but other features don't appear until after age 7
Neurofibromatosis II	Presents ~ age 20
Isolated IgA Deficiency	Doesn't present unless patient receives transfusions/IVIG. Then patients get anaphylaxis
Fabry's	Often not dx until renal or heart disease develops in 20's. Acral pain is earliest finding
Von Hippel-Lindau	Presents in 4th decade
PXE	$2^{nd} – 3^{rd}$ decade (chicken skin)
Buschke-Ollendorff	Childhood to adulthood
Lipoid proteinosis	Birth if hoarse cry, otherwise early childhood
Werner	$3^{rd} – 4^{th}$ decade
Basal Cell Nevus Syndrome	Jaw cysts and BCCs in childhood. Could dx at birth only if skeletal anomalies recognized (not a derm dx)
Muir-Torre	$5^{th} – 6^{th}$ decade. Internal malignancies precede skin cancers, but dx usually missed until skin cancers
Dyskeratosis Congenita	1st decade (nail and skin changes)

Table 9.6: Genoderms that Present after Early Childhood

Cowden	$2^{nd} – 3^{rd}$ decade
MEN-1	Skin tumors start in teens, but dx often not until 3rd decade
Birt-Hogg-Dubé	3rd decade
EBS, Weber-Cockayne	$1^{st} – 3^{rd}$ decade, often after prolonged running/marching results in blisters
Hartnup	1st decade
Alkaptonuria	Childhood (black cerumen and stained underwear). If dx missed, doesn't present until blue skin and arthropathy in adulthood
Wilson's	Adulthood
Hemochromatosis	5th decade
Klinefelter	Childhood to puberty
Porphyria Cutanea Tarda	3rd to 4th decade
Variegate Porphyria	After puberty
Hereditary Coproporphyria	3rd to 4th decade
Dyschromatosis Symmetrica Hereditaria	Age 6 to puberty
Alkaptonuria	Presents in adulthood primarily with joint symptoms
Lipoprotein metabolism disorders	Adulthood (except for Familial LPL Deficiency, which presents with pancreatitis in childhood)
Pachydermoperiostosis	Late adolescence
Reed Syndrome	Presents in late 20s with cutaneous and uterine leiomyomas

Capillary Malformation-AVM Syndrome

- AD; *RASA1* → encodes p120-Ras-GAP protein (signaling by growth factor receptors)
- Single AVM or Parkes Weber Syndrome + multiple small, round capillary malformations with ill-defined borders often on extremities

Cobb Syndrome (Cutaneomeningospinal Angiomatosis)

- Dermal capillary malformation + **spinal cord vascular lesion**
- Spinal anoxia/compression causes pain, weakness, atrophy, hypesthesia, flaccid mono-or paraplegia

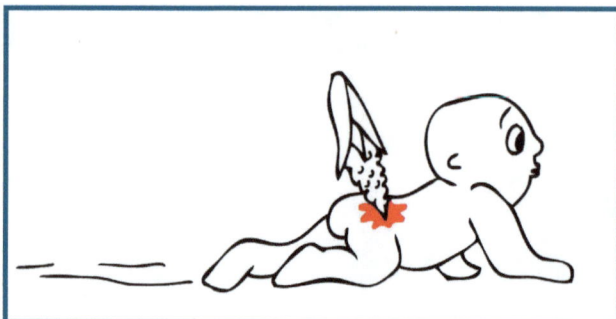

Cobb Syndrome

Picture an infant with a corn cob stabbing him in the spine, creating a bloody vascular stain on his skin. The infant is dragging a paralyzed leg behind him.

Bonnet-Dechaume-Blanc Syndrome (Wyburn-Mason Syndrome)

- (Not genetic)
- Segmental AVM extending from craniofacial to orbital region & brain
- Seizures +/- hemiparesis/hemiplegia

Syndromes with Lymphangiomas

Table 9.7: Syndromes with Lymphangiomas

Lymphangiomatosis
Gorham-Stout Syndrome

Lymphangiomatosis

- Rare disease with diffuse multifocal lymphatic malformations
  - Either soft tissue or parenchymal organs
- Clinical manifestations:
  - Fluctuant and spongelike progressive swellings of the affected limb/area
  - ± overlying skin changes (vesicles, hyperpigmentation and/or verrucous changes)
  - Prognosis: very poor when visceral organs and bones are involved
  - DDx: angiosarcoma (atypical endothelial cells)

- Skin lymphatic malformations in only 2%
- Gorham-Stout Syndrome (Vanishing Bone Disease, Cystic Angiomatosis of Bone)
  - Intramedullary lymphangiomatosis, leading to progressive bone collapse
  - Single or multiple bones, self-limited, no neoplastic formation
  - Can be fatal, with death from chylothorax or hemorrhage into serous cavities
  - Tx: no good treatment

Syndromes with Lymphedema

Table 9.8: Syndromes with Lymphedema

Congenital Lymphedema	Milroy's Disease (Hereditary Lymphedema)
Lymphedema Praecox (puberty)	Meige Lymphedema
	Lymphedema-Distichiasis
	Yellow Nail Syndrome
Very rare forms	Hennekam Syndrome
	Njolstad Syndrome
	Aagenaes Syndrome
Other syndromes w/ lymphedema	WILD Syndrome
	Noonan Syndrome

Milroy Disease (Familial Lymphedema, Hereditary Lymphedema I)

- AD; *FLT4* mutation, which encodes VEGFR-3
  - Some *GJC2* (Connexin 47) mutations
- Congenital Lymphedema

Meige Lymphedema (Hereditary Lymphedema II, Lymphedema Praecox)

- AD; *FOXC2*
- Lymphedema Praecox = lymphedema that presents around puberty
- Meige, Lymphedema-Distichiasis, and Lymphedema-Yellow Nail Syndrome are allelic and have phenotypic overlap

Lymphedema-Distichiasis

- AD; *FOXC2*
- Lymphedema Praecox (presents around puberty)
- Distichiasis (94%) = double row of eyelashes
- Risk of renal disease and diabetes

J. Finch & M. Payette

Lymphedema-Yellow Nail Syndrome (Yellow Nail Syndrome)

- AD; *FOXC2*
- Lymphedema Praecox (presents around puberty)
- Triad of yellow nails, lymphedema, and respiratory tract involvement

Hypotrichosis-Lymphedema-Telangiectasia

- *SOX18*
- Normal nails and teeth
- Lymphedema Praecox (onset at puberty)

Hennekam Lymphangiectasia-Lymphedema Syndrome

- *CCBE1*
- Severe congenital lymphedema + intestinal lymphangiectasia + MR

Aagenaes Syndrome (Cholestasis-Lymphedema Syndrome)

- AR; mutation in 15q
- Leg edema and recurrent cholestatic jaundice

WILD Syndrome

- AD; GATA2 mutation
- **W**arts (disseminated), **I**mmunodeficiency, primary **L**ymphedema, anogenital **D**ysplasia

Miscellaneous Vascular Disorders

CADASIL

- **C**erebral **A**utosomal **D**ominant **A**rteriopathy with **S**ubcortical **I**nfarcts and **L**eukoencephalopathy
- AD mutation in *Notch-3* gene
- Not a derm disorder per se, but relevant because skin biopsy allows early detection
  - Skin biopsy allows early diagnosis by demonstration of **GOM on electron microscopy** (granular osmiophilic material)

CLOVE Syndrome

- **C**ongenital **L**ipomatous **O**vergrowth, **V**ascular malformations, and **E**pidermal nevi
- Caused by somatic mosaicism for postzygotic activating mutations in the *PIK3CA* gene
- LM + VM + CM +/- AVM + lipomatous overgrowth
- See Overgrowth Syndromes section

Neonatal Purpura Fulminans

- AR; mutation in Protein C (*PROC*) or Protein S (*PROS1*) resulting in hypercoagulability and neonatal DIC
- Diffuse retiform purpura, limb necrosis, cerebral thrombosis, retinal vessel occlusion
- Death unless treated with protein C and warfarin

CCM1 (Hyperkeratotic Cutaneous Capillary-Venous Malformations Associated with Cerebral Capillary Malformations)

- AR; mutation in *CCM1* gene, encoding KRIT1 protein
- Venous/capillary malformations with overlying hyperkeratosis
- Cerebral cavernous malformations

10. Hair and Nail Disorders

Genoderms with Hair/Nail Abnormalities

Menkes Disease

- XLR; mutation in **ATP7A copper transporter**
  - Note: *ATP7B* mutation causes Wilson's Disease (↑ copper)
- Hair: **Pili torti** (steel wool-like hair), also trichorrhexis nodosa
- Hypopigmented, doughy skin (tyrosine is a copper-dependent enzyme, so impaired melanin synthesis)
- Cupid's bow upper lip, pudgy cheeks
- Neuro: progressive CNS deterioration, lethargy, seizures, MR
- Musculoskeletal
  - Occipital horns (Allelic with Occipital Horn Syndrome)
  - Long bone spurs and fractures
- Labs: low copper and ceruloplasmin
- Prognosis: poor, death by age 2

Monilethrix (Beaded Hair)

- Defects in hair cortex-specific keratin genes
  - AD: K81, K83, K86
  - AR: Dsg-4
- Alternating normal thickness/constrictions
- Shortly after birth develop fragile hairs that break (eyebrow, lash, and nail [koilonychia] sometimes)
- Associated perifollicular erythema hyperkeratosis

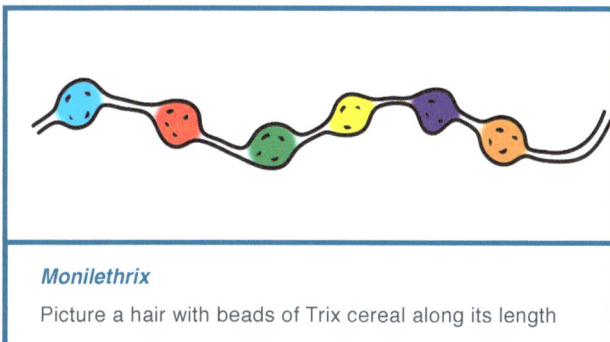

Monilethrix

Picture a hair with beads of Trix cereal along its length

Björnstad Syndrome

- AR; *BCS1L* mutation
- Pili torti + deafness

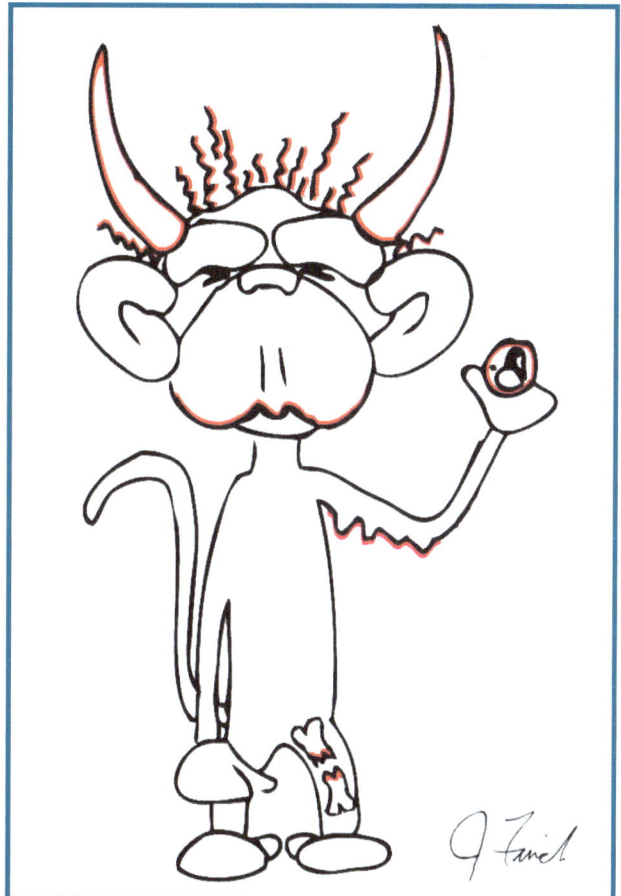

Menkes Disease

Picture the Menkes monkey holding a copper penny (copper transporter mutation), with broken bones, cupid's bow upper lip, saggy skin (cutis laxa), horns (occipital horns) and Pili torti

Björnstad Syndrome

Picture a deaf ear with twisted hairs coming out of it

Trichothiodystrophy (PIBIDS)

- AR; mutation in TFIIH/XPD-XPB complex, transcription/DNA repair function
- Brittle hair. ↓ cysteine (↓ sulfur) in hair matrix causes defective cross-linking.
- Trichogram shows transverse fractures (fig 10.5) (**trichoschisis**). Polarized light shows "**tiger tail**" abnormality (pathognomonic) alternating light and dark bands (fig 10.1)

- Clinical—**PIBI(D)S**
  - **P**hotosensitivity (in 50%, mostly with XPD mutations)
  - **I**chthyosis (collodion membrane)
  - **B**rittle Hair
  - **I**ntellectual Impairment: MR, microcephaly
  - **D**ecreased Fertility
  - **S**hort stature
  - Other: receding chin, protruding ears, sideroblastic anemia, eosinophilia, liver angioendotheliomas

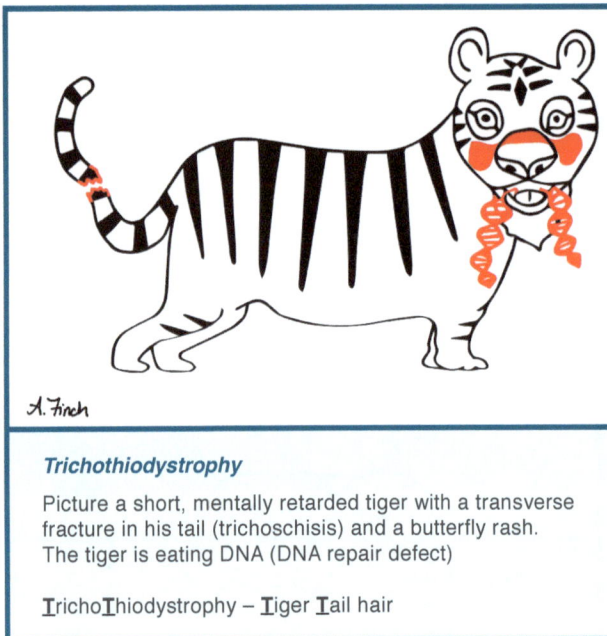

Trichothiodystrophy

Picture a short, mentally retarded tiger with a transverse fracture in his tail (trichoschisis) and a butterfly rash. The tiger is eating DNA (DNA repair defect)

Tricho**T**hiodystrophy – **T**iger **T**ail hair

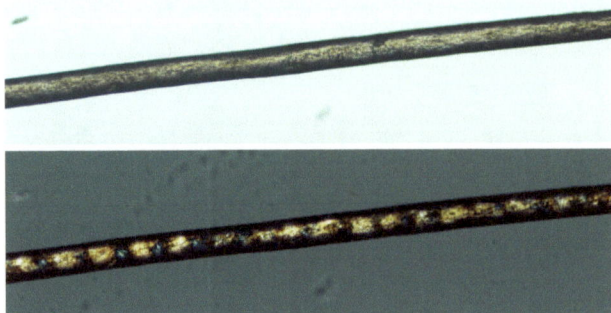

Figure 10.1: Top: Non-Polarized Microscopy; Bottom: "Tiger Tail" Hair with Alternating Light and Dark Bands on Polarized Microscopa

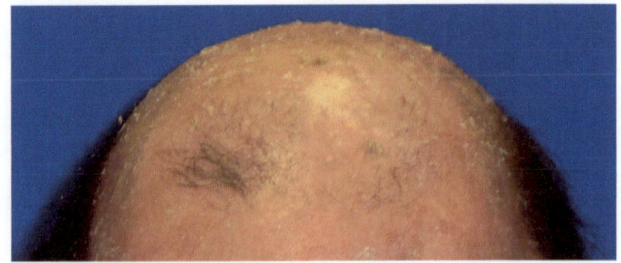

Figure 10.2 Trichothiodystrophy Presenting with Ichthyosis, Photosensitivity, and Brittle Tiger-Tail Hair

Cartilage-Hair Hypoplasia
- AR; *RMRP* mutation
- Form of short-limbed dwarfism with **immunodeficiency** (especially HSV and VZV infections) and **non-infectious skin granulomas**
- Fine, sparse, hypopigmented hair
- Doughy skin

Argininosuccinic Aciduria
- AR; mutation in *ASL* gene encoding argininosuccinate lysase
- **Trichorrhexis nodosa**
- Hepatomegaly and liver failure
- Seizures, MR
- Tx: restricted protein diet

Marie-Unna Hereditary Hypotrichosis
- AR; hairless gene (*HR*) mutation or *U2HR* (upstream regulator of *HR*)
- Slowly progressive atrophy of hair follicles beginning at puberty. Hair-limited disorder (no systemic findings)

Atrichia with Papular Lesions
- AR; hairless gene (*HR*) mutation (irreversibly destroyed hair follicles)
- Natal hair falls out after birth and never regrows
- <1mm monomorphic skin colored papules cover most of the body
- Note: mutation in *VDR* gene (Vitamin D receptor) causes <u>Vitamin D-Dependent Rickets</u>, with nearly identical phenotype. Patients are usually born with hair that is shed over first 2-3 years of life

Böök Syndrome
- AD; unknown gene
- Premature graying of hair, hyperhidrosis, premolar aplasia

Racquet nails
- AD trait, gene unknown
- "Racquet nail" = width of nail plate > length

J. Finch & M. Payette

Table 10.1: Genoderms with Hair Color Abnormalities

Genoderms with Blonde/Red Hair vs Those with Gray or Silver Hair

Blonde/Red Hair

- MC1R (melanocortin receptor) mutation = red hair
- Phenylketonuria
- Homocystinuria
- Oasthouse Disease
- Menkes
- Albinism
- X-Linked Reticulate Pigmentary Disorder

Gray Hair

- Progeria
- Werner Syndrome
- Rothmund-Thomson
- Böök Syndrome

Silver Hair

- Griscelli Syndrome
- Chédiak-Higashi Syndrome

Hair Shaft Abnormalities with Fragility

Trichorrhexis Nodosa

- M.C. hair shaft abnormality
- "Two brushes pointing toward one another"; damaged cuticular cells and intercellular cement of the hair shaft (fig 10.3)
- Congenital
  - **Argininosuccinuria**
- Acquired
  - Proximal (after years of hair straightening)
  - Distal (acquired cumulative cuticular damage)
  - Mitochondrial disorders

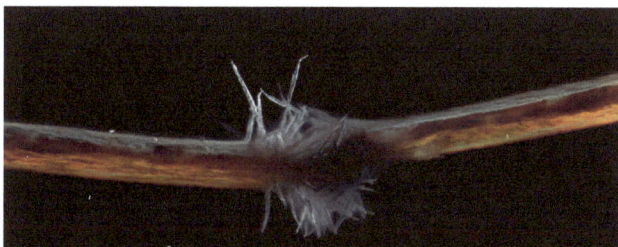

Figure 10.3: Trichorrhexis Nodosa (dark field microscopy, 10x)

Pili Torti

- Flattened hair shaft twists on its own axis; twists occur in groups giving it a glimmering look (fig 10.4); soon after birth hair becomes fragile; sparse/absent body hair

- Associated syndromes:
  - **Menkes Disease** (see p. 67)
  - **Bazex Syndrome** (Bazex-Dupré-Christol) (see p. 98)
  - **Argininosuccinic aciduria** (p. 47) and other urea cycle defects
  - **Ectodermal dysplasias**
  - **Hypotrichosis with juvenile macular dystrophy**
  - **Laron Syndrome (GH insensitivity)**
  - **Mitochondrial disorders**
  - **Björnstad Syndrome** (see p. 67)
- Acquired disorder:
  - Anorexia nervosa
  - Oral Retinoid therapy

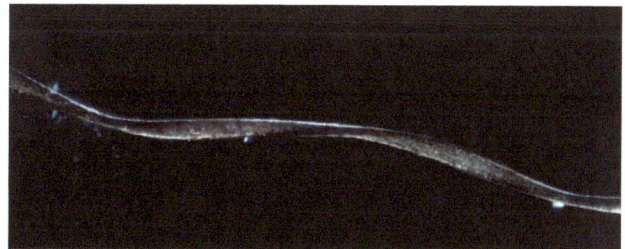

Figure 10.4: Pili Torti (dark field microscopy, 10x)

Trichorrhexis Invaginata (Bamboo Hair)

- Defective cornification → intussusception of proximal hair shaft (socket) into distal end (ball)
  - Associated with **Netherton Syndrome** (see p. 12)

Beaded Hair (Monilethrix)

- See p. 67
- Alternating normal thickness/constrictions
- Defects in hair keratin genes

Trichoschisis

- Transverse hair fractures seen in **Trichothiodystrophy** (p. 67)

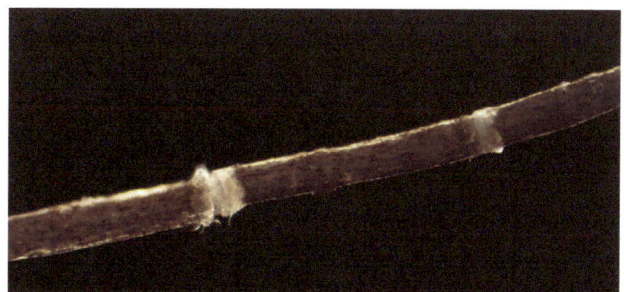

Figure 10.5: Trichoschisis (dark field microscopy, 10x)

Hair Shaft Abnormalities without Fragility

Pili Annulati ("Ringed Hair")

- Periodically occurring air-filled cavities (appear black under microscopy), giving hair light and dark bands ("rings")
- AD or sporadic

Pili Trianguli et Canaliculi (Uncombable Hair Syndrome, Spun Glass Hair)

- AR; mutation in *PADI3, PGM3, PCHH*, genes that encode or modify trichohyalin
- Abnormal keratinization of the IRS → angulated hair shaft; one side with a longitudinal groove on scanning electron microscopy

Woolly Hair

- May be seen as an isolated circumscribed patch ("wooly hair nevus"), or as part of a syndrome
- Woolly Hair Nevus
  - AD or AR
  - Congenital patch of hairs with axial twisting & elliptical cross-sections; occasional T. nodosa
- Associated syndromes:
  - **Naxos Syndrome**
    - (see p. 14, Palmoplantar Keratodermas)
  - **Carvajal Syndrome**
    - (see p. 14, Palmoplantar Keratodermas)
  - **Noonan Syndrome**
    - (see p. 113, Chromosomal Abnormalities)
  - **Cardio-Facio-Cutaneous Syndrome**
    - *KRAS/BRAF/MEK1/MEK2* genes encode proteins in MAP kinase pathway

- Macrocephaly, prominent forehead, bitemporal constriction, heart malformations especially pulmonary valve stenosis, delayed growth, mental retardation, psychomotor retardation, extra toe or fusion of two or more toes

Ectodermal Dysplasias

- Huge group of disorders with almost 200 types

Hypohidrotic/Anhidrotic Ectodermal Dysplasia, (Christ-Siemens-Touraine Syndrome)

- **XLR** variant (M.C. type) = mutation in **ectodysplasin-A** (*EDA*)
- AD variant = mutation in ectodysplasin-A receptor (*EDAR*)
- AR variant = encodes intracellular adaptor protein associated with ectodysplasin-A receptor (*EDARADD*)
- Clinical findings:
  - No eccrine glands → hypohidrosis, severe risk of overheating
  - Hypo-anodontia, peg-shaped/conical incisors (fig 10.7), hypoplastic gums
  - Sparse scalp hair, absent eyebrows, mild nail dystrophy
  - **Characteristic facies**, with frontal bossing, prominent supraorbital ridge, periorbital wrinkles and hyperpigmentation, saddle nose

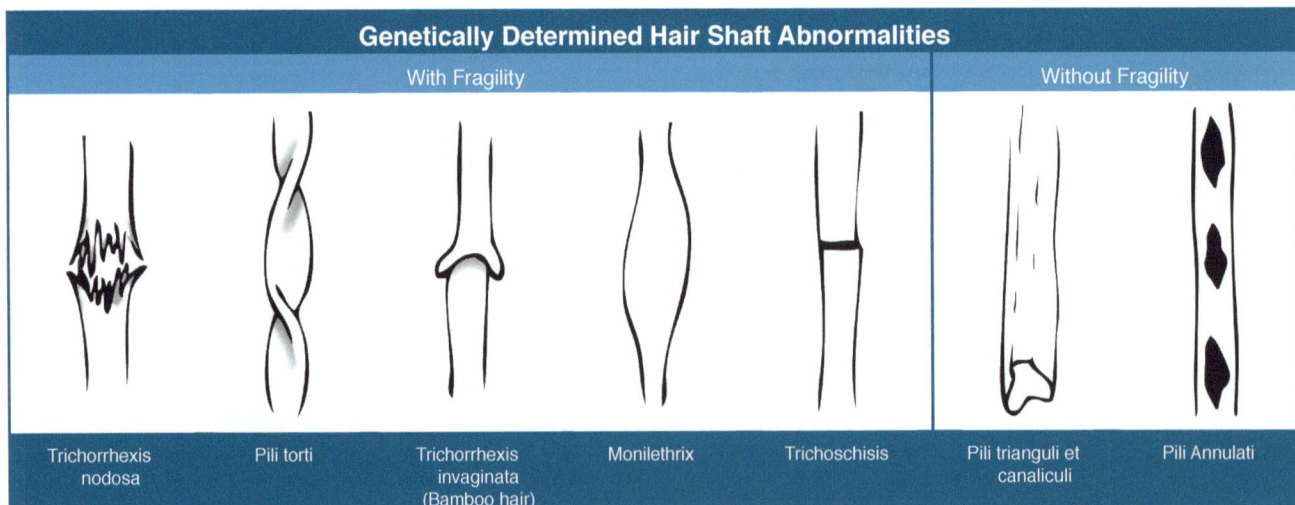

Genetically Determined Hair Shaft Abnormalities

With Fragility: Trichorrhexis nodosa | Pili torti | Trichorrhexis invaginata (Bamboo hair) | Monilethrix | Trichoschisis

Without Fragility: Pili trianguli et canaliculi | Pili Annulati

Figure 10.6: Genetically Determined Hair Shaft Abnormalities

J. Finch & M. Payette

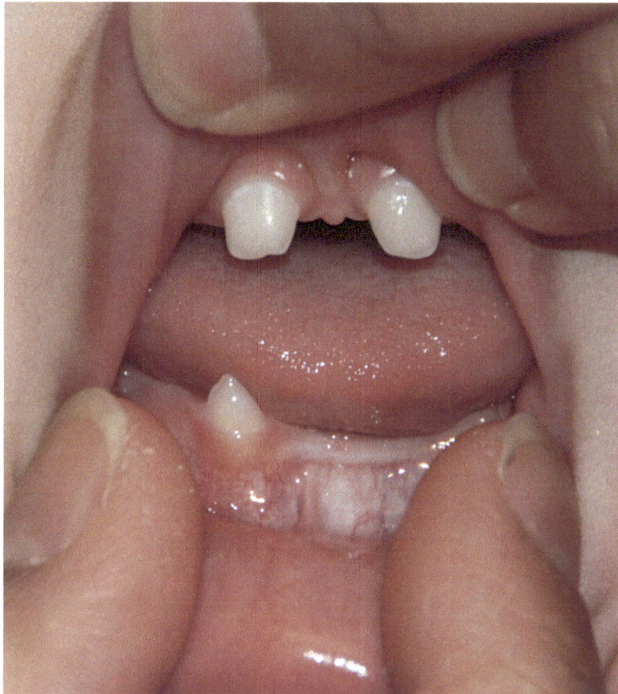

Figure 10.7: Pegged Teeth in a Child with Anhidrotic Ectodermal Dysplasia

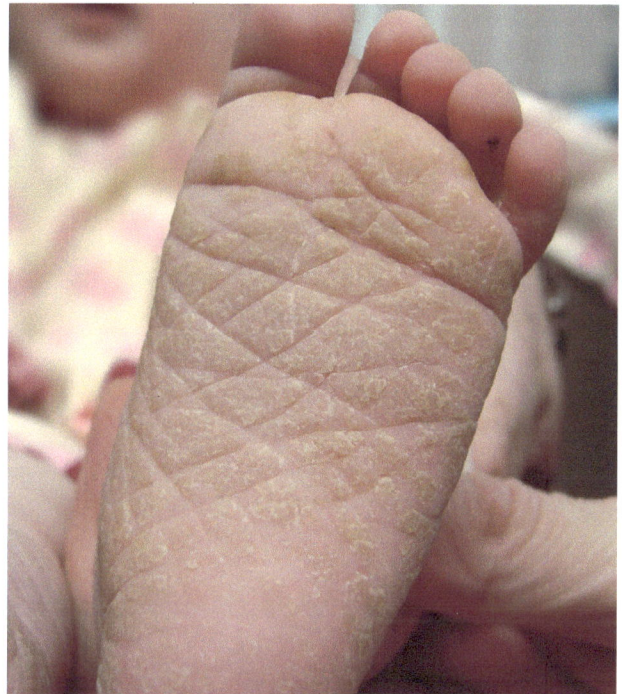

Figure 10.8: PPK with Transgrediens in an Infant with Hidrotic Ectodermal Dysplasia

Hidrotic Ectodermal Dysplasia (Clouston Syndrome)

- AD; *GJB6* encodes **connexin 30**
- Sparse/absent hair, **PPK** with transgrediens (fig 10.8), tufting of terminal phalanges and thickened skull bones
- Nail dystrophy with micronychia, partial anonychia, hyperconvexity of nail plate
- Other gap junction syndromes:
  - **Keratitis-Ichthyosis-Deafness (KID) Syndrome** = AD/AR; *GJB2* mutation (connexin 26)
  - **Vohwinkel Syndrome** = *GJB2* mutation → sensorineural deafness, mutilating PPK
  - **Erythrokeratodermia Variabilis** = *GJB3, GJB4* (connexin 31, 30.3) → transient erythematous patches & hyperkeratotic plaques

EEC Syndrome (Ectrodactyly-Ectodermal Dysplasia-Cleft Lip/Palate Syndrome)

- AD; most cases due to partial loss of *p63* function (needed for limb, craniofacial, epidermal morphogenesis)
- Sparse hair, lacrimal duct abnormalities, cleft lip/palate
- Ectrodactyly = Lobster-claw deformity (also seen in Goltz)
- Hypodontia, conductive deafness, premature tooth loss, dystrophic nails, hydronephrosis

AEC Syndrome (Ankyloblepharon Filiforme Adnatum-Ectodermal Dysplasia-Cleft Palate Syndrome, Hay-Wells, Rapp-Hodgkin)

- AD; partial loss of *p63* function
- Collodion membrane at birth
- **Chronic severe erosive scalp dermatitis**
- Sparse hair, dystrophic/absent nails
- Ankyloblepharon (fusion of eyelids), cleft lip/palate, anodontia/hypodontia
- Chronic otitis media with hearing loss

Pachyonychia Congenita

- 20 nail dystrophy, subungual hyperkeratosis, increased transverse curvature (**pincer nails**) (fig. 10.9), recurrent S*taph*/*Candida* paronychia, **focal PPK**, follicular hyperkeratosis, hyperhidrosis
  - Type 1 = *Jadassohn-Lewandowsky*
    - AD; *K16* and *K6a* mutated
    - **Leukoplakia** (not premalignant) (fig 10.9)
    - **More PPK**
  - Type 2 = Jackson-Lawler
    - AD; *K17* and *K6b* mutated
    - **Steatocystoma** multiplex, epidermoid cysts, natal teeth
    - Milder PPK

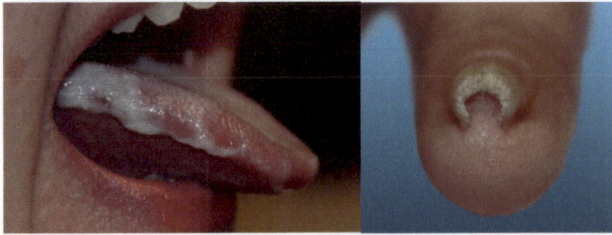

Figure 10.9: Pachyonychia Congenita Type I – Leukoplakia and Pincer Nails

Nail-Patella Syndrome (Hereditary Osteo-Onychodysplasia, HOOD)

- AD mutation in *LMX1B* gene, which encodes a transcription factor required for dorsal/ventral patterning
- Nails: **triangular lunulae**, **absent or hypoplastic nails**, longitudinal nail plate fissures
- Bone: absent/small patellae, **posterior iliac horns**, radial head dysplasia (fig. 10.10)

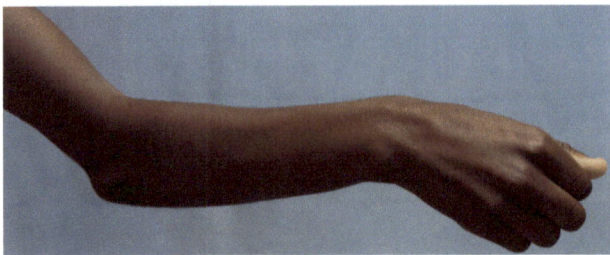

Figure 10.10: Radial Head Dysplasia in Nail-Patella Syndrome

- Eye: **Lester iris** (hyperpigmentation of pupillary margin of iris) (fig 10.11), cataracts
- Kidney: renal dysplasia and glomerulonephritis
  - Caused by Contiguous Gene Syndrome
  - *LMX1B* gene [9q34] is next to *COL5A1* gene [9q33], which encodes collagen component of glomerular basement membrane

> Think "you knee your patellas to ride a BMX" to remember *LMXB* gene

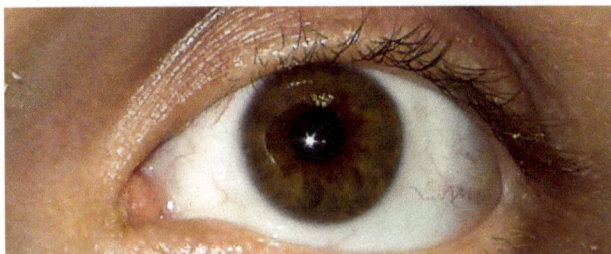

Figure 10.11: Lester Iris, Demonstrating Hyperpigmentation of the Pupillary Margin

Table 10.2: Genoderms with Prominent Tooth and Oral Findings

Tooth Findings	
Anodontia	Hypomelanosis of Ito
Hypodontia (Oligodontia)	Goltz Familial Tooth Agenesis (Witkop) AEC Syndrome EEC Syndrome Schöpf-Schulz-Passarge Odonto-Onycho-Dermal Dysplasia
Supernumerary teeth	Gardner Syndrome
Natal teeth (Erupted teeth at birth)	Pachyonychia Congenita Hallermann-Streiff
Early eruption of teeth	Rabson-Mendenhall
Delayed eruption of teeth	KID, Progeria
Retention of primary teeth	Job Syndrome Familial Tooth Agenesis (Witkop)
Brown teeth	Congenital Erythropoietic Porphyria
Pegged teeth	AED Incontinentia Pigmenti
Pegged, supernumerary, yellow spots	Naegeli-Franceschetti-Jadassohn Syndrome
Premolar aplasia	Böök Syndrome
Dentinogenesis imperfecta	OI Type I
Enamel pits	Tuberous Sclerosis Junctional EB

Tongue Findings	
Leukoplakia, premalignant	Dyskeratosis Congenita
Leukoplakia, non-premalignant	Pachyonychia Congenita I Howel-Evans
Absent fungiform papillae on tongue	Riley-Day (Familial Dysautonomia)
Cobblestone tongue	Cowden, Darier's
Scrotal tongue	Bazex Down Tuzun Melkersson-Rosenthal
Macroglossia	Beckwith-Wiedemann Down Amyloidosis Lipoid Proteinosis Mucopolysaccharidoses
Mucosal neuromas	MEN 2b
Oral ulcers	Hyper-IgM Immunodeficiency (XHIM)

Other Mouth Findings	
Periodontitis	Papillon-Lefèvre Syndrome, EDS
High arched palate	Marfan
Jaw cysts	Gorlin's Syndrome (odontogenic cysts)
Odontomas (teeth-like concretions)	Gardner Syndrome
Telangiectasias	HHT

J. Finch & M. Payette

Familial Tooth Agenesis (Witkop Syndrome)

- AD; *MSX1* mutation
- Hypodontia
- Dysplastic, brittle, slow-growing, spoon-shaped nails

Dyskeratosis Congenita

- Nails: longitudinal ridging and pterygium
- See p. 84

Yellow Nail Syndrome
(Lymphedema-Yellow Nail Syndrome)

- See p. 65 (Syndromes with Lymphedema)

Darier's Disease

- Candy cane nails, V-nicking
- See p. 13 for full discussion

Congenital Hypertrichosis

Hereditary Disorders with Generalized Hypertrichosis

- Universal Hypertrichosis:
  - "Wolf boy" phenotype, with thick hair everywhere. Mexicans
- Congenital Hypertrichosis Lanuginosa:
  - AD; *HTC1* mutation
  - Fine, downy lanugo hair. May shed during first year. Shorter than Universal Hypertrichosis
- X-Linked Congenital Generalized Hypertrichosis:
  - XLD; *HTC2* gene mutation in Mexicans
  - Like Universal Hypertrichosis, but hair is shorter and more associated anomalies
- Ambras Syndrome:
  - Like Universal Hypertrichosis, but hair is silkier and longer. Face and shoulders
  - Due to chromosomal inversion at 8q22

Disorders with Associated Gingival Hyperplasia, Facial Dysmorphism, Skeletal/ocular Anomalies, MR:

- Note: congenital hypertrichosis (above) is also frequently associated with gingival hyperplasia
- Gingival fibromatosis with hypertrichosis:
  - AD
  - Dark terminal hair on peripheral face, central back and extremities
  - Gingival hyperplasia, coarse facies, MR, seizures

- Cantú Syndrome:
  - AD; gingival hyperplasia, coarse facies, osteochondrodysplasia, macrostomia at birth, cardiomegaly
- Zimmermann-Laband Syndrome:
  - AD; gingival hyperplasia, coarse facies, hypoplastic nails and distal phalanges, joint hyperextensibility macrostomia at birth, HSM, MR
- Barber-Say Syndrome:
  - AD; skin laxity, ectropion, macrostomia, coarse facies, hypoplastic nipples, GR
- Schinzel-Giedion Syndrome:
  - AR; midfacial vascular stain, midfacial retraction, hyperconvex nails, hypoplastic distal phalanges and dermatoglyphs, GU anomalies, GR, MR
- Gorlin-Chaudhry-Moss Syndrome:
  - AR; craniofacial dysostosis, with midfacial hypoplasia, hypoplastic distal phalanges, ocular and dental anomalies, genital hypoplasia, GR
- Adducted Thumb Syndrome:
  - AR; arthrogryposis, craniosynostosis, myopathy
- Acromegaly + Hypertrichosis (single family):
  - AD
- Leigh Syndrome:
  - Neurodegenerative disorder. Highly genetically heterogeneous (>12 genes identified), many of which are mitochondrial. But only AR *SURF-1* mutations get derm findings (hypertrichosis of face and limbs)
- CAHMR Syndrome (single family):
  - AR; cataracts, hypertrichosis, MR
- Amaurosis congenita, cone-rod type, with hypertrichosis:
  - AR; photophobia, visual impairment due to retinal dystrophy

Table 10.3: Genoderms with Hair in Weird Locations		
Genoderms with Hypertrichosis		
Cornelia de Lange	Low anterior hairline, synophrys, trichomegaly	
Rubinstein-Taybi	Lateral face hypertrichosis, thick eyebrows, trichomegaly	
Porphyrias	Sun exposed areas	
Lipodystrophy Syndromes	Face, neck, extremities	
Erythrokeratodermia variabilis	Trunk, extremities	
Dystrophic EB	Areas of previous blistering	
Ichthyosis bullosa	Extremities	
Mitochondrial disorders (e.g. Leigh Syndrome)	Face and limbs	
Mucopolysaccharidoses (Hunter & Hurler)	Face and limbs	
Congenital Hypothyroidism		
Sclerodermoid disorders		
Synophrys (unibrow)		
Note: Usually an isolated finding Waardenburg Cornelia de Lange Zimmermann-Laband (AD generalized hypertrichosis) Amaurosis Congenita (AR generalized hypertrichosis) Mucopolysaccharidoses		
Trichomegaly (long eyelashes)		
Oliver-McFarlane Syndrome Cornelia de Lange Syndrome Rubinstein-Taybi Syndrome Congenital Hypertrichosis Lanuginosa Syndrome Hermansky-Pudlak Syndrome Fetal Alcohol Syndrome (not a genoderm)		
Distichiasis (double row of eyelashes)		
Lymphedema-Distichiasis Syndrome Setleis Syndrome		

Other Disorders with Hypertrichosis

Rabson-Mendenhall Syndrome
- AR; mutation in **insulin receptor** (*INSR*)
- Early dentition
- Coarse, senile-appearing facies
- Striking hirsutism, acanthosis nigricans, dry skin, thick nails

Congenital Adrenal Hyperplasia
- 21-hydroxylase mutation (95%)
- 11-β-hydroxylase mutation (5%)
- Precocious puberty
- Early androgenetic alopecia
- Baby girls have ambiguous genitalia
- Baby boys have axillary and pubic hyperpigmentation

J. Finch & M. Payette

11. Disorders with Hypopigmentation

Melanin Biology

Embryologic Melanocyte Migration

- Melanocytes migrate from neural crest to: choroid, retina, iris, skin, cochlea, leptomeninges
  - Retina is the only site where melanosome transfer does NOT occur
  - Defects in melanoblast migration cause
    - **Oculocutaneous Albinism (OCA)**
    - **Piebaldism**
    - **Waardenburg**
- Skin color in humans
  - Normal pigment variation in humans is influenced by polymorphisms in *MC1R*, *SLC24A5* and *OCA2* genes
  - Skin color is determined by melanocyte activity, not melanocyte number. All skin types have same # of melanocytes
    - Type I-II skin: fewer melanosomes, smaller, grouped; quicker degradation
    - Type IV-VI skin: more melanosomes, slightly larger, singly dispersed; slow degradation

Melanin Biosynthesis

- (See figure 11.1)
  - Brown-black = eumelanin
  - Yellow-red = pheomelanin
  - Tyrosine is the building block of melanin
  - **Tyrosinase** is required at 3 synthetic steps in the formation of eumelanin
  - Pheomelanin requires less tyrosinase activity
    - Also requires glutathione or cysteine
  - Melanocyte-Stimulation Hormone (MSH)
    - MSH derived from POMC
    - POMC made in keratinocytes (pituitary, testis, endothelium)
  - Melanocortin-1 receptor (MC1-R)
    - MC1-R is a G-protein-coupled receptor
    - MSH binds to MC1-R → ↑cAMP and ↑tyrosinase activity
  - **Agouti protein = antagonist of MCR**
    - Activation causes cyclic striping of hair
    - Induces expression of pheomelanin

- Related Diseases
  - **Phenylketonuria**: diffuse pigmentary dilution of skin and hair because ↑ L-phenylalanine inhibits tyrosinase
  - **Menkes**: diffuse pigmentary dilution due to ↓↓ Cu++ (tyrosinase is a copper-dependent enzyme)
  - **Mccune-Albright**: G-protein activating mutation → cAMP cascade is constitutively "on". Pigment abnormality = CALM
- UV Radiation → ↑ size of melanocytes; ↑ activity of melanocytes; ↑ stage IV melanosomes transferred to keratinocytes
  - Initial pigment darkening: oxidation of preexisting melanin (minutes to hours)
  - Delayed tanning: new pigment production (48-72 hrs)

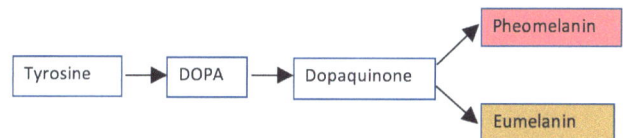

Figure 11.1: Melanin Synthesis

Melanosome Formation

- Melanin Packaging
  - Melanin is packaged into vesicles & combined with matrix proteins (**gp100/Pmel17/silver protein** = stains with **HMB45**)
  - **P protein** = transmembrane protein on intracellular organelle membranes. Helps traffic protein into melanosomes. The ER regulates processing & trafficking of tyrosinase
    - **OCA2** = mutated P protein
    - **Chédiak-Higashi** = mutation in *LYST* gene (involved in melanosome fission)
  - **Adaptor protein-3 (AP-3)** = helps target proteins to intracytoplasmic organelles
    - **Hermansky-Pudlak Syndrome** = mutation in β3A subunit of AP-3

- Melanosome Maturation - Four stages
  - Stage I (premelanosomes): clear vesicles with no melanin
  - Stage II: elongated vesicles with internal membrane, but still no pigment
  - Stage III: **melanin** and internal fibers
  - Stage IV: melanin is so dark that internal fibers cannot be seen

Melanosome Transport

- Proteins involved in melanosome transport (fig. 11.7)
  - Microtubules
  - Kinesin = anterograde transport
  - Dynein = retrograde transport
    - UV exposure → ↑ kinesin and ↓ dynein
  - Myosin Va, *RAB27A*, melanophilin
    - Involved in melanocyte transfer to keratinocyte
    - Mutations in any of these 3 cause **Griscelli Syndrome** and **Elejalde Syndrome**

Tuberous Sclerosis

Tuberous Sclerosis (Bourneville's Syndrome)

- AD mutation (but most are spontaneous)
  - *TSC1* = Hamartin
  - *TSC2* = Tuberin
    - *TSC2* mutations can also cause isolated **Lymphangiomyomatosis**
- Classic triad is MR, seizures, skin findings
- Pathogenesis:
  - *TSC1* and *TSC2* are tumor suppressor genes
  - Downregulate Ras proto-oncogene via hydrolysis of GTP → GDP
  - Ham and Tub form a complex to ↑ hydrolysis of GTP→GDP. Rab and Rheb (GTPase proteins) both need bound-GTP to function, and tub/ham accelerates hydrolysis GTP → GDP
    - Note: similar to neurofibromin in how it downregulates RAS GTPase
- Clinical:
  - 2M = definite TS
  - 1M + 1m = probable TS
  - 1M or 2m = possible TS

- Major criteria (skin):
  - Hypopigmented macules >3 (**earliest skin finding** - birth or soon after); posterior trunk m.c. site
    - a) Thumbprint (polygonal) m.c. (like nevus anemicus/ depigmentosa)
    - b) Ash leaf (lance-ovate)
    - c) Confetti (extremities) **most specific** but rarest, a minor criteria
  - **Facial angiofibromas (adenoma sebaceum) next finding 2-6 years** (fig 11.2) (also seen in MEN1, Birt-Hogg-Dubé)
  - Fibrous cephalic plaque
  - Shagreen patch (connective tissue nevus - also seen in Buschke-Ollendorff)
  - Non-traumatic periungal fibromas

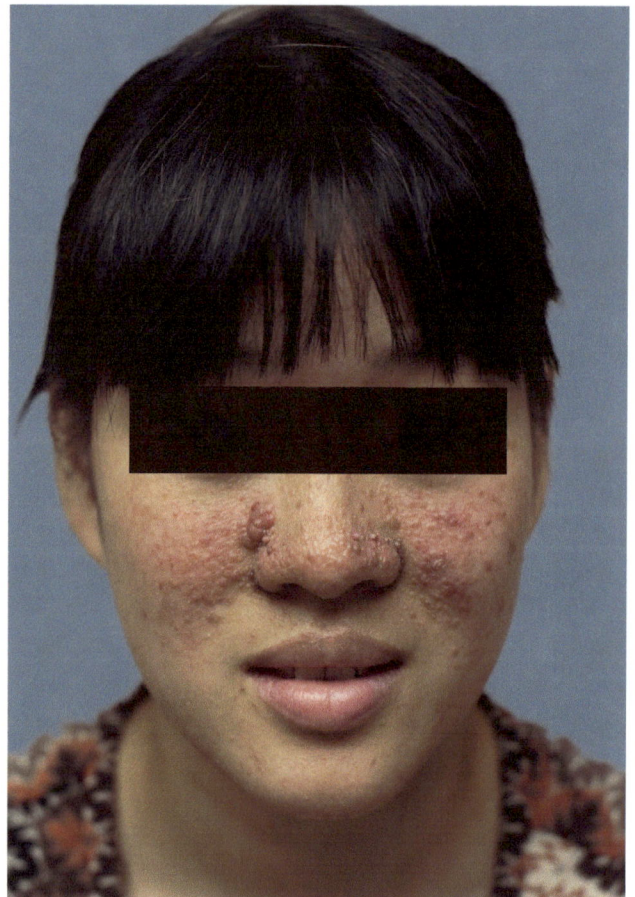

Figure 11.2: Tuberous Sclerosis with Adenoma Sebaceum and Angiofibromas

- Major criteria (non-skin):
  - Multiple retinal hamartomas (gliomas/ phakomas)
  - Subependymal nodule

J. Finch & M. Payette

- Subependymal giant cell astrocytoma
- Cortical tubers
- Cardiac rhabdomyomas - cause arrhythmias, especially WPW. Resolve spontaneously.
- Renal angiomyolipomas
- Lymphangioleiomyomatosis (lungs)
  - Pulmonary angiomyolipomas represent metastatic clones of the renal angiomyolipomas
  - *TSC2* mutations (or rarely *TSC1*) also cause isolated pulmonary lymphangioleiomyomatosis, a rare lung disease with disorderly proliferation of bronchiolar smooth muscle
- Minor criteria:
  - Cutaneous:
    - Dental pits
    - Confetti skin lesions
    - Intraoral fibromas
  - Extracutaneous:
    - Hamartomatous rectal polyps
    - Bone cysts
    - Cerebral white matter radial migration lines
    - Renal cysts (*TSC2* gene is contiguous with polycystic kidney disease *PKD1* gene)
- Other findings (not included in diagnostic criteria):
  - CNS involvement (seizures in 90%, MR in 62%)
- Management:
  - ECHO, renal ultrasound, chest x-ray, brain MRI
  - If 3 or more hypopigmented macules at birth, perform ECHO
  - Sirolimus (an mTOR inhibitor) decreases angiofibroma and angiomyolipoma growth
- DDx:
  - Birt-Hogg-Dubé, MEN-1, Cowden Syndrome, and Tuberous Sclerosis can all get oral papillomas, angiofibromas and collagenomas
  - **Westerhof Syndrome**: congenital hypopigmented macules + MR + growth retardation. May be a forme fruste of TS

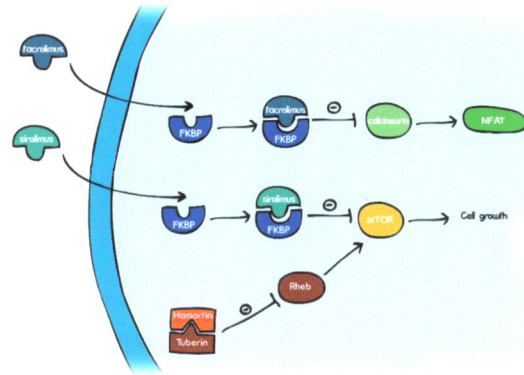

Figure 11.3: Sirolimus and Tacrolimus Mechanism. Sirolimus Acts on the mTOR Pathway

Disorders with Diffuse Pigmentary Dilution

OCA Overview
- All variants of albinism are autosomal RECESSIVE
  - Except for Ocular Albinism (XLR), which does not affect skin
- In OCA1 and OCA3, tyrosinase protein is retained within the lumen of the rough endoplasmic reticulum rather than being transferred to melanosomes

Oculocutaneous Albinism, Type 1A
- AR; mutation in *TYR* gene, with **complete loss of tyrosinase**
- Clinical findings:
  - White hair, white skin, red eyes (fig 11.4)
  - Red nevi (amelanotic)
  - SCC>BCC>Melanoma
  - Eye: miswired optic fibers, causing strabismus, nystagmus, ↓ acuity (even blindness). Unpigmented irides result in photophobia
  - Normal # of melanocytes, but melanocytes only have Stage I and II premelanosomes

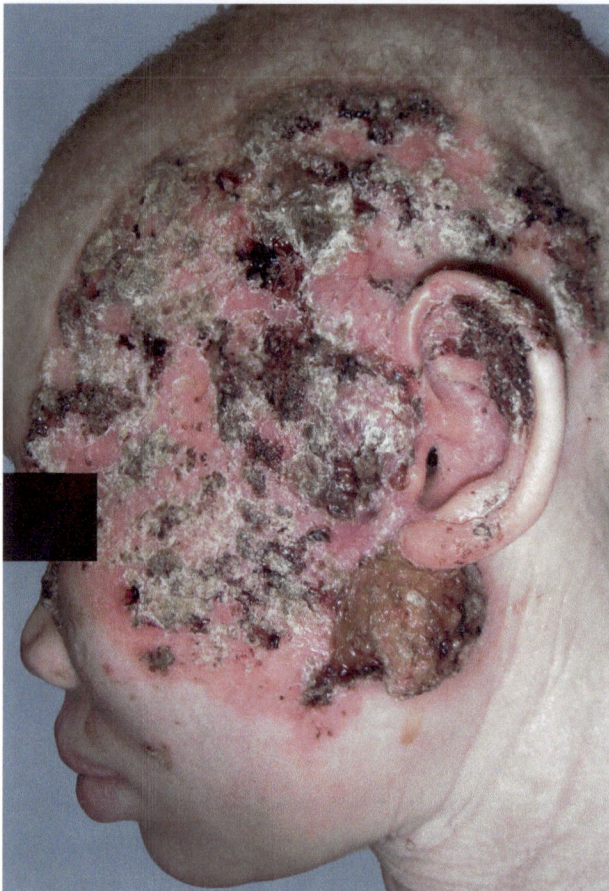

Figure 11.4: Large Squamous Cell Carcinoma in OCA1

Oculocutaneous Albinism, Type 1B

- AR; mutation in *TYR* gene, with ↓ **tyrosinase levels**, but enough residual tyrosinase activity to produce some pheomelanin
- <u>Yellow Mutant phenotype:</u>
  - With age, hair and skin become yellow (due to pheomelanin)
  - Pheomelanin forms because it requires less tyrosinase activity
- <u>Temperature-Sensitive phenotype</u>
  - Mutated *TYR* produces a thermolabile tyrosinase that is inactivated at 35° C
  - White hair axilla, red hair scalp, brown hair arms, dark brown hair legs (like a Siamese cat)

Oculocutaneous Albinism, Type 2

- AR; mutation in *P* gene
  - **Tyrosinase levels are normal**
- M.C. form of OCA, especially in African Americans

- Clinical findings:
  - Skin and hair darken with age
  - Nevi are brown, large lentigines
  - 1% of Prader-Willi (hyperphagia/obesity) and Angelman (puppet like movements, inappropriate laughter) patients have OCA2, because the deleted region in PWS and AS (15q) contains the *P* gene

Oculocutaneous Albinism, Type 3

- AR; mutation in *TYRP* gene
- Slight pigment at birth
  - Skin and hair become red-bronze, blue/brown iris

> **Picture a nerdy kid with red hair.**
> **OCA3 = "the red TwYRP"**

Oculocutaneous Albinism, Type 4

- AR; mutation in *MATP* gene (*SLC45A2* locus)
- Clinical findings like OCA2
- Most common in Japan

Ocular Albinism

- XLR; mutation in *GPR143* gene, encoding a G-protein coupled receptor
- Clinical findings:
  - Severe OA (nystagmus, photophobia, strabismus, photosensitive, no pigment in retina)
  - Macromelanosomes (skin and eyes)
  - Grossly normal skin and hair

Tietz Syndrome

- AD; mutation in *MITF* (allelic with Waardenburg Syndrome 2)
- Clinical:
  - Deafness, **No dystopia canthorum** (same as WS2)
  - Pigmentary dilution of skin, hair and eyes
  - Allelic with WS2 (p. 81), but has:
    - 1) **Generalized hypomelanosis** (not piebald pattern as in WS2)
    - 2) HYPOplasia (vs hyper) of eyebrows

J. Finch & M. Payette

Table 11.1: Oculocutaneous Albinism

TYPE	INH	Gene	Protein	Function
OCA1A	AR	TYR	No tyrosinase	Tyrosinase gets trapped in rER
OCA1B	AR	TYR	↓ Tyrosinase activity	
OCA2	AR	P gene	P protein, a transmembrane-transporter (normal levels of tyrosinase)	Processing/ trafficking of tyrosinase pH regulation glutathione content
OCA3	AR	TRP aka TYRP1	Tyrosine-related protein 1	Stabilizes tyrosinase Tyrosinase gets trapped in rER
OCA4	AR	MATP (SLC45A2)	Membrane-associated transporter protein	Cargo unknown ?sucrose

Hermansky-Pudlak Syndrome

- Overview: HPS phenotype = **oculocutaneous albinism + bleeding diathesis**
  - Pigmentary dilution of skin, eyes, and hair (fig 11.5)
  - Brown nevi
  - Same eye findings as OCA (↓ acuity, nystagmus)
  - Platelet dysfunction, but normal platelet count. Absent platelet granules. Bleeding diathesis. Avoid aspirin
  - Deposition of **ceroid lipofuscin** → pulmonary fibrosis, granulomatous colitis, cardiomyopathy, renal failure
  - Life expectancy 30-50 years
  - Most cases in **Puerto Rico**
- HPS 1 and 4:
  - BLOC3 protein mutations
  - HPS1 = M.C. type, most severe
- HPS 2:
  - HPS1 + **immunodeficiency** (URI, otitis media)
  - *AP3B1* mutation (β3A subunit of AP3)
    - CD1b-binds to AP3 for Ag presentation
- HPS 3, 4, 5, 6, 7, 8:
  - HPS 3, 4, 5, 6, 7, 8 have mild clinical findings, without ceroid lipofuscin problems
  - HPS 3, 5, 6 = BLOC2 protein mutations
  - HPS 7 = BLOC1 protein
  - HPS 8 = dysbindin
- Cross Syndrome:
  - HPS + neurologic problems (ataxia, spasticity)

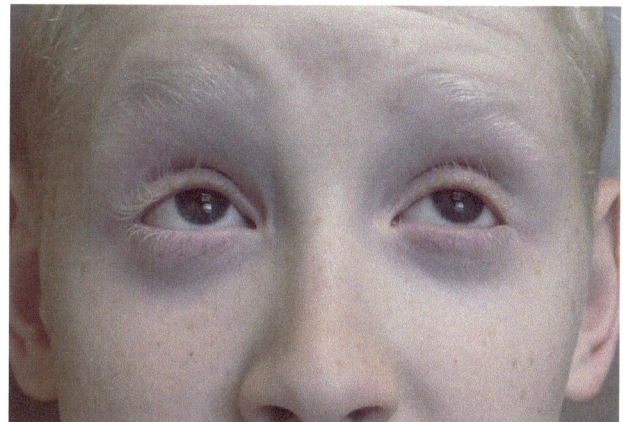

Figure 11.5: Child's Face with Hermansky-Pudlak Syndrome

> Think "Hermansky-Pudlak Syndrome (HPS) Has Pigment and Serum" problems.
> If you see oculocutaneous albinism + bleeding/bruising, think HPS

Table 11.2: Hermansky-Pudlak Syndrome

Disease	Inh	Gene	Protein/Function
HPS1, 4	AR	HPS1, 4	BLOC3 proteins
HPS2	AR	AP3B1	β3A subunit of AP3 (AP-3 traffics proteins from golgi to other organelles)
HPS3, 5, 6	AR	HPS3, 5, 6	BLOC2 proteins
HPS7,8	AR	DTNBP1 BLOC 1S3	BLOC 1 proteins HPS7 = dysbindin
Cross Syndrome		?	

BLOC = biogenesis of lysosome-related organelles complex, involved in trafficking protein from Golgi to lysosomes
HPS = Hermansky-Pudlak Syndrome

Chédiak-Higashi Syndrome

- AR; mutation in *LYST* gene, encoding a microtubule used for fission of lysosomes
- Pigmentary dilution of skin, eyes, and hair. Silver hair
- Normal visual acuity (vs. HPS and OCA), but still have nystagmus
- **Severe immunodeficiency** and bleeding diathesis
- **Hemophagocytic Syndrome** (Lymphocyte-Macrophage Activation Syndrome) (like Griscelli Type 2) in 85%. Results in hemophagocytosis, HSM, CNS deterioration, pancytopenia, bleeding, and death
  - All CHS patients need hematopoietic stem cell transplant or die
  - Survivors get **progressive neurologic deterioration**
- Labs/Path – **Giant organelles** due to vesicle-trafficking defect
  - Giant melanosomes in melanocytes (histo hallmark)
  - **Giant melanin clumps in hair, with regular spacing** (vs irregular in Griscelli)
  - ↓ platelet dense granules and giant non-functional granules in PMNs (fig 11.6)

Chédiak-Higashi

Hemophagocytic Syndrome
Immunodeficiency
Giant melanosomes
Abnormal PMNs
Silver hair
Hypopigmentation

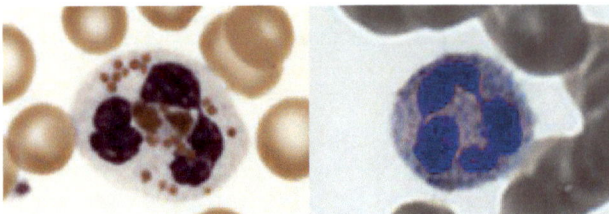

Figure 11.6: Chédiak-Higashi PMN and Normal PMN

The Silver Hair Syndromes:
Chédiak-Higashi & Griscelli/Elejalde

Griscelli Syndrome

- Griscelli Type 1 (Elejalde):
  - AR; *MYO5A* mutation, encoding Myosin 5a
    - One end binds actin skeleton, other binds organelle (fig 11.7)
  - Clinical findings:
    - Silver skin and silver hair
    - **Profound neuro defects** with mental retardation
    - **Hair: irregular clumps of melanosomes** (vs evenly-spaced in CHS)
- Griscelli Type 2:
  - AR; *RAB27A* mutation, encoding Rab27A
    - Ras-like GTPase in melanosomes
  - Clinical findings:
    - **Immunodeficiency/heme disorders**
    - **Accelerated phase hemophagocytic syndrome** (like CHS)
- Griscelli Type 3:
  - AR; *MLPH* mutation, encoding melanophilin
    - Links myosin 5A and Rab 27a (fig 11.7)
  - Clinical findings:
    - Only get melanocyte abnormalities (silver skin/hair); no other findings
- Griscelli PMNs appear normal on peripheral smear (vs huge granules in Chédiak-Higashi)

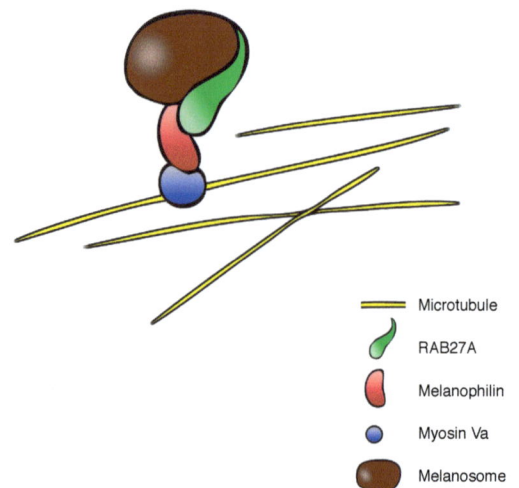

—	Microtubule
	RAB27A
	Melanophilin
•	Myosin Va
	Melanosome

Figure 11.7: Melanosome Transport

P14 Deficiency

- Lysosome defect with phenotype resembling CHS, Griscelli 2, or HPS2
- Pigmentary dilution and immunodeficiency

J. Finch & M. Payette

Table 11.3: Genoderms with Hypopigmentation and Immunodeficiency
Hermansky-Pudlak, Type 2
Chédiak-Higashi
Griscelli Syndrome, Type 2
p14 Deficiency

Disorders with Pigmentary Dilution Discussed Elsewhere

- Phenylketonuria (see p. 46)
  - PKU patients have ↑ L-phenylalanine, which inhibits tyrosinase
- Menkes (see p. 67)
  - Menkes has copper transport abnormality, and tyrosinase requires copper
- Homocystinuria (see p. 34)
- Histidinemia
- EEC Syndrome (see p. 71)
- Apert Syndrome (see p. 108)
- Sialic Acid Storage Disease

Disorders with Circumscribed Leukoderma

Piebaldism

- AD; mutation in *KIT* gene, resulting in inability of KIT receptor to be activated by the steel factor (mast cell growth factor)
  - Note: somatic activating mutations in KIT gene (ckit protein) cause adult onset mastocytosis and some acral melanomas
- Clinical:
  - Poliosis (**forelock in 80-90%**) at birth, with depigmented skin on central anterior trunk, mid extremities, central forehead. Spares hands, feet, back
  - Normal or **hyperpigmented macules within patches of leukoderma**
  - **No systemic findings**. Skin-limited disorder

Waardenburg Syndrome

- Waardenburg Syndrome, Type 1
  - AD; mutation in *PAX3* gene (allelic with WS 3)
  - **Poliosis** (piebald pattern). White forelock = m.c. finding
  - **Synophrys** (medial eyebrow hyperplasia)
  - Deafness
  - Cleft palate

- Ophtho:
  - **Dystopia canthorum** (↑ intercanthal distance with normal interpupillary distance, broad nasal root)
  - **Heterochromia iridis**, but no neuro-ophthalmic problems
  - Short palpebral fissures (blepharophimosis)

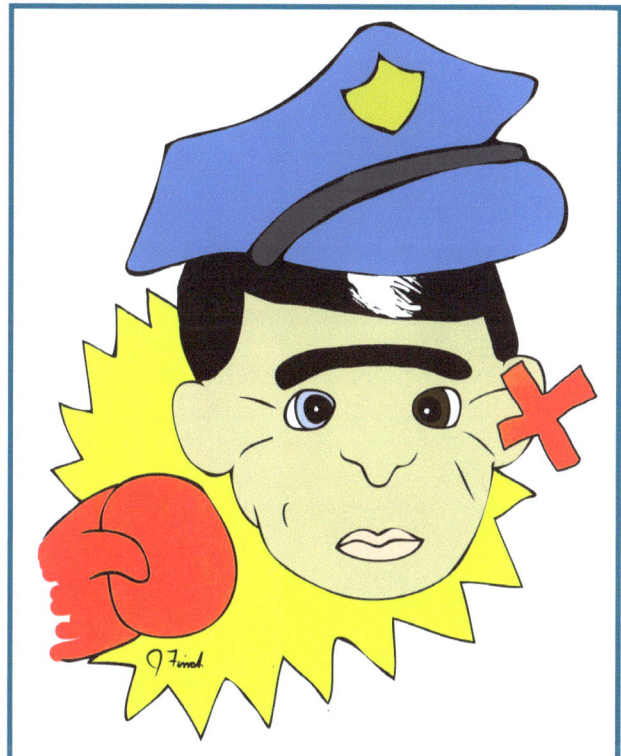

Waardenburg Syndrome

Picture a warden (Waardenburg) getting punched in the face - **"pax a punch,"** causing broad nasal root and dystopia canthorum. The warden has synophrys, piebaldism, heterochromia iridis, deafness. Only PAX3 mutations (WS1 & 3) get dystopia canthorum.

- Waardenburg Syndrome, Type 2
  - AD; mutation in *MITF* or *SLUG* genes
    - Microphthalmia-associated transcription factor
    - Zinc finger transcription factor
  - Like WS1, but no dystopia canthorum (DC)
  - Note: Tietz Syndrome (p. 78) is allelic with WS2, but has generalized hypopigmentation

Think "I might've missed the SLUG" to remember that MITF and SLUG mutations cause Waardenburg 2 and patients do not get dystopia canthorum

- Waardenburg Syndrome, Type 3
  (Waardenburg-Klein)
  - AD; mutation in *PAX3* gene (same as Type 1)
  - **WS1 + upper limb malformations**
    (hypoplasia/syndactyly)
- Waardenburg Syndrome, Type 4
  (Waardenburg-Shah Syndrome)
  - AD mutation in:
    - SRY box 10 (*SOX-10*)
    - Endothelin-3 (*EDN3*)
    - Endothelin-B receptor (*EDNRB*)
  - **WS1 + Hirschsprung Disease**
  - No DC

> Think "Sorry, your endothelium is messed up, too" to remember that Waardenburg 4 is a SRY box & endothelin mutation and gets Hirshsprung's Disease

> Think *"Pack your mittens, pack your socks and underwear"* to remember the gene mutations associated with each Waardenburg subtype
>
> | **Pack** | Pax (Waardenburg 1) |
> | **Mittens** | MITF (Waardenburg 2) |
> | | |
> | **Pack** | Pax (Waardenburg 3) |
> | **Socks** | SOX & Endothelin (Waardenburg 4) |

Albinism-Deafness Syndrome (Woolf Syndrome, Ziprkowski-Margolis)

- **XLR**; defect in *ADFN* gene
- Clinical:
  - Severe piebaldism + deafness
  - Heterochromia iridis
  - Mottled, leopard-like skin
- May be an **XLR** form of Waardenburg Type 2, since nearly clinically identical

Phylloid Hypomelanosis

- Mosaic trisomy 13
- Leaf-like (phylloid) patches of hypopigmentation

12. Disorders with Hyperpigmentation

Blaschkoid Hyperpigmentation

- Dermatoses following these lines are mosaics
- V-shape on back; S-shape on abdomen; swirl on the scalp (fig 12.1)

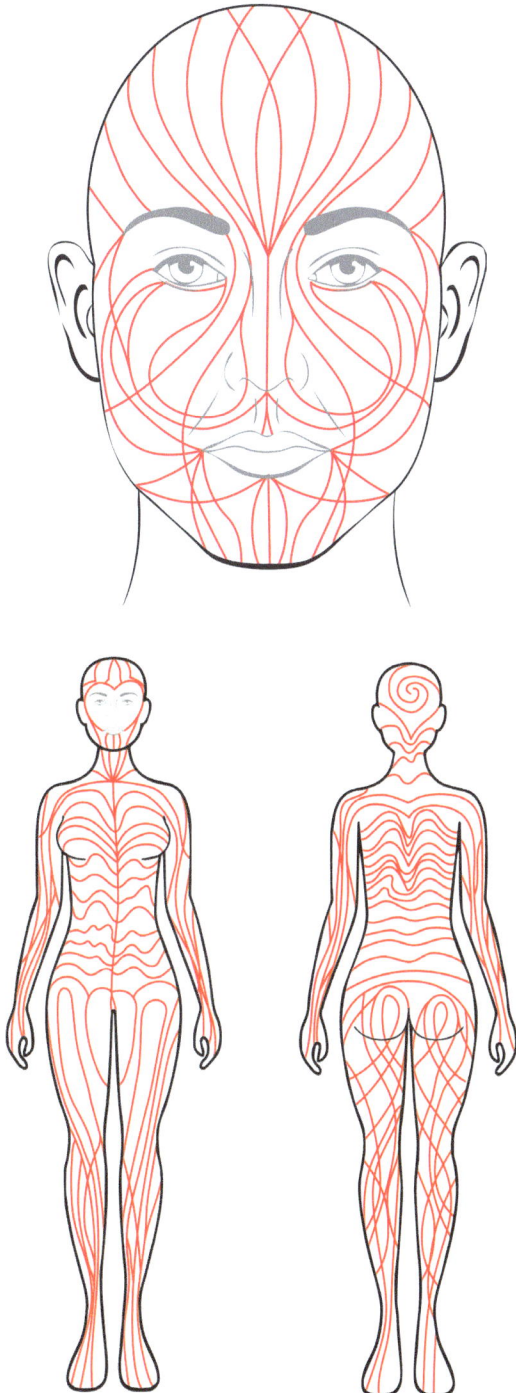

Figure 12.1: Lines of Blaschko

Pigmentary Mosaicism (Linear and Whorled Nevoid Hypermelanosis)

- Sporadic, mosaic disorder of melanoblast migration and clonal expansion
- Clinical:
  - Swirls and streaks of brown hyperpigmentation
  - Most are benign and skin-limited. Rarely, cardiac, neurologic, musculoskeletal defects reported (formerly called Hypomelanosis of Ito)
- Ddx: Stage III IP (melanophages predominantly), early epidermal nevus

Incontinentia Pigmenti (Bloch-Sulzberger Syndrome)

- **XLD;** mutation in NF-κB essential modulator gene (**NEMO**)
- Multisystem disorder in girls (Lethal in males)
- Skin lesions distributed in the lines of Blaschko, evolving through 4 stages:
  - 1) Vesicles – appearing in crops (fig 12.2). Biopsy shows **eos**. Patients have **peripheral eosinophilia** in infancy. Lasts months
  - 2) Verrucous – warty papules in irregular lines, usually on hands/feet. Lasts 1-2 yrs
  - 3) Hyperpigmentation – Blaschkoid hyperpigmentation resembling "Chinese writing figures." Usually presents 3-6 months, progresses until age 2, then fades by adolescence
  - 4) Hypopigmentation – subtle atrophic hypopigmented streaks

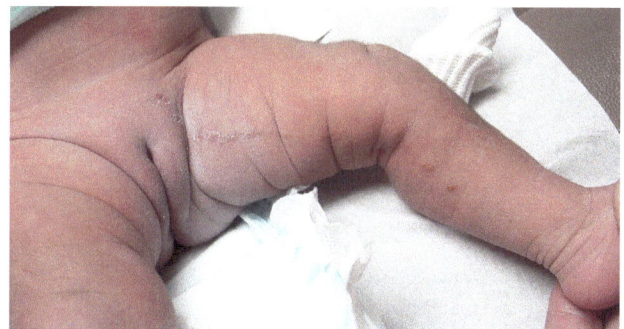

Figure 12.2: Incontinentia Pigmenti, Stage 1 (Image courtesy of Steven Brett Sloan, MD)

- Scarring alopecia, nail dystrophy
- Systemic findings:
  - Pegged teeth, missing teeth (M.C. extracutaneous finding)
  - Seizures
  - Ophtho (1/3): strabismus, atrophy
- Labs: Leukocytosis, eosinophilia

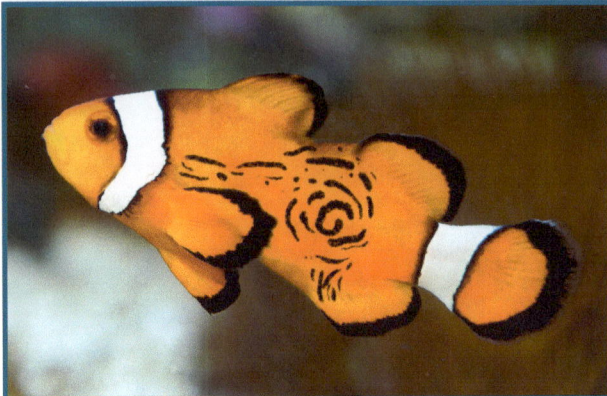

Incontinentia Pigmenti

Picture a clownfish with a Blaschkoid swirl to remember that *NEMO* gene mutation causes Incontinentia Pigmenti

Reticulate Hyperpigmentation

Overview

- Genoderms are rare; think of common dermatoses first:
  - Erythema ab igne
  - Confluent and Reticulated Papillomatosis of Gougerot and Carteaud (CARP)
  - Prurigo pigmentosa
- Examine family history and other signs of ectodermal dysplasia
- Then think of genoderms:
  - **EBS with Mottled Pigmentation**
  - **Dyskeratosis Congenita**
  - **Naegeli-Franceschetti-Jadassohn Syndrome**
  - **X-Linked Reticulated Pigmentary Disorder**
  - **Dowling-Degos Disease**
  - **Reticulate Acropigmentation of Kitamura**
  - **Galli-Galli Disease**
  - **Dermatopathia Pigmentosa Reticularis**

Dyskeratosis Congenita (Zinsser-Engman-Cole)

- 90% males
- Results from **mutations that affect telomerase**
  - **XLR** form (most common) = *DKC1* mutations encoding **dyskerin 1**, resulting in **short telomeres**
  - AD form (rare) = *TERC* (telomerase RNA component)
  - AR form (rare) = *NOLA3*, encoding a protein that interacts with telomerase reverse transcriptase (TERT)
- Clinical features: Highly variable
  - Lacy reticulated pigmentation of neck, chest and upper arms (fig 12.3)
  - **Premature aging** - wrinkled skin
  - Palmoplantar hyperhidrosis & PPK
  - Frictional bullae and acrocyanosis
  - Nails: longitudinal ridging and splitting, pterygium (fig 12.4)
  - **Premalignant leukoplakia** of oral, vaginal, urethral, anal mucosa (adolescence)
  - Malformed, missing teeth
  - Epiphora (continuous lacrimation), lacrimal duct atresia
  - Bone marrow failure (in 80%, 20s-30s)
  - **Malignancies** (**SCC**>MDS, AML, HD, GI carcinomas)

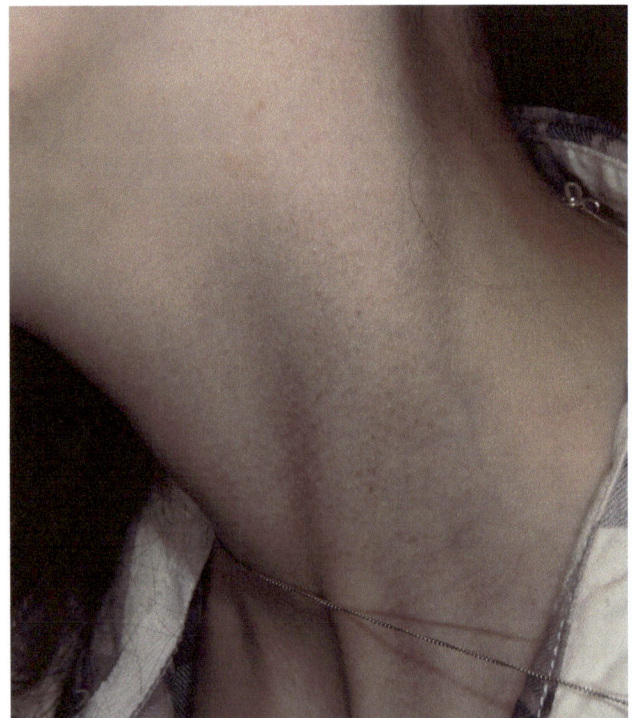

Figure 12.3: Neck Pigmentation in Dyskeratosis Congenita

J. Finch & M. Payette

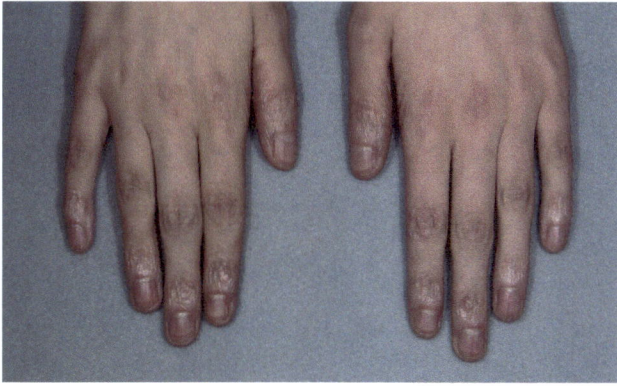

Figure 12.4: Nail Dystrophy in Dyskeratosis Congenita

– Other features: testicular atrophy, pulmonary fibrosis, liver cirrhosis, developmental delay, opportunistic infections

- Death from bone marrow failure
- Phenotypic overlap with <u>Fanconi's anemia</u>:
  – Fanconi's has more generalized hyperpigmentation
  – No nail findings
  – Absent thumbs
  – Earlier onset bone marrow failure
  – Same SCC risk, but more breast and pancreatic CA

Naegeli-Franceschetti-Jadassohn Syndrome

- AD; **K14 gene** (non-helical head); Swiss and British and Anglo-Saxon descent
  – Note: *K14* mutation in alpha-helical rod domain causes EB Simplex
- Clinical features:
  – Reticulated hyperpigmentation beginning by age 2, then fading during adolescence (abdomen, periocular, perioral, neck, trunk, proximal extremities)
  – Bullae on feet in newborn period
  – ↓ sweat gland function, resulting in **heat intolerance**, MAJOR PROBLEM
  – Absent/hypoplastic dermatoglyphs, PPK
  – Severe dental anomalies (pegged, supernumerary, yellow spots)
- Ddx:
  – DKC: in NFJ, no leukoplakia, no bone marrow failure, and no associated malignancies
  – IP: Blaschkoid, preceded by an inflammatory phase
  – X-linked Reticulate Pigmentary Disorder: systemic findings

– Dermatopathia Pigmentosa Reticularis: lack of alopecia, pigmentation fades

Dermatopathia Pigmentosa Reticularis

- AD; *K14* gene (non-helical head)
- Clinical features:
  – Triad: reticulate hyperpigmentation, non-scarring alopecia, onychodystrophy (pterygium)
  – Absent dermatoglyphs, hypo or hyperhidrosis, punctate palmoplantar keratoses
- Ddx:
  – NFJ – no alopecia and fades during adolescence
  – DKC

X-Linked Reticulate Pigmentary Disorder

- **XLR**; mutation in *POL1A* gene
- Males: generalized reticulate hyperpigmentation. Death in infancy or early childhood due to severe systemic anomalies, failure to thrive
- Female carriers: streaky hyperpigmentation (similar to stage 3 of IP). Otherwise normal
- Cutaneous amyloid. No systemic amyloid
- Blonde, unruly hair

Dowling-Degos Disease (Reticulated Hyperpigmentation of the Flexures), Reticulate Acropigmentation of Kitamura, and Galli-Galli Disease

- AD; *K5* mutation (Dowling-Degos; Galli-Galli); ADAM10 mutation (Kitamura)
- Dowling-Degos affects skin folds; Reticulate Acropigmentation of Kitamura is a rarer acral variant
- <u>Dowling-Degos Disease</u>
  – Progressive **reticulate hyperpigmentation of the axilla, groin**, then other body folds
  – Small hyperkeratotic dark brown papules of flexures and great skin folds
  – Comedone-like lesions on the back and the neck
  – Pitted perioral acneiform scars
  – Hidradenitis suppurativa
- <u>Reticulate Acropigmentation of Kitamura</u>
  – Two thirds are Japanese
  – Linear **palmar pits** (irregular breaks in palmar dermatoglyphs) and **atrophic hyperpigmented macules on hands/feet**; appear in childhood

- – Slowly darken and spread during adulthood
- Galli-Galli Disease
  - – Clinically identical to Dowling-Degos, but has **acantholysis** on path
- Ddx: acanthosis nigricans, NF (axillary freckling)

Dyschromatoses

- Dyschromia = hyper <u>and</u> hypopigmentation
- Two forms:
  - – DSH = localized form
  - – DUH = generalized form

Dyschromatosis Symmetrica Hereditaria (DSH, "Reticulate Acropigmentation of Dohi")

- AD; *ADAR* gene mutation; encodes double stranded RNA specific adenosine deaminase
- **Hypo <u>and</u> hyperpigmented macules of dorsal hands** and feet
- Affects Asians, onset by age 6, progresses until puberty, then stabilizes
- Spares palms/soles, mucous membranes

Dyschromatosis Universalis Hereditaria (DUH)

- Similar to Dyschromatosis Symmetrica Hereditaria; gene defect unknown; genetic transmission unknown
- vs DSH:
  - – DUH has earlier onset (by age 1)
  - – DUH affects trunk (not hands/feet)
- Isolated cases associated with systemic manifestations: seizures, deafness, tryptophan metabolism abnormalities, bilateral glaucoma

Hyperpigmentation Syndromes with Ectodermal Dysplasia

Berlin Syndrome

- Generalized gray-brown hyperpigmentation with guttate hypomelanotic macules; sparse eyebrows; delayed dentition
- Mental retardation; 1 family known (Iranian), consanguineous parents

Lucky/Winter Syndrome

- Generalized hyperpigmentation with guttate hypomelanotic macules in flexures
- Scant lightly pigmented hair; enamel hypoplasia; digitized thumbs

Acromelanosis Albo-Punctata

- Diffuse hyperpigmentation with guttate hypopigmented macules on the acral and flexural areas associated with atrophy; keratotic follicular papules
- Pili torti; platonychia

Syndromes with Multiple CALMs

Overview

- Multiple CALMs are relatively rare
- Multiple CALMs seen in:
  - – **RASopathies**
    - **NF1, NF2, Watson, Legius**
  - – **McCune-Albright, Ring chromosome, Bannayan-Riley-Ruvalcaba**
  - – Questionable association: **Bloom, Ataxia-Telangiectasia, Tuberous Sclerosis, Noonan and LEOPARD** (allelic), **Silver-Russell**
- What to do with CALMs:
  - – 1 no significance
  - – >3 f/u for development of disease
  - – >5 monitor for NF1
  - – Bone fractures and/or precocious puberty: look for large CALMs or Blaschko's lines of hyperpigmentation (McCune-Albright)

McCune-Albright Syndrome

- Sporadic post-zygotic **activating mutation** in *GNAS1* gene (allelic with Albright's Hereditary Osteodystrophy, which is an *inactivating* mutation)
- Clinical features:
  - – **Segmental CALM with "coast of Maine" borders**
  - – Endocrine hyperfunction (precocious puberty) (Note: Russell-Silver also has precocious puberty)
  - – **Polyostotic fibrous dysplasia**

J. Finch & M. Payette

Table 12.1: Genoderms with Heart Problems

Pulmonic Stenosis	RASopathies • Noonan • Watson • LEOPARD • Cardiofaciocutaneous Syndrome • NF-1 Carney Complex Cornelia de Lange
Endocardial cushion defects	Down Syndrome
Coarctation	PHACES
Early MI	Fabry's, Werner, Progeria, PXE
Miscellaneous	H Syndrome, Ehlers-Danlos, Cutis Laxa, Homocystinuria, Naxos, Carvajal
Mitral Prolapse	Marfan

Syndromes with Multiple Lentigines

Carney Complex (NAME Syndrome, LAMB Syndrome)

- AD; mutation in *PRKAR1A* (protein kinase A, regulatory subunit 1a) resulting in multiple neoplasias
- Cardiac myxomas (79%)
  - Myxomas can occur in any chamber and embolize, causing necrotic acral lesions
  - Cause of death in 25%
- Skin:
  - Cutaneous myxomas (45%)
  - Lentigines (60%) notably on the medial conjunctiva of eye
  - Blue nevi (65%), especially **epithelioid blue nevus**
- Endocrine overactivity (45%):
  - Pigmented adrenocortical Cushing's Disease
  - Sertoli cell testicular tumors (specifically the rare large-cell calcifying type)
  - Pituitary growth hormone adenoma
- **Psammomatous melanotic schwannomas**
  - Rare skin tumor. 50% are associated with Carney
- Mnemonics:
  - **NAME** = **N**evi (blue), **A**trial myxoma, **M**ucocutaneous Myxoma, **E**phelides/ **E**ndocrinopathy
  - **LAMB = L**entigines, **A**trial myxoma, **M**yxoma (cutaneous), **B**lue nevi

LEOPARD Syndrome

- AD; mutation in *PTPN11* (allelic with Noonan), encodes SHP2 protein
- **L**entigines and **café-noir** macules
- **E**KG conduction defects
- **O**cular hypertelorism
- **P**ulmonary stenosis
- **A**bnormal genitalia
- **R**etardation of growth
- **D**eafness

Table 12.2: Genoderms with Multiple Lentigines

Genoderms with Diffuse Lentigines	
Familial Generalized Lentiginosis	AD; generalized lentigines. Skin-limited
Carney Complex (NAME Syndrome, LAMB Syndrome)	(See above)
LEOPARD Syndrome	(See above)
Genoderms with Mucosal Lentigines	
Peutz-Jeghers Syndrome	AD; mutation in STK11 benign GI polyps Pancreatic and gonad tumors
Laugier-Hunziker Syndrome	Oral lentigines, genital lentigines, longitudinal melanonychia No GI polyps
Genoderms with Localized Lentigines	
Centrofacial Lentiginosis	AD; lentigines in a butterfly distribution on the face
Cowden Disease (PTEN)	Periorificial and acral
Bannayan-Riley-Ruvalcaba (PTEN)	Glans penis > vulva
Cantú	Tiny (1 mm) lentigines on face, forearms, hands, feet
Xeroderma Pigmentosum	Photodistributed
Bloom	Photodistributed
OCA	Photodistributed

13. Immunodeficiency Syndromes

See also Table 18.16: Immunodeficiency Syndromes (p.138)

Immunodeficiency Syndromes

Isolated IgA Deficiency

- *TNFRSF13B* mutation, encodes TACI
- Defect in conversion of B-cell→ IgA-producing plasma cell
- **M.C. immunodeficiency**
- 1:600 in white population is affected
- Can be inherited or acquired (**chemo/phenytoin**)
- ½ are well; ½ get repeated infections
- **Anaphylactic reactions to transfusions/IVIG** (i.e. products containing IgA)
- ↑ association of Celiac Disease, UC, regional enteritis; also SLE, DM, scleroderma, thyroiditis, RA, Sjögren's
- Increased risk of malignancy

Common Variable Immunodeficiency (CVID)

- Second M.C. immunodeficiency
- Heterogeneous group of disorders, mostly acquired, but 10-20% have family history of immunodeficiency
- Six genetic mutations identified: *ICOS*, *TACI* (*TNFRSF13B*), *CD19*, *BAFFR* (*TNFRSF13C*), *CD20*, *CD81*
- Warts
- Recurrent sinopulmonary infections
- Low levels of most immunoglobulin classes
- Abnormal B cell differentiation
- Abnormal T cell function. ↑ Th-1 phenotype and IL-12 expression
- Predisposed to vitiligo and alopecia areata

X-Linked Agammaglobulinemia (Bruton Syndrome, Sex-Linked Agammaglobulinemia)

- **XLR**; *BTK* tyrosine kinase mutation
- Rare, apparent after 3-6 months
- Defect in conversion of pre-B-cells to B-cells, *RPTK* defect
- Increased susceptibility to **Gram (+) pyogenic** infections
- Affected boys prone to atopic dermatitis, vasculitis and urticaria

- Growth failure, **chronic diarrhea**, absence of palpable lymph nodes
- Absence of IgM, A, D, E
- Cell mediated immunity (T-cells) intact
- Unusual susceptibility to **enteroviruses**→death from fatal encephalitis
- Vaccine related Poliomyelitis or Dermatomyositis/ Meningoencephalitis Syndrome

Isolated IgM Deficiency

- Likely due to a defect in IgM-secreting plasma cells
- **Eczema**
- Increased susceptibility to meningococcemia, pneumococci, *H. flu*
- ↓ IgM and IgD, ↑ PMNs, IgA, IgG, IgE
- **Verrucae** in great numbers

Hyper-IgM Immunodeficiency (XHIM)

- **XLR;** mutation in *CD40LG* (*TNFSF5*) gene, resulting in **abnormal CD40 Ligand** on T-cells
  - Normally, binding of CD40-Ligand on T-cell to CD40 on B-cell triggers isotype switching from IgM to IgG. In XHIM, mutated CD40L is unable to bind CD40, and thus B-cells overproduce IgM
- ↑ IgM, IgD; undetectable IgG, E, A
- **Oral ulcers** and therapy resistant **warts** are classic
- (Also diarrhea, respiratory infections, otitis)

Thymic Hypoplasia (DiGeorge Syndrome, CATCH-22)

- Deletion in chromosome 22. *TBX1* gene responsible for most findings
- CATCH 22
  - **C**ardiac abnormality (especially Tetralogy of Fallot, also coarctation)
  - **A**bnormal facies (notched, low-set ears, micrognathia, short philtrum and hypertelorism)
  - **T**hymic aplasia
  - **C**left palate

– **H**ypocalcemia (due to parathyroid aplasia)
  – Deletion in chromosome **22**
- Absent cell-mediated immunity
- Recurrent viral and fungal infections

Severe Combined Immunodeficiency (SCID)

- Heterogeneous group of disorders (at least 20) with defects in cell-mediated and humoral immunity
  - **XLR; *IL-2Rγ*** (γ chain IL-2 receptor); M.C. type (45%)
  - AR; *ADA* (Adenosine deaminase deficiency) (2nd M.C., 20%) part of purine salvage pathway
  - AR; *JAK3* (Janus kinase 3)
- Clinical features:
  - Aplastic thymus, **no T cells**
  - SCID is typically categorized into B+ and B- SCID; some forms have normal B and NK cells, some forms have ↓ B and NK cells (tables 13.1 and 13.2)
  - Low immunoglobulins
  - Various cutaneous eruptions:
    - **Maternofetal GVHD**, with engraftment of maternal T cells, presenting as morbilliform eruption
    - Seborrheic dermatitis
    - Infections with *Pseudomonas*, *Staph*, *Candida*
    - AR SCID caused by *ADA* mutation gets **DFSP tumors**
  - **Triad: candidiasis (oropharynx, skin), pneumonia, diarrhea**
  - Without hematopoietic stem cell transplant, death by age 1

Omenn Syndrome

- AR form of SCID with unique phenotype of **erythroderma and alopecia**
- *RAG-1* or *RAG-2* "Recombination Activating Gene" mutation, which normally activates V(D)J recombination of T-cell receptors. Omenn patients therefore have nonfunctional T-cell receptors
- Clinically, Omenn **resembles acute GVHD**, because T-cells are auto-reactive

Table 13.1: B+ SCID

Gene	Inh	Protein Product/ Function	Lymph Profile	Freq
IL2RG	**XLR**	γ chain of IL-2 receptor **M.C. form of SCID**	T- B+ NK-	45%
JAK3	AR	Janus Kinase 3	T- B+ NK-	6%
IL7R	AR	IL-7 receptor	T- B+ NK+	1%
CD45	AR	Leukocyte Common Antigen (LCA)	T- B+ NK+	1%
CD3D	AR	OKT3 δ-chain (T-cell Ag receptor)	T- B+ NK+	1%

Table 13.2: B-SCID

Gene	Inh	Protein Product/ Function	Lymph Profile	Freq
ADA	AR	Adenosine Deaminase	T- B- NK-	20%
Artemis gene (*DCL-RE1C*)	AR		T- B- NK+	15%
RAG1 *RAG2*	AR	**Omenn Syndrome** Recombination Activating Gene; Activates V(D)J recombination	T- B- NK+ T- B- NK+	15%

Wiskott-Aldrich Syndrome

- **XLR**; *WAS* defect, encoding the WASp protein involved in **actin cytoskeleton** of hematopoietic cells; important in high affinity IgE receptor
- Classic triad: bleeding, **eczema**, recurrent infection
  - Presents first as a bleeding problem. Petechiae = earliest sign
  - **Pyoderma/otitis media** and other infections with encapsulated organisms
- **Lymphoma** in 20%, esp NHL
- Intrinsic platelet abnormality resulting in TTP with HSM
- Labs:
  - ↑ IgA, IgD, IgE, ↓ **IgM**
  - T cells progressively decline in # and activity
- Management: splenectomy
- Prognosis: death by age 6 from infection; otherwise hemorrhage or lymphoreticular malignancies

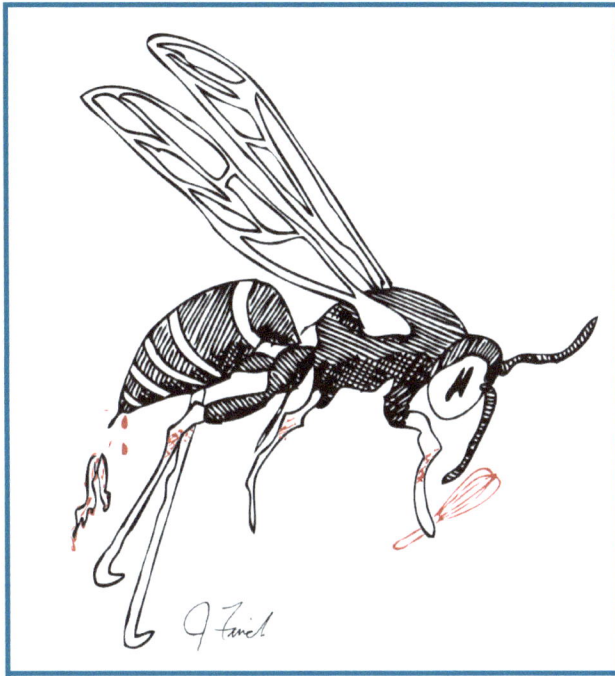

Wiskott-Aldrich Syndrome

Picture a wasp (*WASP* protein) with bloody diarrhea and eczema, holding a whisk (Wiskott-Aldrich)

On board exam kodachromes, Eczema + Petechiae = Wiskott-Aldrich

Hyper IgE Syndrome (Job Syndrome)

- **AD; *STAT3* mutation**
- **AR; *DOCK8* mutation (dedicator of cytokinesis 8)**
  - **AR form gets severe viral infections (especially eczema herpeticum, molluscum, HPV), SCCs and autoimmune diseases**
- AR; *TYK2* mutation (tyrosine kinase 2) → **atypical mycobacterial infections**
- AR; *PGM3* mutation (rare) → leukocytoclastic vasculitis and neuro anomalies (esp low IQ and ataxia)
- Skin findings:
  - Eczematous dermatitis
  - Sometimes get PPK
  - Ichthyosis, urticaria, asthma
  - Retention of primary teeth (presents as double row of teeth), no secondary teeth
  - **Hands/feet resemble ACD**
  - Coarse facies, scoliosis, high arched palate

- Infections
  - **Cold abscesses** (pyogenic infections)
  - Lung infections
  - Chronic mucocutaneous candidiasis
- Labs:
  - **Eosinophilia**, ↑↑ **IgE** (>2000), ↑ IgD and IgE to *Staph.* IgE normalized by adulthood
  - Impaired chemotaxis of PMNs and monocytes
  - ↑ TGF-β and IFN-γ
  - ↓ IL-6 and IL-10
  - AR form: ↓ IL-12
  - AD form: ↓ IL-17 and IL-22
- Tx: anti-staph antibiotics, IFNγ, γ-globulin, cimetidine (immune regulation)
  - DOCK8 Deficiency: hematopoietic stem cell transplant

IL 12/23 Deficiency

- Mutations in p40 subunit of IL-12 and IL-23 (*IL12β* gene) or its receptor (*IL12Rβ* gene)
  - Note: same molecule targeted by ustekinumab
- Disseminated *Salmonella* and *Bacille Calmette-Guérin (BCG)* infection

Table 13.3: Genoderms with Extensive Warts
EDV
WHIM
SCID
CVID
Wiskott-Aldrich
GATA2 Deficiency (MonoMAC, Emberger, WILD Syndrome)
Hyper IgE (DOCK8 deficiency)
Hyper IgM (XHIM)
Netherton
Costello Syndrome (nasolabial warts)

Table 13.4: Genoderms with High IgE
Hyper IgE Syndrome
Wiskott-Aldrich
Netherton
Omenn
DiGeorge
IRAK-4 Deficiency

Ataxia-Telangiectasia (Louis-Bar Syndrome)

- Severe immunodeficiency, both humoral and cell-mediated
- See page 97 (Disorders of Malignant Potential)

Chronic Granulomatous Disease

- Caused by defects in the four subunits of phagocyte **NADPH oxidase**, resulting in inability to produce respiratory burst needed to kill catalase positive organisms after phagocytosis
  - **XLR;** mutations in *CYBB* (cytochrome subunit)
    - M.C. mutation (70%) and most severe phenotype
    - **Female carriers have discoid lupus, aphthous stomatitis and infections**
  - AR mutations in *CYBA* (cytochrome subunit), *NCF-1* and *-2* (neutrophil cytosol factor)
- Clinical:
  - Recurrent pyoderma (*S. aureus*), periorificial dermatitis, ulcerative stomatitis, gingivitis, suppurative lymphadenopathy (cervical M.C.) with abscesses and fistulas (perianal M.C.)
  - Pneumonia with empyema, cavitations (Aspergillosis)
  - Hepatosplenomegaly with granulomas, abscesses, chronic diarrhea (nonbloody)
  - Osteomyelitis (**Serratia marcescens** M.C.)
- Dx: **nitroblue tetrazolium** reduction assay
  - Normal leukocytes reduce the dye, causing yellow → blue color change
  - Abnormal leukocytes cannot reduce dye
- Normal life span but poor quality

Think "Catalase (+) organisms make SPACE in the SKY" to remember the infections in Chronic Granulomatous Disease

Staph, **S**erratia
Pseudomonas
Aspergillus
Candida
Enterobacter
Shigella, **S**almonella
Klebsiella
Yersinia

Leukocyte Adhesion Deficiency

- Three disorders affecting ability of PMNs, monocytes, and lymphocytes to adhere to vascular endothelium (and then migrate into tissues)

- Shared features
  - Gingivitis and periodontitis
  - Poor wound healing; **delayed separation of umbilical stump**
  - Pyoderma-like necrotic ulcers
  - Life-threatening bacterial and fungal infections
  - Marked peripheral neutrophilia (10x normal)
- Leukocyte Adhesion Deficiency 1
  - AR; *ITGB2* mutation, encoding β2 integrin subunit of LFA-1, CR-3, and p150
  - Most severe, death by age 5
- Leukocyte Adhesion Deficiency 2
  - *SLC35C1 (FUCT1)* mutation, encoding Sialyl-Lewis X ligand of E selectin on vascular endothelium
  - Mental retardation, dysmorphic facies, "Bombay" RBCs (lacking H antigen)
- Leukocyte Adhesion Deficiency 3
  - *RASGRP2* mutation, encoding RAS guanyl releasing protein 2 (defective integrin activation)
  - Bleeding

Chronic Mucocutaneous Candidiasis

- Can be seen in a broad group of disorders; not a single disease. E.g. DiGeorge, SCID, APECED, IPEX, Hyper IgE
- Most represent a **T-cell deficiency**
- Severe *Candida* infections of skin, mouth, nails

Leiner's Disease

- Mutation in *C5* gene, leading to complement deficiency
- **Severe seborrheic dermatitis** (often erythrodermic)
- Recurrent infections, diarrhea, failure to thrive
- Presents in first few months of life
- **Hereditary deficiency of any of the terminal complement components C5-C9 results in susceptibility to meningococcal meningitis**

Think "DISC" to remember the findings in Leiner's Disease

Diarrhea and wasting
Infection
Seborrheic Dermatitis
C5 dysfunction

Hereditary Angioedema

- AD mutation in C1-inh gene (*SERPING1*), resulting in **C1 esterase inhibitor (C1-INH) deficiency**
- Recurrent attacks involving the skin, subcutaneous tissue, upper respiratory tract, or GI tissue
- Lasts 2-3 days, followed by refractory period
- Type I (HAE-1) (85%)
  - **Low or no C1-INH**, allowing C2 and C4 cleavage to perpetuate unchecked
  - C1-INH, C2, and C4 levels are low
  - C4 levels are low during an attack; they may be normal in between attacks
  - C1q normal
- Type II (HAE-2) (15%)
  - **High levels of nonfunctional C1-inh**
- Estrogen-dependent HAE (formerly HAE-3)
  - **AD** mutation in **Factor XII** (*F12* gene)
    - Transcription regulated by estrogen, so mainly affects women
  - Normal complement levels
  - Normal function and levels of C1-inh
  - Exacerbated by pregnancy or OCPs
- Treatment of HAE
  - Tx of choice: **stanozolol or danazol** (anabolic steroids)
  - Prophylaxis with aminocaproic or tranexamic acid (antifibrinolytics)
  - **High-dose C1-inh concentrate** or **FFP** for acute attacks
  - rhC1INH for HAE-1-Recombinant human C1 esterase inhibitor
  - Poor response to antihistamines, epinephrine or steroids

Properdin Deficiency

- **XLR**; mutation in properdin (*PFC* gene), a molecule that stabilizes C3 convertase in the alternative complement pathway
- Susceptibility to **fulminant meningococcal infection**

APECED (Autoimmune Polyendocrinopathy)

- AR; *AIRE* gene (autoimmune regulator gene, responsible for deletion of auto-reactive T cells)
  - Or rarely, AD mutation associated with hypothyroidism

- **A**utoimmune **P**oly**E**ndocrinopathy (APE), **C**andidiasis (C), and **E**ctodermal **D**ystrophy (ED)
- Ectodermal dystrophy in APECED is tooth enamel hypoplasia
- Endocrine: **hypoparathyroidism** (90%), **Addison's Disease** (60%), hypogonadism (45%), hypothyroid (15%)
- **Autoimmune skin conditions** (alopecia areata, vitiligo)
- **Chronic mucocutaneous candidiasis**

GATA2 Deficiency

- AD; *GATA2* mutation
- Encompasses five related syndromes with much phenotypic overlap:
  - MonoMAC, DCML Deficiency, Emberger Syndrome have skin findings
  - Familial Myelodysplastic Syndrome has few skin manifestations
  - **WILD Syndrome** [**W**arts (disseminated), **I**mmunodeficiency, primary **L**ymphedema, anogenital **D**ysplasia]
- ↓↓ dendritic cell, monocyte, B cell, NK cell
- Disseminated non-TB mycobacterial infection, **extensive HPV**
- Erythema nodosum in 1/3
- Lymphedema
- Myelodysplasia or AML in 70%

WHIM Syndrome

- AD; GOF mutation in *CXCR4* chemokine receptor gene or *GRK3* (*ADRBK2*) β-adrenergic receptor kinase
- **W**arts, **H**ypogammaglobulinemia, **I**nfections, **M**yelokathexis
- **Myelokathexis** = inability of PMNs to exit bone marrow (causing neutropenia)
- Tx: **plerixafor** blocks *CXCR4* signaling → ↑ cell counts and ↓ infxn

PLAID Syndrome

- AD; *PLCγ2* (PLCγ2-associated **A**ntibody **D**eficiency and **I**mmune **D**ysregulation)
- Cold urticaria, inflammatory lesions on fingers, toes, nose
- Recurrent infections, granulomas

IPEX Syndrome

- **XLR**; *FOXP3* mutation, a key gene in development of T-regulatory cells. Mutation leads to immune dysregulation and $\downarrow \downarrow$ T$_{reg}$
- **I**mmune dysregulation, **P**olyendocrinopathy, **E**nteropathy, **X**-linked
- Eczema, chronic mucocutaneous candidiasis, diarrhea, diabetes, hemolytic anemia
- $\uparrow \uparrow$ IgE, eosinophilia

Mammalian Sterile 20-Like Kinase 1 Deficiency

- AR; *MST1* (*STK4*) mutation
  - *MST1* is a regulator of *FOXP3*, so patients get autoimmune phenomena like IPEX Syndrome
- Mucocutaneous candidiasis, bacterial and viral infections
- Heart malformations

Disorders with Hypopigmentation and Immunodeficiency

Chédiak-Higashi Syndrome

- See p. 80 (Hypopigmentation)

Griscelli Syndrome, Type 2

- See p. 80 (Hypopigmentation)

p14 Deficiency

- See p. 80 (Hypopigmentation)

Hermansky-Pudlak, Type 2

- See p. 79 (Hypopigmentation)

Other Immunodeficiency Disorders

Cartilage-Hair Hypoplasia

- See p. 68
- Short-limbed dwarfism with immunodeficiency and granulomatous skin inflammation

Ataxia-Telangiectasia (Louis-Bar Syndrome)

- See p. 92

Down Syndrome

- See p. 118

Papillon-Lefèvre Syndrome

- See p. 16

Dyskeratosis Congenita (Zinsser-Engman-Cole)

- See p. 84

Secondary Immunodeficiency

- EB
- Infantile Systemic Hyalinosis (ISH)

J. Finch & M. Payette

Table 13.5: Workup of Suspected Primary Immunodeficiency		
Test	Disease	Test Result
Quantitative Immunoglobulins	Wiskott-Aldrich Syndrome	↑ IgA, IgD, IgE, ↓ **IgM**
	Hyperimmunoglobulin-E Syndrome	↑↑ IgE (>2000), ↑ IgD and IgE to Staph
	X-linked Hypogammaglobulinemia	Absence of IgM, A, D, and E
	Common Variable Immunodeficiency	Low levels of most immunoglobulin classes
	Hypogammaglobulinemia with Hyper-IgM Syndrome	↑ IgM, IgD; undetectable IgG, E, A
	IgM Deficiency	↓ IgM and IgD, ↑ PMNs, IgA, IgG, IgE
CBC with diff	Wiskott-Aldrich Syndrome	Thrombocytopenia
	Leukocyte Adhesion Deficiency	Neutrophilia
Examination of peripheral smear	Chédiak-Higashi Syndrome	Abnormal large granules within PMNs
Hair shaft examination	Chédiak-Higashi Syndrome	Large clumps of melanin
Nitroblue tetrazolium reduction assay	Chronic Granulomatous Disease	Normal leukocytes reduce the dye, causing yellow → blue color change. Abnormal WBC's cannot reduce dye
Flow cytometry for B and T cells	SCID	No T cells. B cells vary depending on subtype of SCID

14. Disorders of Malignant Potential

BCC Syndromes

Basal Cell Nevus Syndrome (Gorlin Syndrome)

- AD; mutation in **PTCH1** *(patched 1)* tumor suppressor gene, but 50% are new mutations
- Pathogenesis:
  - PTCH1 encodes a transmembrane protein in the sonic hedgehog pathway
  - ↓patched → ↑ smoothened → uncontrolled cell proliferation through Gli 1-3 transcription factors (important in controlling cell fate, patterning and growth) (fig 14.1)
- Key features:
  - Skin: epidermoid cysts, milia, BCCs, **palmoplantar pits**
  - Skeletal: **odontogenic jaw cysts** (pain, swelling and drainage; radiolucent); **frontal bossing**, bifid ribs, vertebral fusion, kyphoscoliosis
  - CNS: agenesis of the corpus callosum, **calcified falx**, medulloblastoma, meningioma, MR (uncommon)
  - Eyes: congenital blindness, cataracts, colobomas, strabismus, hypertelorism
  - Genitourinary: ovarian fibromas (fibrosarcomas); cardiac fibromas
- >65% frequency
  - Odontogenic keratocysts
  - Calcified falx cerebri
  - Macrocephaly, frontal bossing, hypertelorism
  - Palmar/plantar pits
- 50% or greater frequency
  - Multiple BCCs
  - Facial milia
  - Cutaneous epidermoid cysts
  - High-arched palate
  - Rib anomalies (e.g. bifid, splayed or fused)
  - Hemi- or fused vertebrae
  - Calcified diaphragma sellae
  - Hyperpneumatization of paranasal sinuses
- < 50% frequency
  - Ventricular asymmetry (CNS)
  - Calcified tentorium cerebelli
  - Short fourth metacarpals, poly- or syndactyly
  - Flame-shaped lucencies of hand bones
  - Kyphoscoliosis
  - Spina bifida occulta (cervical, thoracic vertebrae)
  - Narrow sloping shoulders
  - Pectus excavatum or carinatum
  - Prognathism
  - Cleft lip/palate
  - Strabismus
  - Hamartomas (e.g. retinal)
  - Medulloblastomas
  - Meningiomas
  - Calcified ovarian fibromas
  - Cardiac fibromas
  - Generalized overgrowth
- Tx:
  - Avoid radiation therapy
  - Sun avoidance, proper use of sunscreens, and regular skin exams starting as a child
  - Annual dental panoramic x-ray (odontogenic cysts)
  - Annual MRI until age 8 (medulloblastoma)
  - Excise odontogenic keratocysts due to potential for aggressive nature

> **Gorlin Syndrome**
>
> Picture Al Gore (Gorlin) with a patch over his eye (PTCH gene), frontal bossing, lots of BCCs, palmoplantar pits, and jaw cysts, and a calcified falx

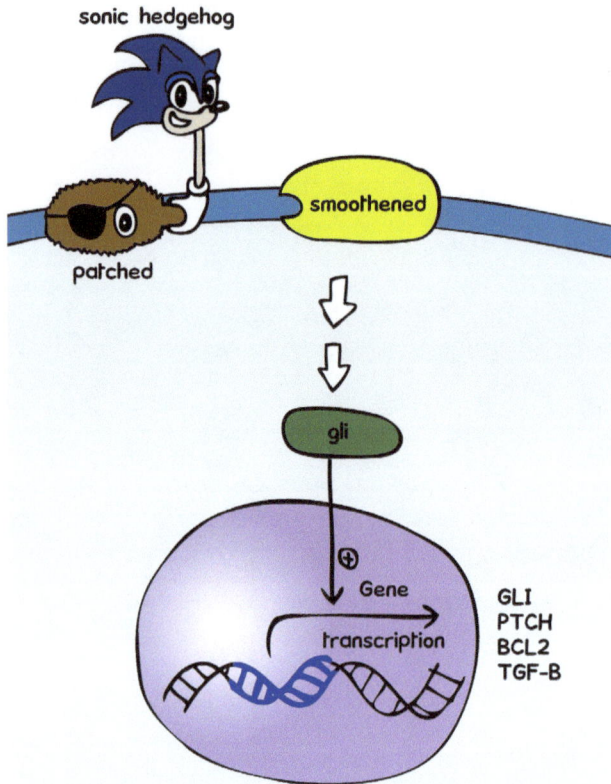

a) Normal Function of Sonic Hedgehog is to Bind Patched, Allowing Activation of Smoothened

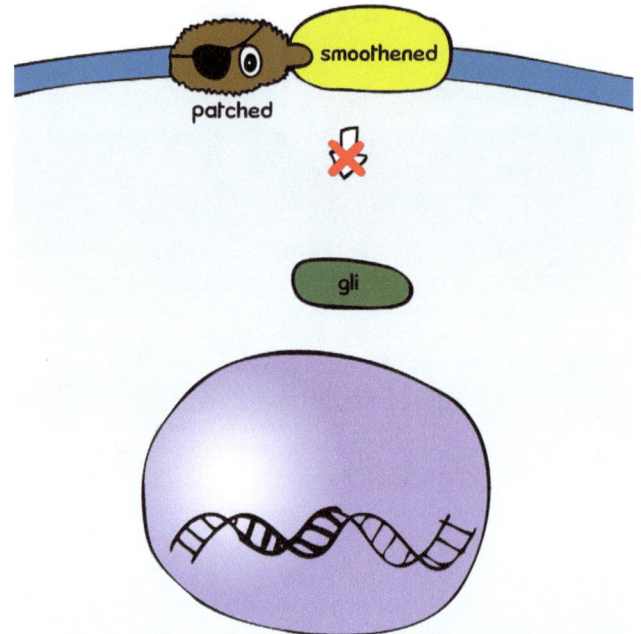

b) Patched Binds Smoothened, Inhibiting Signal Transduction

Figure 14.1: Sonic Hedgehog Pathway

Bazex Syndrome (Bazex-Dupré-Christol)

- **XLD**; unknown gene
- Key features – very similar to Rombo:
  - **BCCs**
  - **Follicular atrophoderma** (dorsal hands/ feet, extensor surfaces, face), ulerythema ophryogenes (fig 14.2), spiny hyperkeratosis
  - **Hypotrichosis**, pili torti
  - **Hypohidrosis** of face, facial hyperpigmentation, milia
  - Multiple genital trichoepitheliomas, scrotal tongue
- NOTE: do not confuse with Acrokeratosis Paraneoplastica of Bazex
  - Psoriasiform plaques on acral skin and helices, psoriatic nails
  - SCCs of upper aerodigestive tract

Basaloid Follicular Hamartoma Syndrome

- AD; mutation in *PTCH1* (allelic with Basal Cell Nevus Syndrome)

Rombo Syndrome

- AD; unknown gene
- Key features:
  - Multiple BCCs, trichoepitheliomas, atrophoderma vermiculatum, hypotrichosis, cyanosis of the hands and feet, milia, telangiectasia
  - No hypohidrosis (vs Bazex)

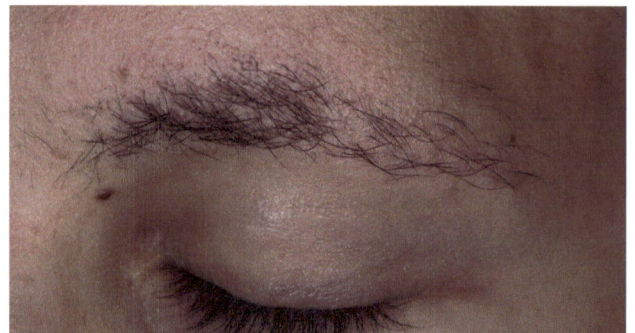

Figure 14.2: Ulerythema Ophryogenes

J. Finch & M. Payette

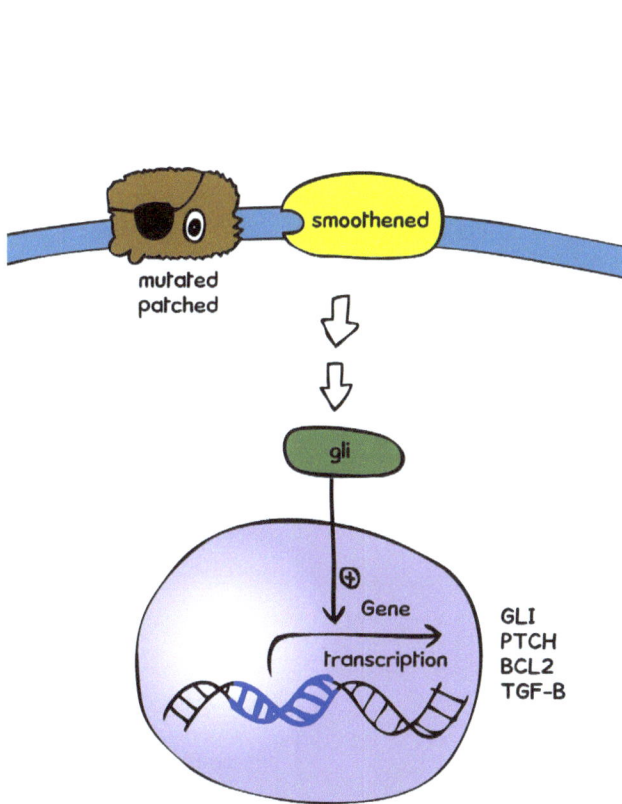

c) Mutated Patched Can't Bind Smoothened, Resulting in Ongoing Activation of Pathway

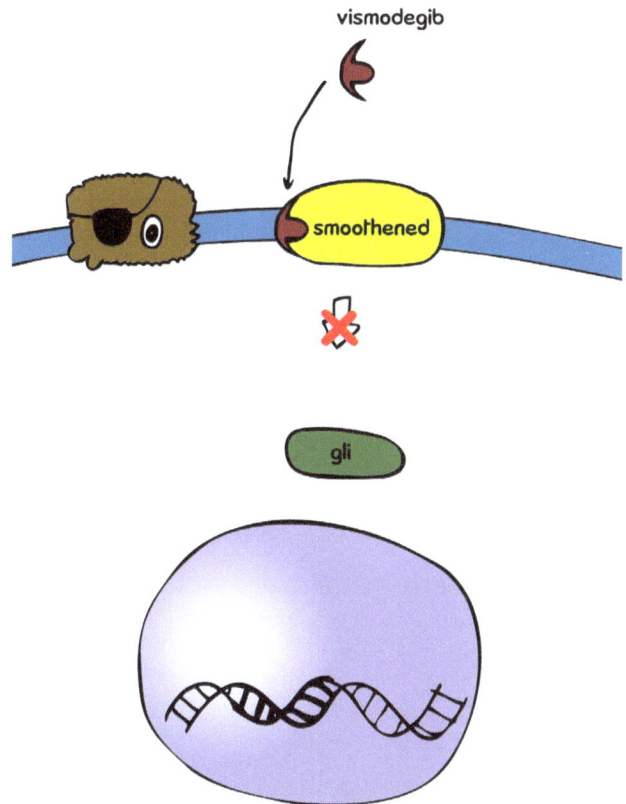

d) Vismodegib Binds and Inhibits Smoothened (Note: Mutated Patched Has Frontal Bossing and Jaw Cysts)

Figure 14.1: Sonic Hedgehog Pathway

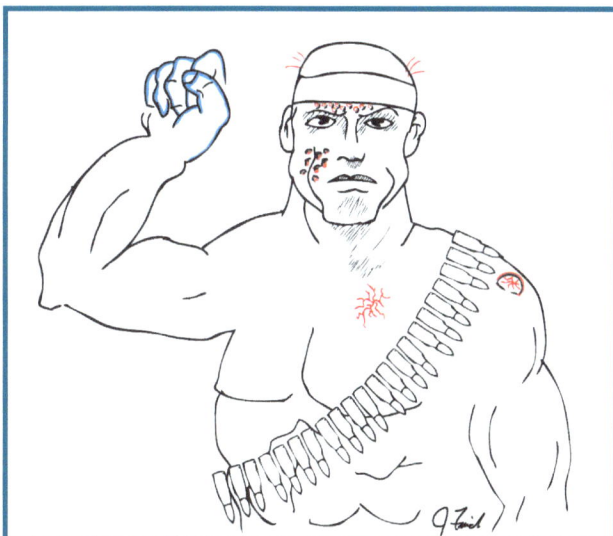

Rombo Syndrome

Picture Rambo with hypotrichosis, telangiectasias on his chest, BCCs, and atrophoderma vermiculatum. Rambo is sweaty (euhidrotic, vs Bazex is hypohidrotic)

Keratoacanthoma Syndromes

Muir-Torre Syndrome

- Variant of Hereditary Non-Polyposis Colorectal Cancer (Lynch Syndrome) caused by AD mutation in *MSH-2* (86%), *MLH-1* (11%) *MSH-6* (3%)
  - DNA mismatch repair genes
- Presents in 4th-5th decade with internal malignancies, but usually not diagnosed until skin lesions present >10 yrs later
- Key features:
  - Skin – multiple **sebaceous gland tumors** (M.C. = **sebaceous adenomas**; also hyperplasia, BCC with sebaceous differentiation, KAs)
  - Malignancies – proximal colon cancer (M.C.), other GI, other GU, lung, breast, hematologic malignancies
- Management: biopsy of sebaceous adenoma → consult genetics, GI, and Internist

Ferguson-Smith

- AD; loss-of-function mutation in *TGFβR1*
- Multiple eruptive **self-healing KAs** beginning in **childhood**

Grzybowski Syndrome

- Eruptive KAs in **adulthood** (not a genoderm, but included with other KA syndromes for completeness)

Other Tumor Syndromes

Birt-Hogg-Dubé

- AD mutation in *FLCN* gene encoding folliculin
- Key features:
  - Skin – trichodiscomas, fibrofolliculomas, skin tags
    - Less commonly, multiple facial angiofibromas
  - Kidney – RCC (bilateral), renal cysts
  - Lung – spontaneous pneumothoraces

Gardner Syndrome

- AD; mutation in *APC* gene (Adenomatous Polyposis Coli)
- Pathogenesis – Tumor suppressor gene regulating β-catenin, an adherens junction protein controlling cell growth
- Key features:
  - Skin – EICs (scalp, toe, and shin)
    - **Pilomatricomas**
  - Musculoskeletal – osteomas (jaw)
  - GI – colorectal polyposis with 100% transformation to adenocarcinoma
  - Eyes – congenital hypertrophy of retinal pigment epithelium (CHRPE)
  - Teeth – odontomas, supernumerary teeth
- Tx:
  - Radiographic survey of the facial skeleton
  - Colonoscopy and barium studies (or videocapsule photography) of the small intestine
  - Prophylactic colectomy

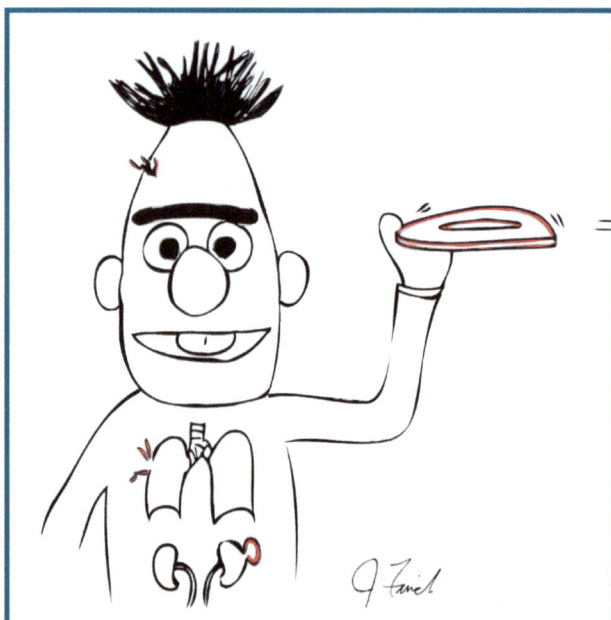

Birt-Hogg-Dubé Syndrome

Picture a puppet catching a disc (trichodiscomas), with fibers coming out of his forehead (fibrofolliculomas). He has a pneumothorax and renal cell carcinoma

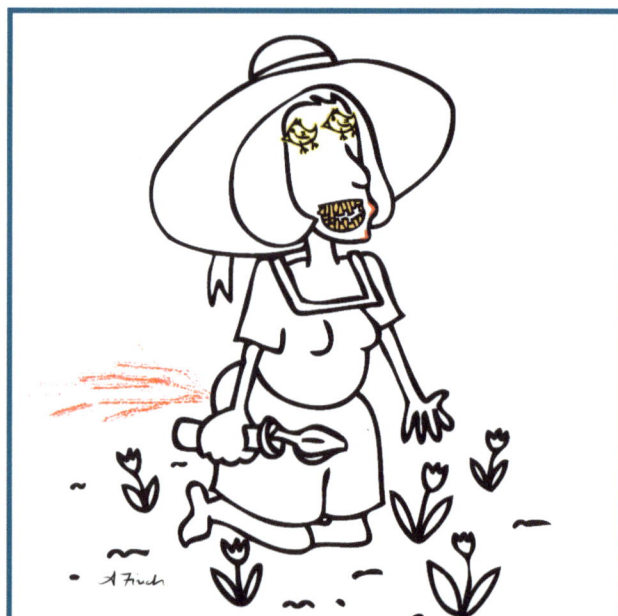

Gardner Syndrome

Picture a gardener with bumps on her face (epidermoid cysts, pilomatricomas, osteomas, birds for eyes (CHRPE), supernumerary teeth, and pooping blood (GI adenocarcinoma)

Think "Birds CHRP in the Garden"

J. Finch & M. Payette

Peutz-Jeghers Syndrome

- AD; mutation in serine/threonine kinase-11, *STK11*
- Pathogenesis – tumor suppressor gene likely involved in cell cycle progression
- Key features:
  - Skin – periorificial lentiginosis (100%, first sign) (fig 14.3), also on digits, palms, nails, soles, and any mucosal surface
  - GI – hamartomatous polyps (only in 13%) small intestine > large intestine, GI bleeding, anemia, intussusception, obstruction
  - Neoplasm – breast, GI (40% by age 40s), ovarian, pancreas

> **Think "Bopped in the Spotted Tongue and Kisser"**
> **BOP = Breast, Ovarian, Pancreas cancers**
> **STK = Spotted Tongue and Kisser**

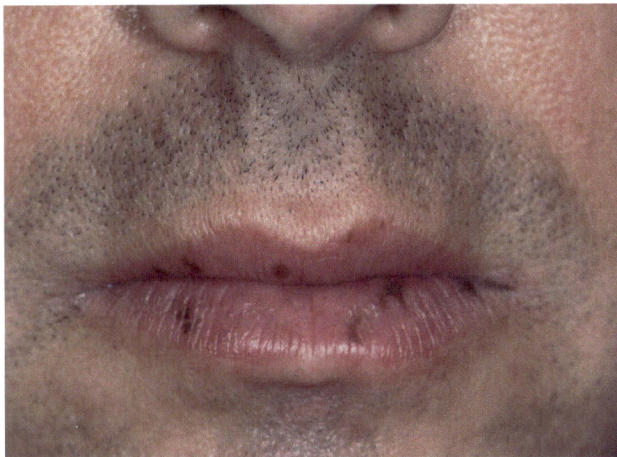

Figure 14.3: Oral Lentigines in Peutz-Jeghers Syndrome

Ataxia-Telangiectasia (Louis-Bar Syndrome)

- AR; mutation in **ATM** (ataxia-telangiectasia mutated) gene
  - Encodes phosphatidylinositol-3-like kinase; regulates cell cycle, DNA repair, p53
- **Truncal ataxia (1st sign) in infancy.** Wheelchair-bound by teenage years
- Telangiectasias: **ocular telangiectasias first** (age 2-5), then sun-exposed skin
- **Severe immunodeficiency**, both humoral and cell-mediated
  - Chronic sinopulmonary infections. ↓ IgE, IgG, IgA
- Hematologic malignancies, T-cell > B-cell

- Malignancy rate 1200x
- Even carriers at high risk (Female carriers get breast Ca)
- **Death from bronchiectasis** (55%) or malignancy (15%)
- Labs: ↑ αFP

> *Think "CAMP TICCI" to remember the findings in Ataxia-Telangiectasia*
>
> **C**erebellar ataxia
> **A**D
> **M**ental retardation
> **P**ulmonary infections/progeria
>
> **T**elangiectasia
> **I**nfancy
> **C**ancer (esp. lymphoma)
> **C**afé-au-lait spots/conjunctival erythema
> **I**gA deficiency

Epidermodysplasia Verruciformis

- AR; mutation in *EVER1* or *EVER2* (*TMC6* or *TCM8*)
  - Encode endoplasmic reticulum transmembrane proteins
  - EDV-like phenotype also seen with homozygous *RHOH, MST-1, COR1A*, and *IL-7* mutations
- Results in ↑ susceptibility to **HPV 5 and 8**
- Widespread warts (fig 14.4), AKs by age 30, SCCs in >50% patients
- Path: keratinocytes have characteristic blue-grey pallor (fig 14.5)

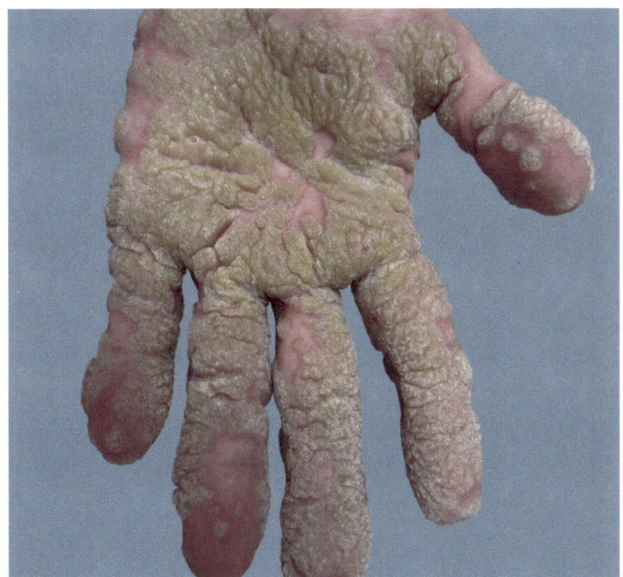

Figure 14.4: Innumerable Warts in Epidermodysplasia Verruciformis (image courtesy of Steven Brett Sloan, MD)

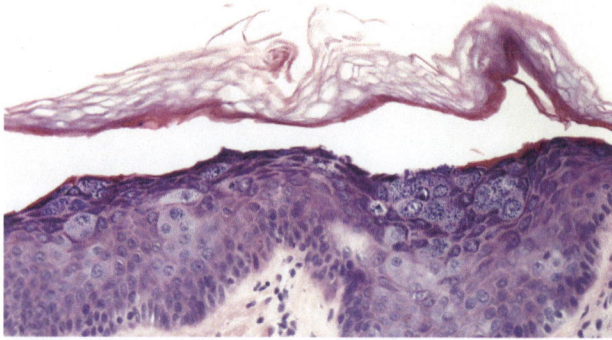

Figure 14.5: Epidermodysplasia Verruciformis (40x)

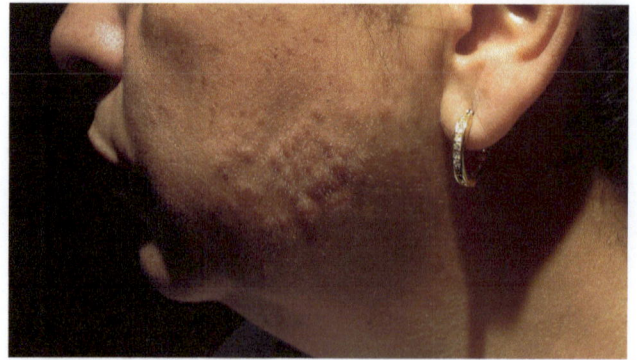

Figure 14.6: Cutaneous Leiomyomas in Reed Syndrome

Familial Atypical Mole-Malignant Melanoma Syndrome (FAMMM, Dysplastic Nevus Syndrome)

- AD; *CDKN2A* mutation
  - *CDKN2A* (9p21) encodes both p16 and p14 (in an alternate reading frame). Both regulate cell cycle progression proteins
  - p16 is a tumor suppressor gene in **retinoblastoma (Rb) pathway**. Normally inhibits CDK2 and 4, thereby arresting G_1 to S transition of the cell cycle
  - $p14^{ARF}$ is a tumor suppressor in the **p53 pathway**. Normally inhibits MDM2, thereby promoting p53-induced cell cycle arrest and apoptosis
- **Melanoma** (60-80%)
- **Pancreatic cancer** (17%)

Hereditary Leiomyomatosis and Renal Cell Cancer (Reed Syndrome)

- AD; **fumarate hydratase** deficiency (*FH*)
- Multiple cutaneous and uterine leiomyomas (fig 14.6)
  - Both are painful
  - Onset in late 20s; usually hysterectomy in early 30s
- **Renal cell cancer**
- Tx:
  - Calcium channel blockers to ↓ pain associated with smooth muscle spasm
  - Annual contrast MRI of kidneys beginning age 10

Multiple Endocrine Neoplasia

MEN 1 (Wermer)

- AD; mutation in *MEN1* gene; encodes menin protein
- Key features:
  - Skin – angiofibromas, collagenomas, CALMs, lipomas, hypopigmented macules, gingival macules
  - Neoplasia – parathyroid, pancreatic, and pituitary

MEN 2A (Sipple Syndrome)

- AD; mutation in *RET* proto-oncogene
- Key features:
  - Skin – **lichen and macular amyloidosis**
  - Neoplasia:
    - Parathyroid
    - Pheochromocytoma, medullary thyroid carcinoma (shared with MEN2B)

MEN 2B (Multiple Mucosal Neuromas)

- AD; mutation in *RET* proto-oncogene
- **Multiple mucosal neuromas** (100%)
  - Asymptomatic, soft, papules of the lips and tongue
  - Earliest finding (1st decade), often presents to dermatologist!
- **Medullary thyroid carcinoma** (> 90%)
  - 1st or 2nd decade of life
  - 75% have metastases at the time of diagnosis
- **Marfanoid** habitus
- GI ganglioneuromatosis
- Pheochromocytoma

Table 14.1: Comparison of Multiple Endocrine Neoplasias

MEN 1 (Wermer Syndrome)	MEN 2A (Sipple Syndrome)	MEN 2B
Parathyroid hyperplasia/ adenoma	Parathyroid hyperplasia/ adenoma	
	Medullary thyroid carcinoma	Medullary thyroid carcinoma
	Pheochromocytoma	Pheochromocytoma
Pancreatic islet cell tumors		
Pituitary gland tumors		Multiple mucosal neuromas

PTEN Hamartoma Tumor Syndromes (PHTS) and Other Overgrowth Syndromes

- Spectrum of clinical syndromes that share features including hamartomatous polyps of the gastrointestinal tract, vascular mucocutaneous lesions, and increased risk of developing neoplasms (fig 14.7)
- Includes
  - Cowden
  - SOLAMEN (Type 2 segmental Cowden)
  - Proteus
  - Bannayan-Riley-Ruvalcaba
  - CLOVE
    - Caused by mutation upstream of PTEN

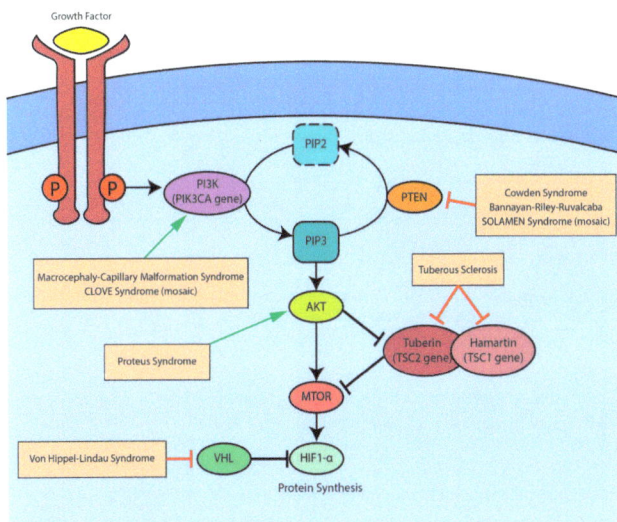

Figure 14.7: PTEN Hamartoma Tumor Syndromes and Overgrowth Syndromes

Cowden Syndrome

- AD; mutation in **PTEN** gene (phosphatase and tensin homologue)
- Pathogenesis – tumor suppressor gene encoding a tyrosine phosphatase. Mutation leads to epidermal, GI, mucosal, thyroid and breast tissue adenomas
- Key features – benign facial hamartomas, **breast (#1) and thyroid (#2) cancer**
  - Skin – **trichilemmomas**, oral papillomas (cobblestone tongue), sclerotic fibromas (aka storiform collagenoma), acral keratotic papules of the dorsal hands, punctate keratoses of the palms, lipomas and angiomas
  - Breast – Fibrocystic Disease, fibroadenomas, adenocarcinoma, gynecomastia (males)
  - Thyroid – goiter, adenomas, thyroglossal duct cysts
  - Gastrointestinal – benign hamartomatous polyps
  - GU – ovarian cysts, menstrual irregularities, vaginal hypertrophy
  - Cerebellar gangliocytoma (Lhermitte-Duclos Disease)
  - Craniofacial – adenoid facies, high arched palate
- **SOLAMEN Syndrome** = Type 2 segmental Cowden (Mosaic *PTEN* mutation)
  - **S**egmental **O**vergrowth, **L**ipomatosis, **A**V**M**, **E**pidermal **N**evus
  - Clinically very similar to Proteus Syndrome

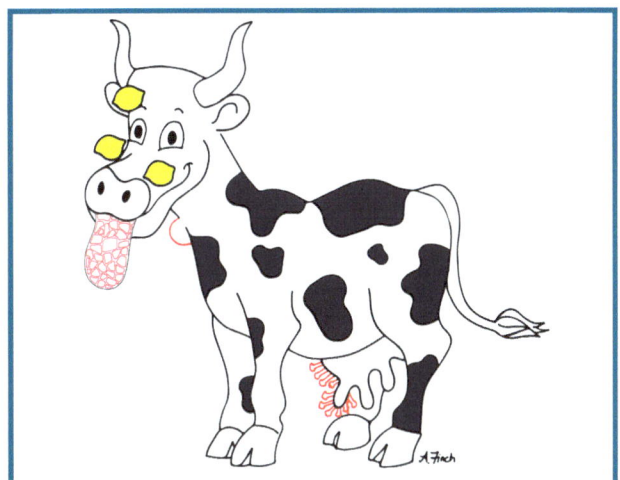

Cowden Syndrome

Picture a cow with lemons on its face (trichilemmomas), cobblestone tongue (oral papillomas), goiter (duct cysts, follicular adenocarcinoma), big boobs (breast fibroadenomas, adenocarcinoma), benign ovarian and GI polyps (especially colon), and 10 penises (PTEN) Think <u>cow</u>den's get trichile<u>moo</u>mas

Proteus Syndrome

- Tissue **overgrowth syndrome** caused by sporadic *AKT1* mutation, part of the PTEN pathway
- Activating mutation in oncogene *AKT1* and *AKT* phosphorylation results in tissue overgrowth and hamartomas
- SQ masses (vascular malformations), lipomas, CMNs, linear epidermal nevi, **cerebriform plantar hyperplasia**, soft tissue/bony hypertrophy

Table 14.2: Genoderms with Colon Polyps
Gardner
Cowden
Familial Polyposis Coli
Peutz-Jeghers
Birt-Hogg-Dubé
Bannayan-Riley-Ruvalcaba

Bannayan-Riley-Ruvalcaba Syndrome

- AD; *PTEN* mutation
- AVM + VM
- Lipomas + hemangiomas + macrocephaly
- Lentigines on penis/vulva
- Shares features with Cowden's: warty papules that histologically are trichilemmomas

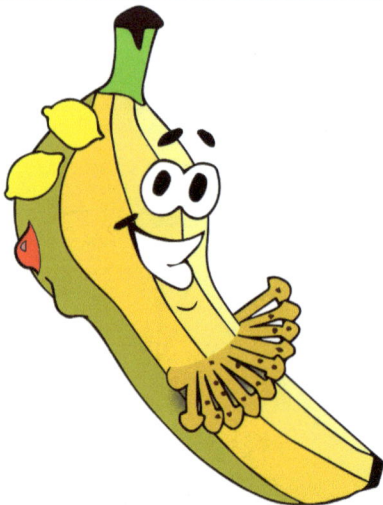

Bannayan-Riley-Ruvalcaba Syndrome

Picture a banana (Bannayan) with brown spots (genital lentigines) on his ten penises (PTEN), macrocephaly trichilemmomas, lipomas, and hemangiomas

CLOVE Syndrome

- **C**ongenital **L**ipomatous **O**vergrowth, **V**ascular malformations, and **E**pidermal nevi
- Caused by somatic mosaicism for postzygotic activating mutations in the *PIK3CA* gene (upstream of PTEN)
- LM + VM + CM +/- AVM + lipomatous overgrowth

Beckwith-Wiedemann Syndrome

- *Epigenetic* overgrowth syndrome caused by abnormalities in imprinting of several genes within 11p15 (*CDKN1C, H19, IGF2,* and *KCNQ1OT1*)
    - 11p15 genes are over-methylated and thus over-activated. By contrast, Russell-Silver (p. 116) is caused by *hypo*-methylation of this same location
- Organomegaly, **macroglossia**, **neonatal hypoglycemia**, omphalocele, **facial capillary malformation**
- Circular depression on rim of posterior helices, linear earlobe crease
- Malignancies: **Wilms' tumor** (nephroblastoma) > hepatoblastoma > adrenocortical CA, rhabdomyosarcoma
- Management
    - Labs: blood glucose, serum alpha-fetoprotein (hepatoblastoma screen)
    - Abdominal and renal U/S every 3 months
- Normal intellect if hypoglycemia is well-controlled; typically large adults leading normal lives

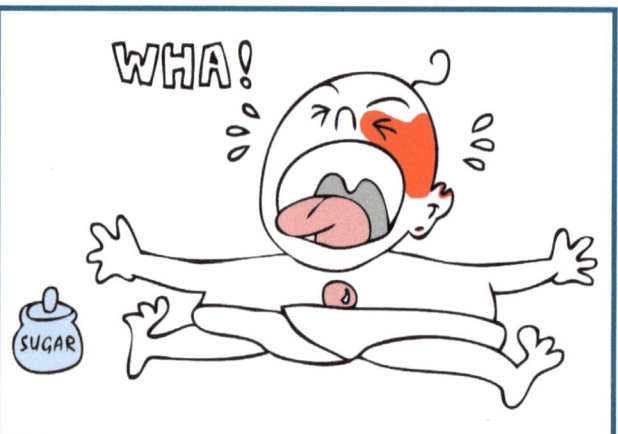

Beckwith-Wiedemann Syndrome

Picture a wide man (Wiedemann) with posterior helical ear pits and earlobe creases crying '**WHA**' (Wilms' > hepatoblastoma > adrenal) from hypoglycemia. The baby has a large tongue (macroglossia), facial PWS, and omphalocele

J. Finch & M. Payette

Porokeratosis

- Group of disorders with AD inheritance
- Keratotic papule or plaque with a thin rim of scale, corresponding to cornoid lamella on pathology (fig 14.8)
- Very low risk of malignant transformation to SCC
- Porokeratosis of Mibelli (Plaque-type)
  - Starts as a small papule that expands centrifugally
  - Predilection for hands, feet, ankles
- Disseminated Superficial Porokeratosis (DSAP)
  - AD; *SART-3* mutation
  - Tiny red-brown porokeratoses in photodistribution
- Linear Porokeratosis
  - Highest risk of malignant transformation
- Porokeratosis Palmaris, Plantaris, et Disseminata
  - Onset in 20's. First on palms, soles, sometimes extending over entire body
  - Initially looks like nevus comedonicus

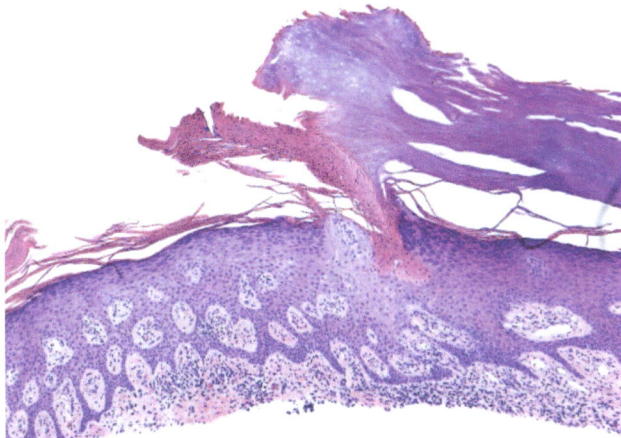

Figure 14.8: Porokeratosis (100x)

Disorders with Cancers, Covered Elsewhere

Huriez Syndrome (sclerotylosis)
- See p. 17 (Palmoplantar keratoderma)

Howel-Evans
- See p. 17 (Palmoplantar keratoderma)

PPK with Cutaneous SCC and Sex Reversal
- See p. 14 (Palmoplantar keratoderma)

Xeroderma Pigmentosum (XP)
- See p. 57 (Genoderms with Photosensitivity)

Rothmund-Thomson Syndrome
- See p. 55 (Genoderms with Photosensitivity)

Bloom Syndrome
- See p. 55

Dyskeratosis Congenita
- See p. 84

Tuberous Sclerosis
- See p. 76

Neurofibromatosis Type I (NF1)
- See p. 111 for full discussion
- AD; mutation of **neurofibromin**; 50% spontaneous mutations
  - Penetrance approaches 100% by age 20
- Need 2 of the following 7 criteria:
  - **Neurofibromas**: 2+ neurofibromas or 1 plexiform neurofibroma (60-90%)
  - **Crowe's sign**: freckling of the groin or axilla (80%)
  - **CALMS**: 6+, > 5mm prepuberty or > 15mm postpuberty (90%)
  - Skeletal abnormalities: sphenoid dysplasia or thinning of cortex of long bones
  - **Lisch nodules** (hamartomas of iris) (90%)
  - **Optic glioma** (15%)
  - **First degree relative with NF** (50%)
- M.C. feature = CALMs (>90%), Lisch nodules (>90%)
- Earliest sign = CALMs

GATA2 Deficiency
- See p. 93 (Immunodeficiency)

Wiskott-Aldrich
- See p. 90 (Immunodeficiency)

Epidermolysis Bullosa
- SCC
- See p. 19

Maffucci's Syndrome
- See p. 61

Table 14.3: Genoderms Associated with Malignancy

Genoderm	Malignancy
Autosomal Dominant	
Bannayan-Riley-Ruvalcaba	No clear risk, but screen same as Cowden
Basal Cell Nevus Syndrome (Gorlin Syndrome)	Skin BCCs, medulloblastoma (10%)
Birt-Hogg-Dubé	Renal cell cancer (12%)
Carney Complex	Myxomas, sertoli testicular cancer
Cowden Syndrome	Breast, thyroid
Ferguson-Smith	Skin keratoacanthoma
Gardner Syndrome	Colorectal
Howel-Evans	Esophagus
Huriez Syndrome (Sclerotylosis)	Skin SCC, bowel adeno
Maffucci	Chondrosarcoma
MEN 1 (Wermer)	Parathyroid, gastrinomas, anterior pituitary
MEN 2a (Sipple Syndrome)	Medullary thyroid carcinoma, pheo, parathyroid
MEN 2b (Multiple Mucosal Neuromas)	Medullary thyroid carcinoma, pheo
Muir-Torre Syndrome	Colorectal
Neurofibromatosis Type I (NF1)	Optic glioma
Peutz-Jeghers Syndrome	Colorectal
Porokeratosis	Skin SCC
Reed Syndrome	Uterine leiomyoma, renal
Rombo Syndrome	Skin BCC
Tuberous Sclerosis	Intracranial tubers, cardiac rhabdo, renal angioleiomyoma
Autosomal Recessive	
Ataxia-Telangiectasia (Louis-Bar Syndrome)	Leukemia/lymphoma, breast (in heterozygotes)
Bloom Syndrome	ALL, lymphoma, GI
Chédiak-Higashi	Lymphocyte-Macrophage Activation Syndrome
Epidermodysplasia Verruciformis	Skin SCC
Fanconi Anemia	AML

Table 14.3: Genoderms Associated with Malignancy

Genoderm	Malignancy
Griscelli	Lymphocyte-Macrophage Activation Syndrome
PPK With Cutaneous SCC and Sex Reversal	Skin SCC, bowel adenocarcinoma (same as Huriez)
Rothmund Thomson Syndrome	Osteogenic sarcoma
Werner Syndrome	Sarcomas (soft tissue, bone), thyroid
Xeroderma Pigmentosum	Ocular, lung, GI
Epidermolysis Bullosa, Dystrophic	Skin SCC
Beckwith-Wiedemann	Wilms', hepatoblastoma
XLD	
Bazex Syndrome (Bazex-Dupré-Christol)	Skin BCC
XLR	
Dyskeratosis Congenita	Mucosal SCC
Wiskott-Aldrich	Lymphoreticular (esp Hodgkin's)
X-Linked Ichthyosis	Testicular (from cryptorchidism)
Misc	
Familial Atypical Mole-Malignant Melanoma Syndrome (FAMMM, Dysplastic Nevus Syndrome)	Melanoma, pancreas

J. Finch & M. Payette

15. Auto-Inflammatory Syndromes

Periodic Fever Syndromes

Periodic fever syndromes encompass eight disorders, including three associated with cryopyrins:

- Cryopyrin-associated periodic syndromes
  - Familial cold autoinflammatory/urticaria syndrome (FCAS)
  - Muckle–Wells
  - CINCA Syndrome (aka NOMID)
- Familial Mediterranean Fever
- Hyper-IgD with Periodic Fever Syndrome
- Tumor Necrosis Factor Receptor Associated Periodic Syndrome (TRAPS)
- PFAPA Syndrome
- DIRA Syndrome

Cryopyrin-Associated Periodic Syndromes (CAPS)

- Continuum of diseases with AD mutations in *NLRP3* (formerly *CIAS1*), which encodes NALP3, a pyrin-like protein
- NALP3 **processes IL-1β** via caspase-1
- All get **urticarial**-like lesions, but are not itchy
- All can get amyloidosis (amyloid A, an acute-phase reactant)
- Path: neutrophilic infiltrates with minimal if any mast cells
- Tx: **IL-1 antagonists**
  - Canakinumab: anti-IL-1β
  - Rilonacept: fusion protein IgG$_1$ + IL-1 receptor
  - Anakinra: recombinant non-glycosylated human IL-1RA (receptor antagonist), from *E. coli*

Familial Cold Autoinflammatory/Urticaria Syndrome (FCAS)

- Urticaria-like eruptions, limb pain, recurrent fever, **amyloidosis**, flares with generalized cold exposure (local ice cube test is NEGATIVE)
- **Normal hearing**

Muckle–Wells

- FCAS + **deafness**
- Compared to FCAS, Muckle-Wells gets more **amyloidosis**, hyperpigmented sclerodermoid lesions, and lacks flares with cold exposure

CINCA Syndrome (NOMID Syndrome)

- **C**hronic **I**nfantile **N**eurological, **C**utaneous, and **A**rticular Syndrome
- **N**eonatal **O**nset **M**ultisystem **I**nflammatory **D**isease
- Triad of **arthritis mutilans**, **urticaria**, and **CNS abnormalities** (HA, seizure)
- May have deafness, visual disturbance, recurrent fever, amyloidosis

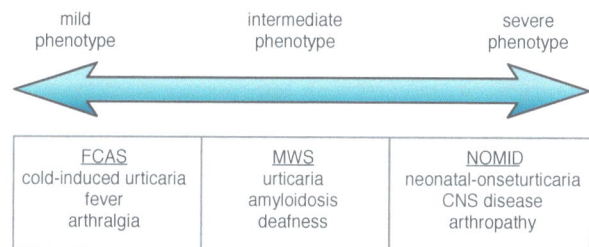

mild phenotype	intermediate phenotype	severe phenotype
FCAS cold-induced urticaria fever arthralgia	MWS urticaria amyloidosis deafness	NOMID neonatal-onseturticaria CNS disease arthropathy

Figure 15.1: Spectrum of Periodic Fever Syndromes

Familial Mediterranean Fever

- AR/AD; mutations in **pyrin** protein (*MEFV*)
- Erysipelas-like erythema particularly on the legs
- Recurrent fever (lasting hours to several days), polyserositis, amyloidosis, and renal failure
- Path: neutrophilic dermatosis

> **Both Familial Mediterranean Fever and Hyper IgD Fever have been associated with Henoch–Schönlein Purpura and Erythema Elevatum Diutinum**

Hyper-IgD with Periodic Fever Syndrome

- AR; mutations in mevalonate kinase (*MVK*), an enzyme involved in cholesterol metabolism
- Recurrent fever (lasting 3-7 days), abdominal pain, diarrhea, HA, arthralgias, cervical LAD
- Small erythematous macules and papules and mevalonic aciduria during attacks
- Path: vasculitis and/or Sjögren's Syndrome-like findings

TRAPS (Familial Hibernian Fever)

- **T**NF **R**eceptor-**A**ssociated **P**eriodic **S**yndrome
- AD; mutation in TNF receptor 1 (*TNFRSF1A*)
- Recurrent fever (lasting 1 to 3 weeks), myalgias with overlying migratory erythema, pleurisy, abdominal pain, conjunctivitis, periorbital edema, **amyloidosis**, renal failure

- Serpiginous, edematous, purpuric, or reticulated lesions on the extremities
  - Histopathology: interstitial and perivascular mononuclear cell infiltrates, vasculitis, and panniculitis

> **TRAPS and MWS are the most common to get amyloidosis (15-25%)**

DIRA Syndrome

- AR; mutation in *IL1RN*, resulting in **D**eficiency in **I**L-1 **R**eceptor **A**ntagonist
- Subcorneal pustules (pustular psoriasis-like rash) + sterile osteitis + recurrent fevers
- Occurs in Puerto Ricans
- Tx: anakinra

DITRA Syndrome

- AR mutation of *IL36RN* (IL-36 receptor antagonist)
- Identical skin findings to DIRA Syndrome, but no osteitis

PFAPA Syndrome

- **P**eriodic **F**evers, **A**phthous stomatitis, **P**haryngitis, and cervical **A**denopathy
- AD; mutation in *PSTPIP1* (allelic with PAPA)
  - Mutated PSTPIP1 binds pyrin protein more strongly
- Usually onset by age 2 and resolves by age 10

CANDLE Syndrome

- AD; mutation in *PSMB8*
- **C**hronic **A**typical **N**eutrophilic **D**ermatitis with **L**ipodystrophy and **E**levated temperature
- Clinical features:
  - Generalized annular erythematous plaques
  - **Progressive lipodystrophy**
  - **Eyelid edema**
  - Arthralgias, periodic fevers

Acne Syndromes

PAPA Syndrome (PASH Syndrome)

- *PSTPIP1* gene (aka *CD2BP1*) – allelic with PFAPA Syndrome (periodic fevers)
- **PAPA = P**yogenic **A**rthritis, **P**yoderma gangrenosum, **A**cne
- **PASH = P**yogenic arthritis, severe **A**cne, **S**uppurative **H**idradenitis

Apert Syndrome

- AD; *FGFR2* mutation (allelic with Beare-Stevenson Cutis Gyrata Syndrome)
- Diffuse acne, treatment-resistant
- Disfiguring synostoses of hands/feet, vertebrae, cranium
- Mosaic *FGFR-2* mutations have been called "Munro's acne nevus" and "nevus comedonicus"

Other Autoinflammatory Syndromes

Blau Syndrome

- AD; mutation in *NOD2/CARD15* gene
- **Sarcoidal granulomas**, granulomatous arthritis, dermatitis and uveitis (fig 15.2)

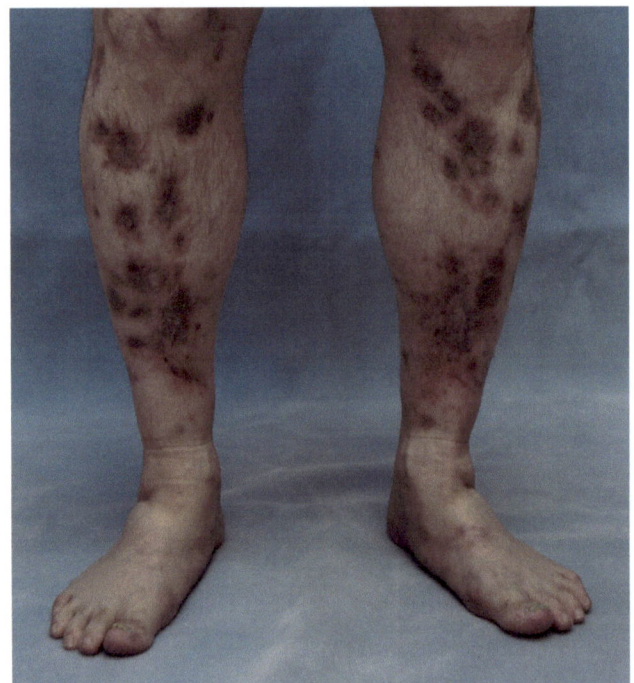

Figure 15.2: Blau Syndrome

Majeed Syndrome

- AR; mutation in Lipin2 (*LPIN2*)
- **Recurrent Sweet's Syndrome** + multifocal osteomyelitis
- Also congenital dyserythropoietic anemia, fever
- Complications:
  - Poor growth and permanent joint contractures
  - Cryptorchidism (80%)
  - Congenital heart defects (35%)

> **Majeed Syndrome**
>
> Picture a middle eastern child holding his head saying "my head, my head!" (Majeed) because he is lightheaded (anemia) and febrile. He has 2 lapel pins (LPIN2). He is surrounded by candy (Sweet's). He has swollen, red joints (osteomyelitis)

Familial Chilblain Lupus

- AD; *TREX1* mutations

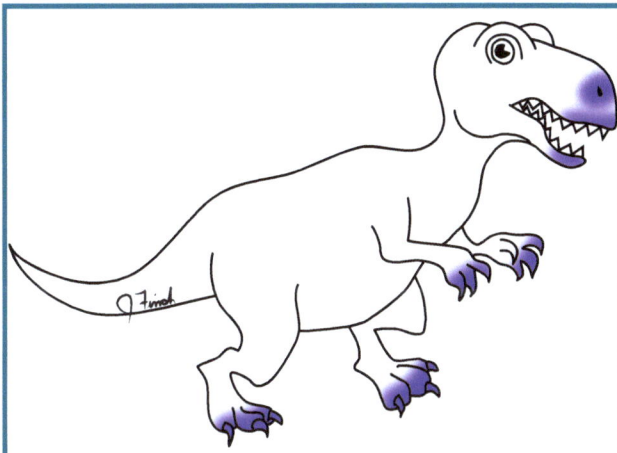

> **Familial Chilblain Lupus**
>
> Picture a tyrannosaurus rex (T-REX) with blue toes

ADA2 Deficiency

- AR; mutation in *ADA2* (adenosine deaminase)
- Causes childhood-onset **polyarteritis nodosa** and some cases of **Sneddon Syndrome**
- Clinical: livedo racemosa, recurrent fever, recurrent ischemic stroke, myalgias
- Path: vasculitis

16. RASopathies

Overview

- Ras is a family of GTPases, including Hras, Nras, and Kras
- All the RASopathies (formerly called Neurocutaneous Syndromes) result from **Ras-MAPK mutations**
  - All have cardiac manifestations, most commonly **pulmonary valve abnormalities**
- Neurocutaneous Syndromes (discussed here)
  - Neurofibromatosis
  - Watson Syndrome
  - Legius Syndrome
  - Noonan Syndrome
  - LEOPARD Syndrome (Noonan with Multiple Lentigines Syndrome)
  - Cardio-Facio-Cutaneous Syndrome
  - Costello Syndrome
- Other Ras-MAPK mutations (discussed elsewhere)
  - Capillary Malformation–Arteriovenous Malformation
  - Cerebral Capillary Malformations (Familial)
  - Leukocyte Adhesion Deficiency (Type III)
  - Somatic mutations in RAS (usually HRAS or KRAS) cause Schimmelpenning Syndrome (mosaic nevi + rickets)

Neurofibromatosis Type I

- Mutation of **neurofibromin**
- AD; 50% spontaneous mutations
  - Penetrance approaches 100% by age 20
- Exact function unknown. May be a GAP (GTPase activating protein) involved in negative regulation of *Ras* proto-oncogene (accelerates hydrolysis of GTP → GDP)
- Need 2 of the following 7 criteria:
  - **Neurofibromas**: 2 neurofibromas or 1 plexiform Neurofibroma (60-90%, starts at puberty) (fig 16.1 and 16.2)

Table 16.1: RASopathies

Disease	Gene
Noonan	PTPN11, KRAS, NRAS, SOS1, RAF1, BRAF, SHOC2
LEOPARD	PTPN11, RAF1
NF-1	NF1
Legius	SPRED1
Capillary malformation-AVM	RASA1
Cardio-Facio-Cutaneous	BRAF, MAP2K1, MAP2K2, KRAS
Costello	HRAS
Gingival Fibromatosis 1	SOS1
Autoimmune Lymphoproliferative Syndrome	NRAS
Leukocyte Adhesion Deficiency (Type III)	KIND3
Keratinocytic Epidermal Nevus	Mosaic NRAS, HRAS, PIK3CA, FGFR3

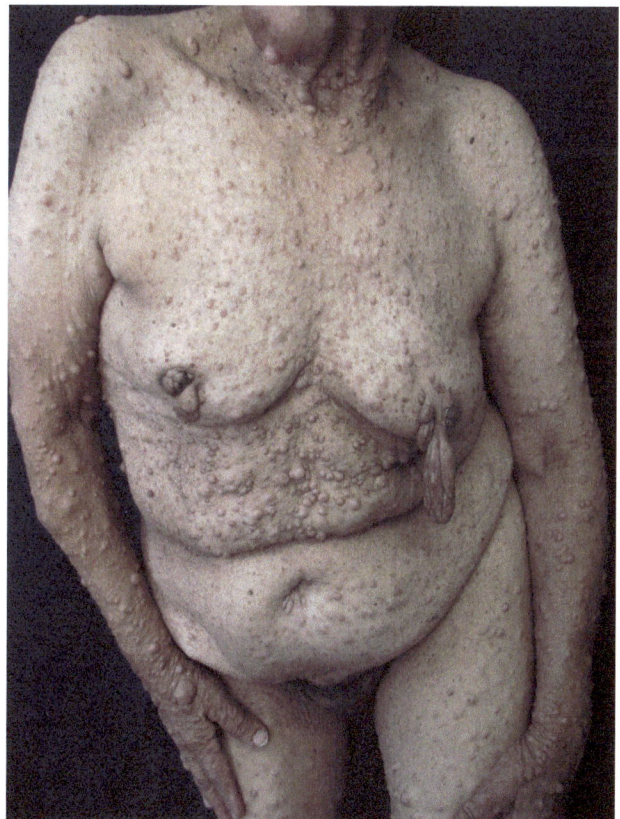

Figure 16.1: Numerous Neurofibromas, a Plexiform Neurofirboma (Neck), and Scoliosis in Neurofibromatosis

- **Crowe's sign**: freckling of the groin or axilla (80%) (fig 16.2)
    - **CALMS**: 6+, > 5mm prepuberty or > 15mm postpuberty (90%, infancy)
    - Skeletal abnormalities: sphenoid dysplasia or thinning of cortex of long bones
    - **Lisch nodules**: hamartomas of iris (90%, age 7) (fig 16.3)
    - **Optic glioma** (15%)
    - **First degree relative with NF** (50%)

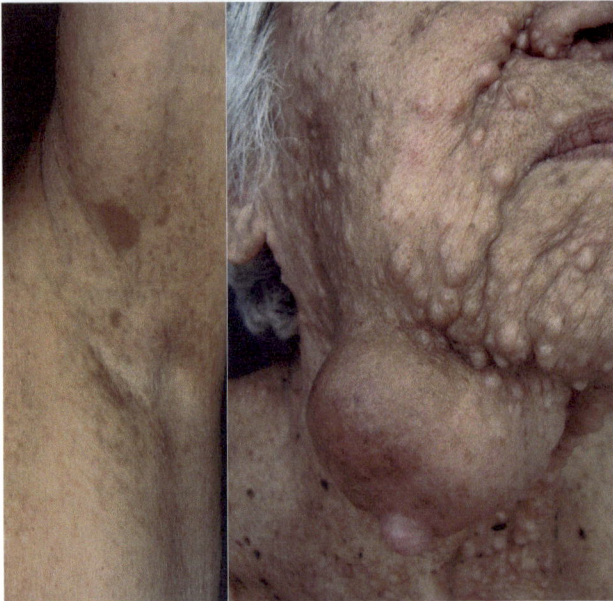

Figure 16.2: Crowe's Sign Along with CALM in Neurofibromatosis (left), Plexiform Neurofibroma (right)

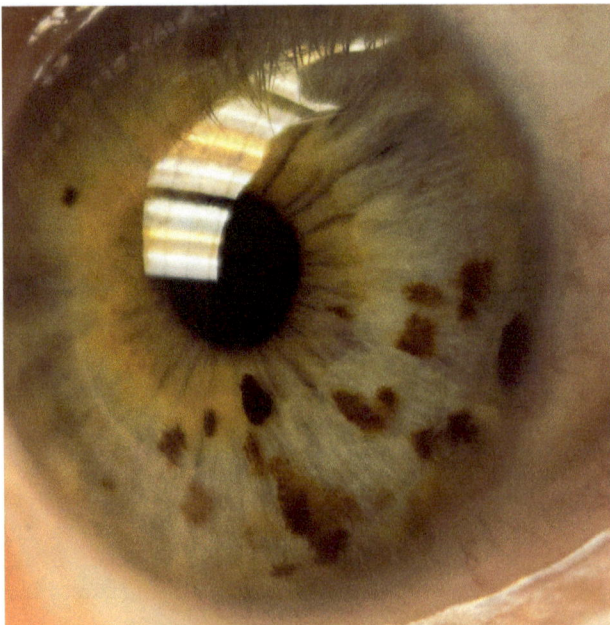

Figure 16.3: Lisch Nodules of Neurofibromatosis

- Common skin findings:
    - M.C. feature = CALMs (>90%), Lisch nodules (>90%, but presents after age 7)
    - First sign = CALMs
    - Most specific feature = Crowe's sign **nearly pathognomonic** (DDx: Dowling-Degos)
    - NFs appear around puberty, ↑ growth in pregnancy
    - Plexiform NFs
        - Feel like a "bag of worms"
        - Occur in ~1/3 of NF1 patients. Are congenital and present by age 5
        - ~10% of NF1 patients develop **Malignant Peripheral Nerve Sheath Tumor,** which **usually arises from a preexisting plexiform NF**
- Uncommon findings:
    - **NF1 confers 200-500x risk of juvenile myelomonocytic leukemia (JMML). Screen for presenting features: hepatosplenomegaly, lymphadenopathy, pallor, petechiae**
    - Juvenile xanthogranuloma (JXG) present in 1% of NF1
        - **NF1 + JXG** confers a 32x risk of (JMML) vs NF1 alone (24 reported cases of "triple association")
    - **Glomus Tumor**: small blue-red papule/nodule; marked pain and cold intolerance, M.C. location = subungual finger
    - **Melanoma**: frequency 0.1% -5.4%; patients more likely female, younger, higher Breslow thickness
    - **Blue-Red Macules:** soft to palpation
        - Path: thickened blood vessel walls with widened lumina and tumor-like neurogenic tissue in the papillary and reticular dermis, neurofibromatous tissue infiltrates vascular structures
    - **Pseudoatrophic Macules:** oval, slightly depressed lesions, softer than surrounding skin
        - Path: ↓ collagen in reticular dermis, ↑ perivascular neuroid tissue
    - **Nevus Anemicus**: correlation unclear, few reports
- DDx:
    - **Legius Syndrome**
    - Familial CALMs (formerly called NF-6)
        - AD; no other manifestations of NF1; no ↑ risk of developing classical NF1

- – Segmental NF1
  - • Can have pigmentary changes alone (background hyperpigmentation, CALMs, and freckling), neurofibromas alone, or both pigmentary changes and neurofibromas, or isolated plexiform neurofibromas
  - – Axillary Freckling: Dowling-Degos

Neurofibromatosis Type 2

- • AD; mutation in **NF-2 gene (Merlin, Schwannomin)**
- • Bilateral acoustic schwannomas (8th cranial nerve), brain meningiomas
- • 60% get skin tumors. M.C. = peripheral schwannoma

Table 16.2: Genoderms with Eye Findings

Spoke-like ("whorled") corneal opacities	Fabry
Heterochromia iridis	Nail-Patella, Waardenburg, Ziprkowski-Margolis
Lester iris	Nail-Patella
Retinitis pigmentosa	Sjögren-Larsson, Refsum, Cockayne, Mucopolysaccharidoses
Glaucoma	Sturge-Weber
↑ Red reflex	Chédiak-Higashi (also photophobia)
Lisch nodules	NF-1
Optic glioma	NF-1
Phakoma	TS
Angioid streaks	PXE, Ehlers-Danlos
Downward lens displacement	Homocystinuria
Upward lens displacement	Marfan
CHRPE	Gardner's
Corneal opacities	X-linked ichthyosis
Pinguecula	Gaucher, Alkaptonuria
Kayser-Fleischer rings	Wilson
Brushfield spots	Down Syndrome
Osler's sign	Alkaptonuria
Trichomegaly	Oliver-McFarlane Syndrome Cornelia de Lange Syndrome Rubinstein-Taybi Syndrome Congenital Hypertrichosis Lanuginosa Syndrome Hermansky-Pudlak Syndrome Fetal Alcohol Syndrome Drugs: HIV, IFN-α, latanoprost, minoxidil, phenytoin, psoralen, penicillamine, CsA

Watson Syndrome

- • AD; mutation in *NF1* gene
- • Clinical features – **Neurofibromatosis + pulmonic stenosis**
  - – Pulmonic stenosis, CALMs, low intelligence, and short stature
  - – Lisch nodules, neurofibromas (33%)

Legius Syndrome

- • AD; mutation in **SPRED1** gene, a negative regulator of the Ras-MAPK pathway (similar to neurofibromin)
- • Multiple CALMs, axillary freckling, macrocephaly, and Noonan-like facies
- • Lacks nonpigmentary changes of NF1 (e.g. Lisch nodules, neurofibromas, bony changes)

> Think "Spread your legs" to remember the Legius syndrome is caused by a mutation in the SPRED-1 gene.

Noonan Syndrome

- • AD; *PTPN11* mutation (allelic with LEOPARD) in 50%, 50% sporadic; common (1:1000-2500 live births)
  - – Rarely caused by other Ras-MAPK mutations, including *KRAS, NRAS, RAF1, BRAF, SOS1, SHOC2*
- • Key features:
  - – Skin: lower extremity lymphedema; multiple large nevi; CALMs
  - – Hair: coarse, light-colored, curly
  - – Craniofacial: hypertelorism; low-set ears with thickened helices; micrognathia; **webbed neck** with low posterior hairline (fetal cystic hygroma remnants); high-arched palate; eyelid ptosis, cutis verticis gyrata
  - – Musculoskeletal: short stature; pectus excavatum, cubitus valgus
  - – CV (50-80%): **pulmonic valve stenosis** (M.C.), ASD
  - – CNS: MR (mild-severe)
  - – GU: cryptorchidism; hypogonadism
- • Normal life span if cardiac defects are treated

Table 16.3: Genoderms with Webbed Neck (Pterygium Colli)

Noonan
Turner
Trisomy 21 (Down)
Trisomy 18
Trisomy 13

LEOPARD Syndrome (Noonan with Multiple Lentigines Syndrome)

- AD; *PTPN11* mutation (allelic with Noonan)
- LEOPARD =
  - **L**entigines and **café-noir** macules. Classic finding, characteristically involving face, neck, upper trunk; spares mucosa
  - **E**KG conduction defects
  - **O**cular hypertelorism
  - **P**ulmonary stenosis (40%)
  - **A**bnormal genitalia
  - **R**etardation of growth
  - **D**eafness
- See also p. 83 (Disorders with Hyperpigmentation)

Cardio-Facio-Cutaneous Syndrome

- Caused by sporadic mutations in the **Ras-MAPK pathway**, including *BRAF, KRAS, MEK1 (MAP2K1), MEK2 (MAP2K2)*
  - Phenotypic overlap with Costello, Noonan, and LEOPARD
  - Noonan-like phenotype, but differs from Noonan due to presence of abnormal hair and hyperkeratotic lesions
- Distinctive facial appearance, heart defects (especially pulmonic valve), and MR
- Skin: **sparse and friable hair, hyperkeratotic lesions**, and a generalized ichthyosis-like condition

Costello Syndrome (Faciocutaneoskeletal (FCS) Syndrome)

- AR; *HRAS* mutation, part of the Ras-MAPK pathway
- Phenotypic overlap with Cardio-Facio-Cutaneous Syndrome (*KRAS* mutation)
- **Distinctive hands**: thick, loose skin on hands. Distinctive hand posture, with ulnar deviation of wrist
- **Nasolabial warts**, cutis laxa
- Severe feeding difficulty and failure to thrive
- Gregarious personality, coarse facies, short stature
- Increased risk of rhabdomyosarcoma and bladder cancer
- CV: pulmonic stenosis

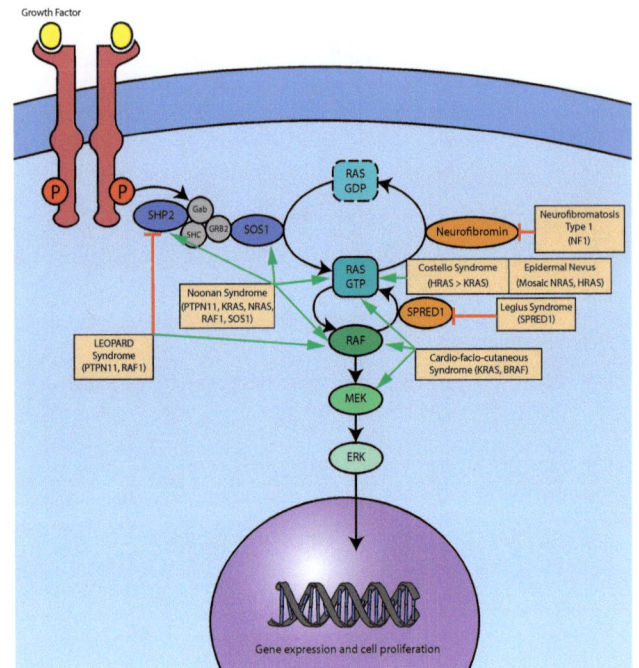

Figure 16.4: Ras-MAPK Pathway

17. Miscellaneous Genoderms

Syndromes with Prominent Lipomas

Benign Symmetric Lipomatosis (Madelung Disease)

- Gene unknown
- Extensive symmetric fat deposits in the head, neck, and shoulder girdle area
- 97% male
- Severe peripheral neuropathy
- Associated with alcohol abuse

Familial Multiple Lipomatosis

- AD; gene unknown

Adiposis Dolorosa (Dercum Disease)

- Most sporadic, some AD; gene unknown
- Obesity, multiple lipomas, chronic pain in all adipose tissue (not just in lipomas)

Lipomas are Also Prominent In:

- PTEN Hamartoma syndromes, including
  - CLOVE
  - Cowden
  - SOLAMEN
  - Proteus
  - Bannayan-Riley-Ruvalcaba Syndrome
- MEN1

Miscellaneous Tumor Syndromes

Brooke-Spiegler Syndrome

- AD; CYLD gene mutation
- Trichoepithelioma + Spiradenoma + Cylindroma (fig 17.1)
- Milia
- Allelic with:
  - Epithelioma Adenoides Cysticum of Brooke = trichoeps only
  - Familial Cylindromatosis = cylindromas only
  - Rasmussen Syndrome = Milia, trichoepitheliomas and cylindromas (gene not reported, but probably same)

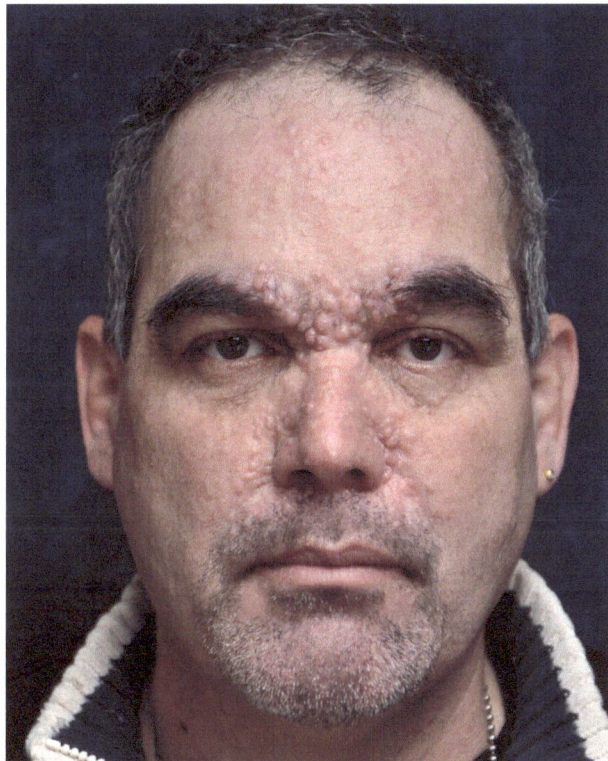

Figure 17.1: Trichoepitheliomas in Brooke-Spiegler Syndrome

Pilomatricoma (Calcifying Epithelioma of Malherbe)

- Rock-hard bluish nodule on the cheek of children. 50% head/neck
- Sporadic *CTNNB1* mutation, encodes **β-catenin**
- Multiple pilomatricomas are a feature of:
  - **Myotonic Dystrophy** (40% have pilomatricomas)
  - **Gardner's Syndrome**
  - **Rubinstein-Taybi**
  - **Turner Syndrome**

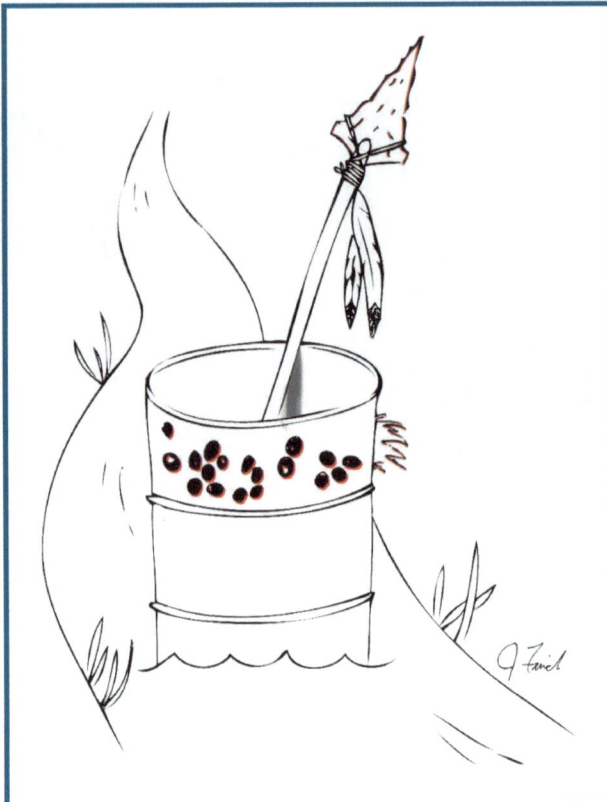

Brooke-Spiegler Syndrome

Picture a brook, down which is floating a cylinder (cylindromas) containing a spear (spiradenoma). The cylinder has trichoepitheliomas growing out of it.

- Path
  - Hair follicle differentiation (matrix)
  - Shadow cells
  - Calcification
  - Basaloid cells

Genoderms with Short Stature

(Genoderms not covered in other areas)

Cornelia de Lange Syndrome

- Mostly sporadic (some familial); variety of chromosomal abnormalities
- Key features:
  - Skin: **cutis marmorata**; hirsutism; hypoplastic nipples and umbilicus
  - Craniofacial: striking and characteristic facies ("Greek tragedy mask") including **synophrys**, **long lashes (trichomegaly)**, small nose/anteverted nostrils, downturned thin lips, late-erupting wide spread teeth, microcephaly, low-set ears, low hair line, short neck

  - Severe MR, short stature
  - GU: cryptorchidism; hypospadius; renal anomalies; bicornuate uterus
  - CV: variety of heart disease
  - Lungs: recurrent infection
- Often premature death due to aspiration and recurrent lung infections

Russell-Silver Syndrome

- Extremely rare; almost all sporadic
- Most cases caused by **epigenetic** DNA alterations. That is, hypomethylation (and thereby under-activation) of 11p15, the same locus that is *over*-methylated in Beckwith-Wiedemann (p. 104)
- Key features:
  - Skin: CALMs
  - OB: severe intrauterine growth retardation, poor postnatal growth
  - Musculoskeletal: triangular shaped face (large cranium, medium upper face, small jaw), short stature
  - GU: variety of anomalies; ± precocious puberty
- Normal life span; impairment depends on severity of asymmetry

Trichorhinophalangeal Syndrome

- Type I – AD; mutation in *TRPS1*, a zinc finger protein
- Type II (Langer-Giedion Syndrome) – contiguous gene deletion syndrome of *TRPS1* and *EXT1*
- Type III – AD; mutation in *TRPS1*, a zinc finger protein
- Clinical features, Type I
  - Distinctive facies, with pear-shaped nose and long philtrum
  - Hair is fine, brittle, and sparse
  - Short stature
- Clinical features, Type II
  - Type I + exostoses
  - Features of both Trichorhinophalangeal Type I (*TRPS* gene) and Multiple Exostoses Type I (*EXT* gene)
- Clinical features, Type III
  - Type I + severely shortened phalanges
- Clinical diagnosis, no treatment

H Syndrome

- AR; mutation in *SLC29A3*, encoding a nucleoside transporter of unknown function

Skin: hyperpigmentation and hypertrichosis
Rosai-Dorfman Disease
Extracutaneous:

- Sensorineural deafness
- Uveitis
- Heart abnormalities
- Hypogonadism
- Hyperglycemia/ Diabetes
- Hallux valgus
- Short Height

Osteoma Cutis

- Occurs in four genetic disorders
  - Albright hereditary osteodystrophy
  - Progressive osseous heteroplasia
  - Plate-like osteoma cutis
  - Fibrodysplasia ossificans progressiva
- FOP is the most severe, but patients do not present to a derm clinic
- The other three all have *GNAS1* mutations (allelic with McCune-Albright) and manifest ossification that begins in the dermis

Albright Hereditary Osteodystrophy

- *GNAS1* mutation (encodes a subunit of stimulatory G protein, regulates adenylyl cyclase activity (may be a negative regulator of bone formation)
- Skeletal findings: brachydactyly, obesity, short stature, short 4th and 5th metacarpals (**Albright's sign)**
- Pseudohypoparathyroidism, hypocalcemia, and ↑PTH levels (PHP Ia)
  - None of the other osteoma cutis disorders have derangements of Ca or PO_4!
- Occasionally MR

Table 17.1: Genoderms with Bone/Musculoskeletal Associations	
Stippled epiphyses (chondrodysplasia punctata)	Conradi-Hünermann Syndrome (XLD CDP) Rhizomelic CDP XLR CDP CHILD Syndrome Neonatal lupus, in-utero warfarin exposure
Osteopoikilosis	Buschke-Ollendorff Syndrome
Dysostosis multiplex (stiff joints)	Mucopolysaccharidoses
Debilitating limb pain	Fabry Disease
Scoliosis	NF-1 Familial Dysautonomia (Riley-Day Syndrome, HSAN 3) Cold-Induced Sweating Syndrome EDS, Classical EDS, Kyphoscoliosis Marfan Basal Cell Nevus Syndrome Hypomelanosis of Ito
Pseudarthrosis of tibia	NF-1
Sphenoid wing dysplasia	NF-1
Congenital hip dislocation	EDS, VII
Leg length discrepancy	Cutis marmorata telangiectatica congenita Klippel-Trenaunay
Chondrosarcoma & endochondroma	Maffucci Syndrome, Olliers
Hypermobile joints ("double jointed")	EDS
Codfish vertebrae, crumpled fractures	OI
Osteopathia striata	Focal dermal hypoplasia
Syndactyly (lobster claw deformity)	Focal dermal hypoplasia EEC Waardenburg 3
Albright's sign	Albright Hereditary Osteodystrophy (AHO) Basal Cell Nevus Syndrome (also get bifid ribs)
Hypoplastic/absent thumbs	Fanconi's Anemia Rothmund-Thomson
Osteomas	Gardner's Albright hereditary osteodystrophy Fibrodysplasia ossificans progressiva Progressive osseous heteroplasia Plate-Like osteoma cutis
Osteosarcoma	Rothmund-Thomson Syndrome
Osteomyelitis	Chronic Granulomatous Disease DIRA
Erlenmeyer Flask Deformity	Gaucher Disease
Clinodactyly of 5th finger	Russell-Silver Syndrome Down Syndrome Orofaciodigital Syndrome 1 Cornelia de Lange Syndrome Turner Syndrome

Table 17.2: Eye Findings

Finding	Associations
Spoke-like ("whorled") corneal opacities	**Fabry**
Heterochromia Iridis	**Nail-Patella** **Waardenburg** **Ziprkowski-Margolis**
Lester Iris	**Nail-Patella**
Retinitis pigmentosa	**Sjögren-Larsson** **Refsum** **Cockayne** **Mucopolysaccharidoses**
Glaucoma	**Sturge-Weber**
↑ Red reflex	**Chédiak-Higashi** (also photophobia)
Lisch nodules	**NF-1**
Optic glioma	**NF-1**
Phakoma	**Tuberous Sclerosis**
Angioid streaks	**PXE** **Ehlers-Danlos**
Downward lens displacement	**Homocystinuria**
Upward lens displacement	**Marfan**
CHRPE	**Gardner's**
Corneal opacities	**X-linked ichthyosis**
Pingueculae	**Gaucher** **Alkaptonuria**
Kayser-Fleischer rings	**Wilson**
Brushfield spots	**Down Syndrome**
Osler's sign	**Alkaptonuria**
Trichomegaly	**Oliver-McFarlane Syndrome** **Cornelia de Lange Syndrome** **Rubinstein-Taybi Syndrome** **Congenital Hypertrichosis Lanuginosa Syndrome** **Hermansky-Pudlak Syndrome** Drugs: HIV, IFN-α, latanoprost, minoxidil, phenytoin, psoralen, penicillamine, CsA Fetal Alcohol Syndrome

Progressive Osseous Heteroplasia

- AD; *GNAS1* mutation
- Rapidly progressive ossification of skin and muscle presenting soon after birth as asymptomatic papules/nodules with "rice grain" texture, F>M
- No associated developmental or endocrine abnormalities

Plate-Like Osteoma Cutis

- AD; *GNAS1* mutation
- Like POH, but only single/limited sites
- No dysmorphic features or Ca/Phosphate abnormalities

Fibrodysplasia Ossificans Progressiva

- AD; *ACVR1* mutation, encodes activin A receptor. Results in ↑ levels of BMP4 (bone morphogenetic protein-4)
- Tumor-like swellings of bone
- No direct skin involvement, but bony swellings can extend to skin
- Dystrophic great toe, bald, MR, deaf
- Extremely poor prognosis, death in childhood

Chromosomal Abnormalities

- Incidence of nondisjunction of chromosomes increases with maternal age

Down Syndrome

- Caused by trisomy 21 (2% caused by translocation of chromosome 21)
- Skin
  - **Syringomas** (20%)
  - **Elastosis perforans serpiginosa**
  - Vitiligo
  - Cheilitis
  - Single palmar crease ("Simian crease", also seen in Basan's Syndrome)
  - Flat nipple
  - Nuchal skin folds in infancy
  - Xerosis
  - Infections
  - Cutis marmorata
  - Hyperkeratosis (keratosis pilaris)
  - Alopecia areata
  - Premature wrinkling
  - Milia-like calcinosis cutis (hands)
- Eyes
  - Epicanthal folds
  - Upslanting palpebral fissures
  - **Brushfield spots**
  - Opacities
  - Strabismus
- Craniofacial: brachycephaly; flat face; short broad neck; small ears with dysplastic/absent earlobes
- Mouth: large scrotal tongue; fissured, thick lips; periodontal disease
- Musculoskeletal: short stature; small hands; many others
- CNS: MR (IQ 30-50); seizures (10%)

- CV: **endocardial cushion defects**
- GI: duodenal atresia M.C.; others
- Heme: AML; transient leukemoid reaction and polycythemia (newborns); immunodeficiency
- Endocrine: autoimmune hypothyroidism > hyperthyroidism

Dermatoses of Down Syndrome "CHEAPS"

Cutis marmorata, **C**heilitis

Hyperkeratosis (keratosis pilaris)

EPS

Alopecia areata

Premature wrinkling

Syringoma (20%)

Diseases with Elastosis Perforans Serpiginosa "RTAP MOPEDS"

Rothmund-
  Thomson
Acrogeria
PXE

Marfan
Osteogenesis Imperfecta
Penicillamine (disrupts elastin crosslinks)
Ehlers-Danlos
Down (#1 cause)
Scleroderma

Turner Syndrome (Gonadal Dysgenesis)
- XO
- Due to nondisjunction or mosaicism
- Multiple anomalies
  - Skin: redundant neck folds/webbed neck (fetal cystic hygroma remnants); multiple large nevi; keloid formation
  - Hair: low-set nuchal hairline
  - Nails: hypoplastic; hyperconvex; deep-set
  - CV: **aortic coarctation**
- Normal life span if congenital anomalies are treated

Klinefelter Syndrome
- XXY
- Common (~1:500 males)
- Presents in childhood-adolescence
- Key features:
  - Varicose veins, arterial and venous **leg ulcers**

- Scant body and pubic hair
- Musculoskeletal: tall with long legs/arms, obesity, gynecomastia
- GU: small testes, small penis, infertile
- CNS: delayed speech as a child, dull mentality, antisocial behaviors
- Labs: markedly ↓ testosterone
- Normal life span with improved secondary sexual characteristics when treated with testosterone

Phylloid Hypomelanosis
- Mosaic trisomy 13

Syndromes with Follicular Atrophoderma

Braun-Falco-Marghescu Syndrome
- PPK, KP, atrophoderma vermiculatum

Tuzun Syndrome
- Atrophoderma vermiculatum and scrotal tongue

Nicolau-Balus Syndrome
- Atrophoderma vermiculatum, eruptive syringomas and milia

Rombo Syndrome
- See p. 98
- Atrophoderma vermiculatum, milia, BCCs, trichoepitheliomas, hypotrichosis, telangiectasias, acral cyanosis

Bazex-Dupré-Christol Syndrome (Bazex Syndrome)
- See p. 98
- Follicular atrophoderma (misnomer because have ice-pick depressions, but no true atrophy)
- Multiple BCCs, hypotrichosis, localized hypohidrosis (above the neck), facial hyperpigmentation, milia, hair shaft dystrophy, multiple genital trichoeps

Keratosis Follicularis Spinulosa Decalvans
- **XLR**; (*MBTPS2* or *SAT1*), rarely AD
- Follicular hyperkeratosis (keratosis pilaris), progressive cicatricial alopecia, and photophobia
- Allelic with and much phenotypic overlap with IFAP Syndrome

Conradi-Hünermann-Happle Syndrome (Chondrodysplasia Punctata)

- Transient blaschkoid ichthyosiform erythroderma at birth that quickly heals with **blaschkoid follicular atrophoderma** by age 1
- See p.11 for full discussion

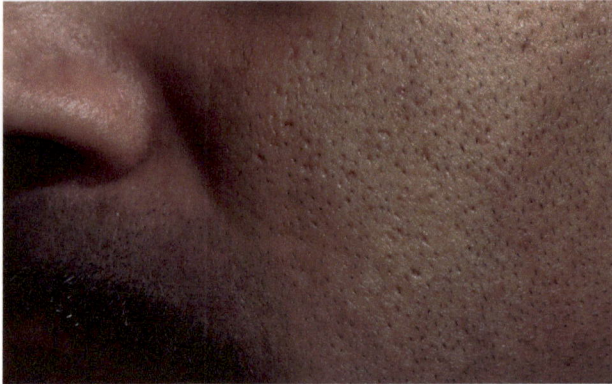

Figure 17.2: Follicular Atrophoderma, Visible as Atrophic Pits on Each Hair Follicle Ostium

Genoderms with Amyloidosis

- Think of genetic disease when macular or lichen amyloid occurs in a child

Primary Localized Cutaneous Amyloidosis 1 (PLCA1)

- AD; mutations in *OSMR* (Oncostatin M receptor-β,) or *IL31RA*, which form the heterodimeric receptor through which IL31 (made by Th2 cells) signals
- Genetic form accounts for 10% of cases of amyloidosis
- Intense pruritus and macular or lichen amyloidosis. No systemic amyloid

MEN-2A (Sipple Syndrome)

- 33% with MEN2A get interscapular lichen amyloidosis
- Think of MEN2A when macular or lichen amyloid occurs in a child
- For full discussion of MEN2A, see p. 102

X-Linked Reticulate Pigmentary Disorder

- Males: generalized reticulate hyperpigmentation. Death in infancy
- Female carriers: Blaschkoid hyperpigmentation (similar to stage 3 of IP). Otherwise normal
- Cutaneous amyloid. No systemic amyloid

Genoderms with Secondary Cutaneous Amyloidosis

- Chronic inflammation results in ↑ hepatic synthesis of the acute phase reactant **Apoprotein (AA)**. Usually deposition in internal organs. Skin findings are rare
- Chronic severe inflammatory disorders (e.g. **periodic fever syndromes**, among which TRAPS and Muckle-Wells have the highest incidence of amyloidosis)

Heredofamilial Systemic Amyloidosis (Familial Amyloid Polyneuropathy)

- Skin findings rare. Neurologic symptoms predominate, including peripheral sensory, motor, and autonomic neuropathies: paresthesias, atrophic ulcers, postural hypotension, impotence, ileus
- Three types
  - **Transthyretin** (*TTR* gene; AD)
    - ATTR amyloid
    - Transthyretin is a serum transport protein for thyroxine and retinol-binding protein
    - Made primarily in the liver, a little in the choroid of the eye
    - Tx: liver transplant for transthyretin mutations
  - **Apolipoprotein A1** (*APOA1* gene; AD)
    - AApoA1 amyloid
  - **Gelsolin** (Finnish-Type Amyloidosis) (*GSN* gene; AD)
    - Encodes an actin-severing protein
    - AGel amyloid
    - Patients get Cutis Laxa and Lattice Corneal Dystrophy Type II

Genetic Disorders with Hyperhidrosis

- Disorders of cornification:
  - **PPKs**
  - **Pachyonychia congenita**
  - **CIE (bullous and non-bullous)**
- Other genoderms:
  - **EB (simplex > junctional)**
  - **Dermatopathia pigmentosa reticularis**
  - **Dyskeratosis congenita**
  - **Pachydermoperiostosis**
  - **Apert Syndrome**
  - **Nail-Patella Syndrome**
  - **Böök Syndrome**

- Hereditary Sensory and Autonomic Neuropathies (HSANs)
  - **Familial Dysautonomia (Riley-Day, HSAN-3)**
  - **Congenital Sensory Neuropathy**
  - **Congenital Autonomic Dysfunction with Universal Pain Loss**

Familial Dysautonomia (Riley-Day Syndrome, HSAN-3)

- AD; mutation in *IKBKAP* gene; common in Ashkenazi Jews (1:3700)
- Autonomic dysfunction
- Key features:
  - Skin:
    - Episodic hyperhidrosis of face and trunk, with blotchy erythema
    - Recurrent burns; cold hands/feet
    - Absence of fungiform papillae on tongue (and absent taste)
  - Dysautonomic crises when stressed (vomiting, HTN), postural hypotension, decreased DTRs, failure to thrive, developmental delay
  - Craniofacial: alert expression; ↓ blink frequency; straight upper lip with smile
  - CNS: hypotonia in infancy; ↓ DTRs; **insensitivity to pain**; labile BP; prolonged bedwetting; breath-holding spells
  - Normal IQ
  - Eyes: ↓ corneal sensation and tear flow → corneal ulceration
  - Excessive saliva and bronchial secretions; recurrent aspirations and infections
  - Musculoskeletal: short stature; kyphoscoliosis; ↑ incidence of aseptic necrosis
  - Labs: inject histamine → get wheal without flare or pain; ↓ ratio of urinary homovanillic acid to vanillylmandelic acid
- High mortality due to lung problems

Cold-Induced Sweating Syndrome

- AR; *CRLF1* mutation or *CLCF1* mutation (cytokine receptor-like factor-1; cardiotrophin-like cytokine factor)
- Facial dysmorphism, flexion deformities, and scoliosis

Granulosis Rubra Nasi

- AD; unknown gene
- Marked sweating of nose, followed by redness, papules, and vesicles

- Occurs in children and resolves by puberty
- Commonly, hyperhidrosis of palms/soles, pernio, and acrocyanosis

Genetic Disorders with Hypohidrosis

- Ectodermal dysplasias:
  - **Hypohidrotic ectodermal dysplasia**
  - **AEC Syndrome (Ankyloblepharon-Ectodermal Dysplasia-Clefting, Hay-Wells, Rapp-Hodgkin)**
  - **Naegeli-Franceschetti-Jadassohn**
- **Bazex-Dupré-Christol**
- **Incontinentia Pigmenti**
- **Fabry** (hyperhidrosis can also occur)
- **Congenital Insensitivity to Pain with Anhidrosis (HSAN-4)**
  - AR; *NTRK1*, encodes neurotrophic tyrosine kinase receptor Type 1
  - Recurrent fevers, self-mutilation, MR
  - Not a derm disease, per se, but can be **diagnosed based on skin biopsy**: IHC stain against **protein gene product 9.5** (axonal marker) = absence of small nerve fibers in epidermis and lack of innervation of sweat glands

Miscellaneous Syndromes

Oral-Facial-Digital Syndrome

- **XLD**; *OFD1* gene mutation
- **EICs on face**, especially ears
- Short metacarpals
- MR in 40%
- Polycystic Kidney Disease

Popliteal Pterygium Syndrome (van der Woude Syndrome)

- AD; mutation in *IRF6* gene
- Lower **lip pits** and fistula, cleft upper lip
- Filiform **eyelid adhesions**
- GU and heart abnormalities

Flegel Disease (Hyperkeratosis Lenticularis Perstans)

- AD; unknown gene
- Red-brown keratotic papules on lower legs and top of feet
- Onset in 50's

Aquagenic Wrinkling of the Palms

- AR; CFTR mutation
- Occurs in 60% of patients with **cystic fibrosis**
- Many patients with AWofP are heterozygous carriers of *CFTR* mutation

18. Ridiculous Tables and Preposterous Lists

Table 18.1: Molecular Classification of Genoderms

Molecular Defect	Skin Disorders That Result
Keratin defects	Bullous CIE (epidermolytic hyperkeratosis, EHK)
	Annular epidermolytic ichthyosis (cyclic ichthyosis with EHK)
	Ichthyosis hystrix of Curth–Macklin
	Ichthyosis bullosa of Siemens
	Epidermolytic PPK
	Non-epidermolytic PPK
	White sponge nevus (of Cannon)
	EBS, Dowling–Meara type
	EBS, Koebner type
	EBS, Weber–Cockayne type
	EBS, With mottled pigmentation
	EBS, With migratory circinate erythema
	EBS, Autosomal recessive type
	Dowling–Degos Disease
	Naegeli–Franceschetti– Jadassohn Syndrome
	Dermatopathia pigmentosa reticularis
	Pachyonychia congenita Type 1 (Jadassohn–Lewandowsky)
	Pachyonychia congenita Type 2 (Jackson–Lawlor)
	Steatocystoma multiplex
	Monilethrix (autosomal dominant)
	'Pure' hair–nail type ectodermal dysplasia
Defects in structural proteins of the cornified cell envelope	Icthyosis Vulgaris Progressive Symmetric Erythrokeratoderma Vohwinkel Syndromes (Variant Form)
Lipid metabolism defects	Various ichthyoses (including CHILD Syndrome, Conradi–Hunermann–Happle Syndrome, Neutral Lipid Storage Disease, non-bullous congenital ichthyosiform erythroderma (defective lipoxygenase 3 or 12R), Refsum Disease, rhizomelic chondrodysplasia punctata, Sjogren–Larsson Syndrome and **XLR** ichthyosis) Various hyperlipidemias Farber lipogranulomatosis Gaucher Disease Type 2 hyperimmunoglobulinemia D with Periodic Fever Syndrome Mari-type hypotrichosis Niemann–Pick Disease

Table 18.1: Molecular Classification of Genoderms

Molecular Defect	Skin Disorders That Result
Transglutaminase defects	Lamellar Ichthyosis Non-Bullous Congenital Ichthyosiform Erythroderma Acral Peeling Skin Syndrome
Protease inhibitor defects	Antithrombin III Deficiency Hereditary Angioedema (Types I & II) Netherton Syndrome
Desmosomal defects	AR Localized Hypotrichosis Carvajal Syndrome Ectodermal Dysplasia/Skin Fragility Syndrome Hypotrichosis Simplex Of The Scalp Lethal Acantholytic EB Monilethrix (Autosomal Recessive) Naxos Disease Skin Fragility/Woolly Hair Syndrome Striate PPK
Connexin defects	Bart–Pumphrey Syndrome PPK with deafness Vohwinkel Syndrome (classic) KID Syndrome (keratitis–ichthyosis–deafness) Hidrotic Ectodermal Dysplasia (Clouston) HID Syndrome (hystrix-like ichthyosis–deafness) Erythrokeratodermia variabilis oculodentodigital dysplasia
Defects in keratinocyte–extracellular matrix (ECM) adhesion	Various forms of epidermolysis bullosa (EB) simplex, junctional EB and dystrophic EB (keratin–ECM linkage) Kindler Syndrome (actin–ECM linkage)
ATP-binding cassette (ABC) transporter defects	Harlequin Ichthyosis Lamellar Ichthyosis Pseudoxanthoma Elasticum Sitosterolemia Tangier Disease/Familial Hypoalphaproteinemia
Calcium pump defects	Darier's Disease Hailey–Hailey Disease Acrokeratosis Verruciformis
Copper transporter defects	Menkes Disease Occipital Horn Syndrome Wilson Disease
Nuclear membrane defects	Buschke–Ollendorff Syndrome/Melorheostosis Mandibuloacral Dysplasia Progeria Partial Lipodystrophy (Familial And 'Acquired' Forms) Restrictive Dermopathy

(Transmembrane Transporter Defects)

Table 18.1: Molecular Classification of Genoderms

Molecular Defect	Skin Disorders That Result
Collagen defects	Dystrophic EB Localized JEB various types of Ehlers–Danlos Syndrome (classical, vascular, arthrochalsia, hypermobility) Ullrich muscular dystrophy Osteogenesis imperfecta
Defects in pyrin/ NOD-family members and related proteins	Blau Syndrome CINCA (NOMID) Syndrome Familial Cold Autoinflammatory Syndrome Familial Mediterranean Fever Muckle–Wells Syndrome PAPA Syndrome PFAPA Syndrome
RecQ DNA helicase defects	Bloom Syndrome Rothmund–Thomson Syndrome Werner Syndrome
Classic DNA repair defects	Various subtypes of xeroderma pigmentosum, trichothiodystrophy and Cockayne Syndrome Muir–Torre Syndrome Childhood Cancer Syndrome with neurofibromatosis Type 1 phenotype Ataxia-Telangiectasia
Protein-tyrosine phosphatase (PTP) defects	Bannayan–Riley–Ruvalcaba Syndrome Cowden Disease LEOPARD Syndrome Noonan Syndrome
RAS-ERK pathway defects	Capillary Malformation–Arteriovenous Malformation Cerebral Capillary Malformations (Familial) Cardio-Facio-Cutaneous Syndrome Costello Syndrome LEOPARD Syndrome Leukocyte Adhesion Deficiency (Type III) Neurofibromatosis Noonan Syndrome
cAMP and AMP-activated protein kinase pathway defects	Albright hereditary osteodystrophy Carney complex McCune–Albright Syndrome Peutz–Jeghers Syndrome Tuberous sclerosis
Defective protein sorting to vesicles	ARC (arthrogryphosis–renal dysfunction–cholestasis) Syndrome Hermansky–Pudlak Syndrome
Defective vesicle trafficking or transport	CEDNIK (cerebral dysgenesis, neuropathy, ichthyosis and keratoderma) Chediak–Higashi Griscelli Ocular albinism Type 1

PPK: palmoplantar keratoderma
EBS: Epidermolysis bullosa simplex

Derm Diseases with Megalencephaly

- With cutaneous findings
  - PTEN Hamartoma Syndromes (Cowden, Bannayan-Riley, Proteus)
  - NF1 (Neurofibromatosis)
- With overgrowth
  - Macrocephaly-Cutis Marmorata Telangiectatica Congenita
  - Sotos Syndrome and Weaver Syndrome (allelic, *NSD1* mutations)
  - Beckwith-Wiedemann Syndrome, Simpson-Golabi-Behmel Syndrome (Bulldog Syndrome) (allelic, *IGF2* mutations)
- Neuro-Cardio-Facial-Cutaneous Syndromes (all are Ras-MAPK Pathway mutations)
  - Noonan, Costello
  - Cardio-facio-cutaneous (CFC)
  - LEOPARD

J. Finch & M. Payette

Table 18.2: Molecular Basis of Ichthyosis

1) Disorders of Keratinocyte Proteins ("bricks")

Defect	Skin Disorder That Results	Gene	Disease
Cytoskeleton			
Keratin intermediate filament disorder	Weakening or collapse of cytoskeleton and decreased mechanical stability of epidermis; affecting lamellar body secretion resulting in paucity of SC lamellar material and corneodesmosome retention	K1/10 K1 K2	EI ICM SEI
Cornified lipid/cell envelope			
TGase-1 deficiency	Weak CE with reduced lamellar membrane and NLPS Weak cornified envelope with reduced lamellar membrane and NLPS	TGM1	LI, CIE, SHCB, BSI
Loricrin disorder	Possible cytotoxic effect through gain of function of mutant loricrin molecules	LOR	LK
Protease/protease inhibitors			
LEKTI deficiency	Increased serine protease activity with premature loss of corneodesmosome and induction of inflammation	SPINK5	NS
Matriptase deficiency	Defective filaggrin processing	ST14	IHS
Cathepsin C deficiency	Impaired innate immune response and desquamation	CTSC	Papillon-Lefévre Syndrome
Keratohyaline			
Filaggrin deficiency	Decreased corneocyte hydration as result of low NMF; high SC pH resulting in increased protease activity	FLG	IV

2) Disorders of Lipid Metabolism, Assembly, and/or Transport ("mortar")

Defect	Skin Disorder That Results	Gene	Disease
Lipid synthesis/modification			
Hepoxilin pathway defect	Defect of different enzymes (or receptors) within lipoxygenase pathway, impaired processing of profilaggrin to monomeric filaggrin (abnormal SC lipid composition likely)	ALOX12B ALOXE3 CYP4F22 NIPAL4	LI, CIE
Steroid sulfatase deficiency	Abnormal SC lipid composition with lamellar/NLPS; inhibition of proteases causes persistence of corneodesmosome	STS	RXLI
Fatty acid transporter defect	Impaired transport and activation of fatty acids (critical fetal/neonatal period), defective SC lipid homeostasis	SLC27A4	IPS
Lipid transport and secretion			
Primary lamellar body defect	Disturbed transport of lipids and proteases, protease inhibitors, and antimicrobial peptides; paucity of SC lamellar structures	ABCA12 (nonsense vs missense)	HI; LI/CIE
Cholesterol biosynthesis and homeostasis disorders			
8-7 sterol isomerase	Defective "Kandutsch" pathway	EBP	CDPX2
C3 sterol dehydrogenase	Interference with sonic hedgehog	NSDHL	CHILD Syndrome
Zinc endopeptidase/site-2-protease defect	Impaired transcription factors (SREBF1and2) affect sterol/ER homeostasis and cell differentiation	MBTPS2	IFAP Syndrome
Triglyceride metabolism			
Neutral Lipid Storage Disease	Abnormal SC lipid composition with lamellar/NLPS	ABHD5	Neutral Lipid Storage Disease with ichthyosis
Lysosomal storage			
Glucocerebrosidase deficiency	Disturbance of SC lipid composition of ceramides, cholesterol, and free fatty acids	GBA	Gaucher Syndrome Type 2
Peroxisomal hydroxylation			
Phytanoyl-CoA hydroxylase deficiency	Phytanic acid excess disturbs cholesterol/ cholesterol sulfate, or alters lipid degradation	PHYH PEX7	Refsum Syndrome
Microsomal oxidation			
Fatty aldehyde dehydrogenase deficiency	SC lamellar phase separation or NLPS	ALDH3A2	SLS
Intracellular membrane trafficking			

Table 18.2: Molecular Basis of Ichthyosis

2) Disorders of Lipid Metabolism, Assembly, and/or Transport ("mortar")

Defect	Skin Disorder That Results	Gene	Disease
Intracellular membrane trafficking			
Secretory (SNARE) pathway defects	Impaired lamellar body function	AP1S1	MEDNIK Syndrome
		SNAP29	CEDNIK Syndrome
		VPS33B	ARC Syndrome

3) Disorders of Cell-Cell Junctions

Defect	Skin Disorder That Results	Gene	Disease
Gap junctions			
Connexin disorders	(?) Increased sensitivity to apoptosis, reactive hyperproliferation, impaired calcium regulation	GJB2 (GJB6)	KID Syndrome
		GJB3/GJB4	EKV
Tight junctions			
Claudin disorders	(?) Impaired regulation of paracellular permeability, defective epithelial polarization	CLDN1	IHSC Syndrome

4) Disorders of DNA Transcription/Repair

Defect	Skin Disorder That Results	Gene	Disease
Nucleus			
Nucleotide excision repair defect	?	C7Orf11 ERCC2/XPD ERCC3/XPB	TTDs/ TFIIH related
Transcription defect (?)	?	C7Orf11	TTD without CI

J. Finch & M. Payette

Table 18.3: Disorders of Keratinization

Disorder	Inheritance	Protein	Gene
Classic Ichthyoses and Erythro-Keratodermas			
Epidermolytic Ichthyosis	AD	Keratin 1	K1
	AD>>AR	Keratin 10	K10
Ichthyosis hystrix Curth–Macklin	AD	Keratin 1	K1
CHILD Syndrome	XD	3b-hydroxysteroid dehydrogenase	NSDHL
Conradi-Hunermann-Happle Syndrome	XD	D8-D7 sterol isomerase (emopamil binding protein)	EBP
Erythrokeratodermia Variabilis	AD	Connexin 31	GJB3
	AD	Connexin 30.3	GJB4
Harlequin Ichthyosis	AR	ATP-binding cassette (ABC), subfamily A, member 12	ABCA12
Ichthyosis Bullosa of Siemens	AD	Keratin 2	K2
Ichthyosis Vulgaris	AD	Profilaggrin	FLG
KID (Keratitis–Ichthyosis–Deafness) Syndrome	AD	Connexin 26 (gap junction protein b2)	GJB2
	AD	Connexin 30 (gap junction protein b6)	GJB6
HID (Hystrix-Like Ichthyosis–Deafness) Syndrome	AD	Connexin 26 (gap junction protein b2)	GJB2
Lamellar Ichthyosis	AR	Transglutaminase 1	TGM1
	AR	ATP-binding cassette (ABC), subfamily A, member 12	ABCA12
	AR	Cytochrome P450, family 4, subfamily F, polypeptide 22	CYP4F22
Non-Bullous Congenital Ichthyosiform Erythroderma	AR	Transglutaminase 1	TGM1
	AR	Epidermal lipoxygenase 3	ALOXE3
	AR	12(R)-Lipoxygenase	ALOX12B
	AR	Ichthyin	ICHTHYIN
Multiple Sulfatase Deficiency	AR	Sulfatase-modifying factor 1	SUMF1
Netherton Syndrome	AR	Serine protease inhibitor, Kazal Type 5 (lymphoepithelial Kazal-type-related inhibitor, LEKTI)	SPINK5
Neutral Lipid Storage Disease (Chanarin–Dorfman Syndrome)	AR	Abhydrolase domain-containing 5 (comparative gene identification 58, esterase-lipase-thioesterase subfamily)	ABHD5 (CGI-58)
Progressive Symmetric Erythrokeratoderma	AD	Loricrin	LOR
Refsum Disease	AR	Phytanoyl-CoA 2-hydroxylase	PHYH (PAHX)
	AR	Peroxin-7	PEX7
Rhizomelic Chondrodysplasia Punctata	AR	Peroxin-7	PEX7

Table 18.3: Disorders of Keratinization

Disorder	Inheritance	Protein	Gene
Sjogren–Larsson Syndrome	AR	Aldehyde dehydrogenase family 3, member A2 (fatty aldehyde dehydrogenase)	ALDH3A2 (FALDH)
X-linked Recessive (XR) Ichthyosis	XR	Steroid sulfatase	STS
Newly Described Icthyosis			
ARC (Arthrogryposis–Renal Dysfunction–Cholestasis) Syndrome	AR	Vacuolar protein sorting 33 homologue B	VPS33B
Autosomal Recessive Congenital Ichthyosis, Non-Lamellar and Non-Erythrodermic	AR	Unknown	Unknown
Autosomal Recessive Congenital Ichthyosis with Hypotrichosis	AR	Matriptase (serine protease)	ST14
Autosomal Recessive Exfoliative Ichthyosis	AR	Unknown	Unknown
CEDNIK (Cerebral Dysgenesis, Neuropathy, Ichthyosis and Keratoderma) Syndrome	AR	Synaptosomal-associated protein, 29 kDa	SNAP29
Dolichol Kinase Deficiency	AR	Dolichol kinase	DOLK
Ichthyosis–Prematurity Syndrome	AR	Unknown	Unknown
Ichthyosis–Sclerosing Cholangitis Syndrome	AR	Claudin 1	CLDN1
Other Keratinocyte Disorders			
Acral Peeling Skin Syndrome	AR	Transglutaminase 5	TGM5
Cardio-Facio-Cutaneous Syndrome	AD	v-Ki-ras2 Kirsten rat sarcoma viral oncogene homologue	KRAS
	AD	v-Raf murine sarcoma viral oncogene homologue B1	BRAF
	AD	Mitogen-activated protein kinase Kinase1	MAP2K1 (MEK1)
	AD	Mitogen-activated protein kinase Kinase2	MAP2K2 (MEK2)
Darier's Disease	AD	Sarcoplasmic/endoplasmic reticulum CA2+ ATPase 2 (SERCA2)	ATPA2
Acrokeratosis Veruciformis of Hopf	AD	Sarcoplasmic/endoplasmic reticulum CA2+ ATPase 2 (SERCA2)	ATPA2
Hailey-Hailey	AD	Human secretory pathyway Ca2+ ATPase 1 (hSPCA1)	ATP2C1
Keratolytic Winter Erythema	AD	Unknown	Unknown
Keratosis Follicularis Spinulosa Decalvans	XR	Spermidine/spermine N(1)-acetyltransferase	SAT1

Table 18.3: Disorders of Keratinization

Disorder	Inheritance	Protein	Gene
Keratosis Pilaris Atrophicans Faciei (Ulerythema Ophryogenese)	AD	Unknown	Unknown
Hailey-Hailey	AD	Human secretory pathyway Ca2+ ATPase 1 (hSPCA1)	ATP2C1
Keratolytic Winter Erythema	AD	Unknown	Unknown
Keratosis Follicularis Spinulosa Decalvans	XR	Spermidine/spermine N(1)-acetyltransferase	SAT1
Keratosis Pilaris Atrophicans Faciei (Ulerythema Ophryogenese)	AD	Unknown	Unknown
Noonan Syndrome	AD	Protein tyrosine phosphatase, non-receptor Type 11	PTPN11
	AD	v-Ki-ras2 Kirsten rat sarcoma viral oncogene homologue	KRAS
	AD	v-Raf-1 murine leukemia viral oncogene homologue	RAF-1
	AD	Son of sevenless homologue 1 (guanine Nucleotide exchange factor)	SOS1
Porokeratosis, Disseminated Superficial Actinic	AD	(?slingshot homologue 1)	(?SSH1)
Craniosynostosis, Anal Anomalies and Porokeratosis Syndrome (CAP)	AR	Unknown	Unknown
Seborrhea-like Dermatitis With Psoriasiform Elements	AD	Zinc finger protein 750	ZNF750
Dyskeratosis, hereditary Benign Intraepithelial	AD	Unknown	Unknown
White Sponge Nevus	AD	Keratin 4	K4
	AD	Keratin 13	K13

Table 18.4: Syndromic Inherited Ichthyoses

Disorder	Inheritance	Gene
X-linked ichthyoses		
Recessive X-Linked Ichthyosis (syndromic)	XLR	*STS* (and others)
IFAP Syndrome (Ichthyosis-Follicularis-Atrichia-Photophobia)	XLR	MBTPS2
Conradi-Hunermann-Happle Syndrome (Chondrodysplasia Punctata, Type 2)	XLD	EBP
Prominent hair abnormalities		
Netherton	AR	SPINK5
Ichthyosis-Hypotrichosis Syndrome (IH)	AR	ST14
Ichthyosis-Hypotrichosis-Sclerosing Cholangitis (IHSC)	AR	CLDN1
Trichothiodystrophy	AR	ERCC2 (XPD) ERCC3 (XPB) GTF2H5 (TTDA)
Trichothiodystophy not associated with Congenital Ichthyosis	AR	C7Orf11 (TTDN1)
Prominent neurologic signs		
Sjogren-Larson	AR	ALDH3A2
Refsum Syndrome (Hereditary Motor and Sensory Neuropathy, Type 4)	AR	PHYH (PEX7)
MEDNIK Syndrome	AR	AP1S1
Fatal diseases course		
Gaucher Syndrome Type 2	AR	GBA
Multiple Sulfatase Deficiency	AR	SUMF1
CEDNIK Syndrome (Cerebral Dysgenesis-Neuropathy-Ichthyosis-PPK)	AR	SNAP29
ARC Syndrome (Arthrogryposis-Renal-Cholestasis)	AR	VPS33B
Other associated signs		
KID Syndrome	AD	*GJB2* (most) *GJB6*
Neutral Lipid Storage Disease with Ichthyosis	AR	ABHD5
Ichthyosis Prematurity Syndrome	AR	SLC27A4

J. Finch & M. Payette

Table 18.5: Non-Syndromic Inherited Ichthyoses

Disorder	Inheritance	Gene	
Common ichthyoses			
Ichthyosis Vulgaris	Autosomal semidominant	FLG	
Recessive X-Linked Ichthyosis (Nonsyndromic presentation)	XLR	STS	
AR Congenital Ichthyosis (ARCI)			
Harlequin Ichthyosis	AR	ABCA12	
Lamellar Ichthyosis	AR	TGM1 NIPAL4 ALOX12B	*ABCA12 loci on 12p11.2-q13*
Congenital Ichthyosiform Erythroderma	AR	ALOXE3 ALOX12B ABCA12 CYP4F22	*NIPAL4 TGM1 Loci on 12p11.2-q13*
Self-Healing Collodion Baby	AR	TGM1 ALOX12B ALOXE3	
Acral Self-Healing Collodion Baby	AR	TGM1	
Bathing Suit Ichthyosis	AR	TGM1	
Keratinopathic Ichthyosis (KPI)			
Epidermolytic Ichthyosis (formerly EHK, Bullous CIE)	AD	K1 K10	
Superficial EI	AD	K2	
Annular EI	AD	K1 K10	
Autosomal Recessive EI	AR	K10	
Ichthyosis Curth-Macklin (formerly Ichthyosis Hystrix)	AD	K1	
Epidermolytic nevi	AR	Somatic mutations in *K1/K10*	
Other forms			
Loricrin Keratoderma (Vohwinkel keratoderma, Camisa variant)	AD	LOR	
Erythrokeratodermia Variabilis	AD	GJB3 GJB4	
Peeling Skin Disease	AR	CDSN	
Congenital Reticular Ichthyosiform Erythroderma	AD?	Locus unknown	
KLICK (Keratosis Linearis-Ichthyosis Congenita-Keratoderma)	AR	POMP	

Table 18.6: Connective Tissue Disorders

Disorder	Inheritance	Protein	Gene
Disorders with Lax Skin			
Cutis Laxa, AD	AD	Elastin	ELN
	AD	Fibulin-5	FBLN5
	AR	Fibulin-5	FBLN5
Cutis Laxa, AR	AR	EGF-containing fibulin-like extracellular Matrix protein 2 (fibulin-4)	EFEMP2 (FBLN4)
Cutis Laxa, X-linked	XR	ATPase, Cu2+-transporting Alpha-polypeptide	ATP7A
Cutis Laxa, Neonatal Marfanoid-type	AD	Laminin polypeptide subunit b1	LAMB1
Arterial Tortuosity Syndrome	AR	Solute carrier family 2 (facilitated Glucose transporter), member 10	SLC2A10
Costello Syndrome	AD	v-Ha-ras Harvey rat sarcoma viral oncogene homologue	HRAS
	AD	v-Ki-ras2 Kirsten rat sarcoma viral oncogene homologue	KRAS
Hereditary Gelsolin Amyloidosis	AD	Gelsolin	GSN
Pseudoxanthoma Elasticum (PXE)	AR	ATP-binding cassette, subfamily C,member 6	ABCC6
PXE-like Disorder with Multiple Coagulation Factor Deficiency	AR	g-glutamyl carboxylase	GGCX
Wrinkly Skin Syndrome	AR	a2 subunit of the V-type H(+)-ATPase	ATP6VOA2
Ehlers-Danlos Syndromes			
Classic EDS (Types I, II)	AD	Collagen V, a1 chain	COL5A1
	AD	Collagen V, a2 chain	COL5A2
	AD	Collagen I, a1 chain, substitution of Non-glycine residue	COL1A1
Hypermobility-type EDS (type III)	AD	Tenascin X	TNXB
	AD	Collagen III, a1 chain	COL3A1
Vascular-type EDS (Type IV)	AD	Collagen III, a1 chain	COL3A1
Kyphoscoliosis-type EDS(Type VI)	AR	Lysyl hydroxylase	PLOD
Arthrochalasia-Type EDS	AD	Collagen I, a1 chain, deletion of N Peptidase cleavage site	COL1A1
	AD	Collagen I, a2 chain, deltetion of N Peptidase cleavage site	COL1A2
Dermatosparaxis-type	AR	Procollagen I N-peptidase	ADAMTS2
Periodontitis-type	AD		
Cardiac Valvular form of EDS	AR	Collagen I, a2 chain	COL1A2
EDS with Periventricular Nodular Heterotopia	XD	Filamin A (actin-binding protein 280)	FLNA

Table 18.6: Connective Tissue Disorders

Disorder	Inheritance	Protein	Gene
Progeroid form of EDS	AR	Xylosylprotein 4b-galactosyltransferase, Polypeptide 7	B4GALT7
EDS due to tenascin-X deficiency	AR	Tenascin X	TNXB
Disorders with Excessive Extracellular Matrix Protein Deposition			
Buschke-Ollendorff Syndrome	AD	LEM domain containing 3 (Man 1, an inner nuclear membrane protein)	LEMD3 (MAN1)
Goeminne Syndrome (torticollis, keloids, cryptorchidism, renal dysplasia)	XD	Unknown	Unknown
Infantile Systemic Hyalinosis	AR	Anthrax toxin receptor 2 (capillary morphogenesis Protein 2)	ANTXR2
Juvenile Hyaline Fibromatosis	AR	Anthrax toxin receptor 2 (capillary morphogenesis protein 2)	ANTXR2
Lipoid Proteinosis	AR	Extracellular matrix Protein 1	ECM1
NAO (nodulosis, arthropathy, Osteolysis) Syndrome	AR	Matrix metalloproteinase 2	MMP2
Winchester Syndrome	AR	Matrix metalloproteinase 2	MMP2
Other Disorders			
Goltz Syndrome (focal dermal hypoplasia)	XD	Porcupine homologue	PORCN
Loeys-Dietz Syndrome	AD	TGF-β receptor 1	TGFRB1
	AD	TGF-β receptor 2	TGFRB2
Marfan Syndrome Type 1	AD	Fibrillin-1	FBN1
Marfan Syndrome Type 2	AD	TGF-β receptor 2	TGFRB2
MIDAS Syndrome (microphthalmia, dermal aplasia, and sclerocornea)	XD	Holocytochrome c Synthase	HCCS
Multiple Pterygium Syndrome	AR	Cholinergic receptor, Nicotinic g	CHRNG
Popliteal Pterygium Syndrome	AD	Interferon regulatory Factor 6	IRF6
Van der Woude Syndrome	AD	Interferon regulatory Factor 6	IRF6
Restrictive Dermopathy	AD	Lamin A/C	LMNA
	AR	Zinc metallopeptidase (STE24 homologue)	ZMPSTE24
Ullrich Disease	AR	Collagen VI, a1 chain	COL6A1
	AR	Collagen VI, a2 chain	COL6A2
	AR	Collagen VI, a3 chain	COL6A3

Table 18.7: Hereditary Disorders of Hair and Nails

Disorder	Inheritance	Protein	Gene
Disorders with Hypotrichosis			
Argininosuccinic Aciduria	AR	Argininosuccinate lyase	ASL
Atrichia with Popular Lesions	AR	Hairless (zinc finger transcriptTion factor)	HR
Bjornstad Syndrome	AR	BCS1-like (mitochondrial Membrane protein)	BCS1L
Cartilage-Hair Hypoplasia	AR	RNA component of mitochondrial RNA-processing endoribonuclease	RMRP
Giant axonal neuropathy with curly hair	AR	Gigatoxin	GAN1
Laron Syndrome (pituitary Dwarfism II)	AR	Growth hormone receptor	GHR
Hypotrichosis, Mari-type	AR	Lipase H	LIPH
Hypotrichosis, Marie-Unna-type	AD	HR, lysine demethylase and nuclear receptor corepressor	U2HR
Hypotrichosis Simplex	AD	APC down-regulated 1	APCDD1
Hypotrichosis Simplex of The Scalp	AD	Corneodesmosin	CDSN
Hypotrichosis w/ juvenile macular dystrophy	AR	Cadherin 3 (P-cadherin)	CDH3
Localized autosomal recessive hypotrichosis	AR	Desmoglein 4	DSG4
Menkes Disease	XR	Cu2+ transporting P-type ATPase 7A	ATP7A
Monilethrix	AD	Keratin 81	K81
	AD	Keratin 83	K83
	AD	Keratin 86	K86
	AR	Desmoglein 4	DSG4
T-cell immunodeficiency and congenital alopecia	AR	Forkhead box N1 (winged helix nude)	FOXN1
Trichothiodystrophy (PIBIDS)	AR	XPB; TFIIH subunit, DNA helicase	ERCC3
	AR	XPD; TFIIH subunit DNA helicase	ERCC2
	AR	General TFIIH	GTF2H5
	AR	Chromosome 7 open reading frame 11	C7orf11
	AR	M-phase-specific PLK1-interacting protein	MPLKIP
Vitamin D-dependent Rickets with Alopecia	AR	Vitamin D receptor	VDR
Disorders with Hypertrichosis			
Hypertrichosis, generalized, X-Linked	XR	Unknown	Unknown
Hypertrichosis universalis congenital	AD	Unknown	HTC1
Leigh Syndrome	Mt	Various components of mitochondrial respiratory chain complexes	(>12 genes identified)
	AR	Surfeit 1	SURF1
Zimmerman-Laband	AD	K+ voltage-gated channel subfamily H member 1	KCNH1

J. Finch & M. Payette

Table 18.7: Hereditary Disorders of Hair and Nails

Disorder	Inheritance	Protein	Gene
Nail Disorders			
Anonychia Congenita	AR	R-spondin family, member 4	RSPO4
Isolated Congenital Nail Dysplasia	AD	Unknown	ICND
Isolated Toenail Dystrophy	AD	Collagen VII, a1 chain	COL7A1
Nail-Patella Syndrome	AD	LIM homeobox transcription factor 1b	LMX1b
Pachyonychia congenita Type 1 (Jadassohn-Lewandowsky)	AD	Keratin 6a	K6a
	AD	Keratin 16	K16
Pachyonychia congenita Type 2 (Jackson-Lawler)	AD	Keratin 6b	K6b
	AD	Keratin 17	K17
Tricho-Rhino-Phalangeal Syndrome	AD	TRPS1 (zinc finger protein)	TRPS1
Yellow Nail Syndrome	AD	Forkhead box C2	FOXC2

Table 18.8: Ectodermal Dysplasias

Disorder	Inheritance	Protein	Gene
AEC (Hay-Wells, Rapp-Hodgkin) Syndrome	AD	Tumor protein p63, sterile Alpha motif (SAM) domain	TP63
EEC Syndrome	AD	Tumor protein p63, sterile Alpha motif (SAM) domain	TP63
ADULT (Acro-Dermato-Ungual-Lacrimal Tooth Syndrome)	AD	Tumor protein p63, sterile Alpha motif (SAM) domain	TP63
Limb-Mammary Syndrome	AD	Tumor protein p63, sterile Alpha motif (SAM) domain	TP63
Cleft Lip/Palate-ED Syndrome	AR	Nectin-1 poliovirus receptor related 1	PVRL1
EED Syndrome	AR	Cadherin 3 (P-cadherin)	CDH3
Ellis-van Creveld (EVC) Syndrome	AR	EVC	EVC
	AR	EVC2 (limbin)	EVC2
Hidrotic ED (Clouston Syndrome)	AD	Connexin 30 (gap jxn prot b6)	GJB6
Hypohidrotic ED	AD	Ectodysplasin A receptor	EDAR
	AR	EDAR	EDAR
	AD	EDAR-assoc death domain	EDARADD
	AR	EDAR-assoc death domain	EDARADD
	XR	Ectodysplasin A	EDA
Hypohidrotic ED w/ immunodeficiency	XR	Inhibitor of k light polypeptide gene enhancer in B cells kinase g (nuclear factor-kB essential modulator)	IKBKG (NEMO)
	AD	Nuclear factor of k light polypeptide gene enhancer in B cells inhibitor a	NFKBIA
Odonto-onycho-dermal dysplasia	AR	Wingless-type MMTV integration site family, member 10A	WNT10A
Pure Hair-Nail Type ED	AR	Keratin 85	K85
Tooth and Nail (Witkop) Syndrome	AD	Muscle segment homeobox 1	MSX1
Trich-Dento-Osseous Syndrome	AD	Distal-less homeobox 3	DLX3

Table 18.9: Cancer Syndromes

Disorder	Inheritance	Protein	Gene
Disorders with Prominent Cancer Proneness			
Bazex-Dupre-Christol	XD	Ubiquitin-conjugating enzyme E2 A	UBE2A
Epidermodysplasia Syndrome	AR	Transmembrane channel-like 6	TMC6
Epidermodysplasia Syndrome	AR	Transmembrane channel-like 8	TMC8
Familial Atypical Mole-Malignant Melanoma (FAMMM) Syndrome	AD	Cyclin dependent kinase inhibitor 2A	CDKN2A
Familial Atypical Mole-Malignant Melanoma (FAMMM) Syndrome	AD	Cyclin-dependent kinase 4	CDK4
Gorlin (nevoid basal cell CA)	AD	Patched homologue 1	PTCH1
Huriez Syndrome (sclerotylosis)	AD	Unknown	Unknown
PPK with cutaneous SCC and sex reversal	AR	R-spondin 1	RSPO1
Xeroderma Pigmentosum Group			
XPA	AR	DNA damage-binding protein and progressivity factor in nucleotide excision repair	XPA
XPB	AR	ERCC3 (TFIIH subunit 3' to 5' DNA helicase in nucleotide excision repair	ERCC3
XPC	AR	DNA damage-binding protein in nucleotide excision repair	XPC
XPD	AR	ERCC2 (TFIIH subunit 5' to 3' DNA helicase in nucleotide excision repair	ERCC2
XPE	AR	DNA damage binding protein 2	DDB2
XPF	AR	ERCC4 (5' endonuclease)	ERCC4
XPG	AR	ERCC5 (3' endonuclease)	ERCC5
XP variant	AR	DNA polymerase	POLH
PTEN Hamartoma-Tumor Syndromes			
Bannayan-Riley Ruvalcaba Syndrome	AD	Phosphatase and tensin homologue	PTEN (MMAC1)
Cowden	AD	Phosphatase and tensin homologue	PTEN (MMAC1)
Proteus-like Syndrome		Phosphatase and tensin homologue	PTEN (MMAC1)
Other Cancer Syndromes			
Ataxia telangiectasia	AR	Ataxia telangiectasia mutated phophatidylinositol 3-kinase like serine/threonin protein kinase	ATM
Birt Hogg Dube	AD	Folliculin	FLCN
Bloom Syndrome	AR	RecQ protein like 3 (DNA helicase)	BLM (RECQL3)
Cowden-like Syndrome	AD	Bone morphogenetic protein receptor Type IA	BMPR1A

Table 18.9: Cancer Syndromes

Disorder	Inheritance	Protein	Gene
Dyskeratosis congenita	XR	Dyskerin	DKC1
Dyskeratosis congenita	AD	Telomerase RNA component	TERC
Dyskeratosis congenita	AD, AR	Telomerase reverse transcriptase	TERT
Gardner Syndrome	AD	Adenomatous polyposis coli	APC
Howel-Evans Syndrome (tylosis-esophageal CA)	AD	Unknown	TOC
Muir Torre Syndrome	AD	MutS homologue 2 (mismatch repair enzyme)	MSH2
Muir Torre Syndrome	AD	MutS homologue 6 (mismatch repair enzyme)	MSH6
Muir Torre Syndrome	AD	MutL homologue 1 (mismatch repair enzyme)	MLH1
Childhood CA Syndrome (CNS, hematologic and GI malignancies) with NF 1 phenotype (formerly Lynch Syndrome)	AR	Postmeiotic segregation increased 2	PMS2
Childhood CA Syndrome (CNS, hematologic and GI malignancies) with NF 1 phenotype (formerly Lynch Syndrome)	AR	MutS homolog 2 (mismatch repair enzyme)	MSH2
Childhood CA Syndrome (CNS, hematologic and GI malignancies) with NF 1 phenotype (formerly Lynch Syndrome)	AR	MutS homolog 6 (mismatch repair enzyme)	MSH6
Childhood CA Syndrome (CNS, hematologic and GI malignancies) with NF 1 phenotype (formerly Lynch Syndrome)	AR	MutL homolog 1 (mismatch repair enzyme)	MLH1
Multiple endocrine neoplasia (MEN1)	AD	Menin	MEN1
MEN2A	AD	Ret-proto-oncogene (cysteine-rich extracellular domain)	RET
MEN2B	AD	Ret proto-oncogene (Met918Thr in substrate recognition pocket)	RET
MEN4	AD	Cyclin dependent kinase inhibitor 1B (p27, Kip1)	CDKN1B
Rothmund Thomson Syndrome	AR	recQ protein like 1 (DNA helicase)	RECQ4
Hereditary Leiomyomatosis and Renal Cell Cancer Syndrome (Reed Syndrome)	AD	Fumarate hydratase	FH

J. Finch & M. Payette

Table 18.10: Disorders with Benign Tumors

Disorder	Inheritance	Protein	Gene
Familial cylindromatosis; Brooke-Spiegler Syndrome	AD	CYLD (deubiquinating enzyme)	CYLD
Multiple familial trichoepitheliomas	AD	CYLD	CYLD
Familial mastocytosis ? gastrointestinal stromal tumors	AD	KIT proto-oncogene (stem cell factor receptor)	KIT
Infantile hemangiomas, hereditary	AD	Kinase insert domain receptor (encodes VEGFR)	KDR
Lipomatosis, familial multiple	AD	Unknown	Unknown
Maffucci Syndrome (multiple enchondromatosis)	somatic	Isocitrate dehydrogenase 1, Isocitrate dehydrogenase 2 (black, not blue)	IDH1, IDH2
Multiple self-healing squamous epitheliomas (Ferguson-Smith Syndrome)	AD	Transforming growth factor beta receptor 1	TGFBR1
Neurofibromatosis 1	AD	Neurofibromin 1 (GTPase activating protein)	NF1
Watson Syndrome; neurofibromatosis	AD	Neurofibromin 1 (GTPase activating protein)	NF1
Noonan Syndrome	AD	Protein-Tyrosine Phosphatase, Nonreceptor-type, 11	PTPN11
Neurofibromatosis 2	AD	Neurofibromin 2 (merlin)	NF2
Steatocystoma multiplex	AD	Keratin 17	K17
Tuberous sclerosis	AD	Hamartin	TSC1
	AD	Tuberin	TSC2

Table 18.11: Disorders of Pigmentation

Disorder	Inheritance	Protein	Gene
Disorders with Pigmentary Dilution			
Albinism, Oculocutaneous Types 1A, 1B (OCA1A, 1B)	AR	Tyrosinase (absent protein (OCA1A) or decreased activity (OCA1B)	TYR
Albinism, OCA 2	AR	P protein (pink eye dilution homologue)	OCA2
Albinism OCA3	AR	Tyrosinase related protein 1	TYRP1
Albinisn, OCA4	AR	Solute carrier family 45, member 2 membrane assoc transporter protein	SLC45A2
Albinism, ocular Type 1 (Nettleship-Falls)	XR	G protein coupled receptor 143	GPR143
Chédiak-Higashi Syndrome	AR	Lysosomal trafficking regulator	LYST
Griscelli Syndrome	AR	Myosin Va	MYO5A
	AR	RAS-assoc protein RAB27A	RAB27A
	AR	Melanophilin	MLPH
Hermansky Pudlak	AR	HPS1 (BLOC3 component)	HPS1
	AR	Adaptor protein 3, b1 subunit	AP3B1
	AR	HPS3 (BLOC-2 component)	HPS3
	AR	HPS4 (BLOC3 component)	HPS4
	AR	Ruby-eye 2 (BLOC-2 component)	HPS5
	AR	Ruby eye (BLOC2 component)	HPS6
	AR	Dysbindin (dystrobrevin binding prot 1)	DTNBP1
	AR	BLOC-1, subunit 3	HPS8
Tietz Syndrome	AD	Microphthalmia assoc transcription factor	MITF
Disorders with Circumscribed Leukoderma			
Piebaldism	AD	KIT proto-oncogene (stem cell factor receptor)	KIT
	AD	Snail homologue 2	SNAI2
Waardenburg Syndrome Type1	AD	Paired box gene 3	PAX3
Waardenburg Syndrome Type 2	AD	Microphthalmia-assoc transcription factor	MITF
	AR	Snail homologue 2	SNAI2
Waardenburg Syndrome Type 3	AD	Paired box gene 3	PAX3
Waardenburg Syndrome Type 4	AD, AR	Endothelin 3	EDN3
	AD	Endothelin-B receptor	EDNRB
	AD	SRY-related HMG-box gene 10	SOX10

Table 18.11: Disorders of Pigmentation

Disorder	Inheritance	Protein	Gene
Albinism, Black Lock, Cell Migration Disorder of the Neurocytes of the Gut and Deafness (ABCD)	AR	Endothelin B receptor	EDNRB
Yemenite Deaf-Blind Hypo-Pigmentation	AD	SRY-related HMG box gene 10	SOX-10
Albinism-Deafness (Ziprkowski-Margolis)	XR	Unknown	Unknown
Disorders with Hyperpigmentation			
Dermatopathia Pigmentosa Reticularis	AD	Keratin 14	KRT14
Naegeli–Franceschetti–Jadassohn Syndrome	AD	Keratin 14	KRT14
Dowling–Degos Disease	AD	Keratin 5	KRT5
Incontinentia Pigmenti	XD	Inhibitor of κ light polypeptide gene enhancer in B cells, kinase γ (nuclear factor-κB essential modulator)	IKBKG (NEMO)
McCune–Albright Syndrome	AD	Stimulatory G protein, αsubunit (G$_s$α; activating mutations)	GNAS
X-linked Reticulate Pigmentary Disorder, Partington-type	XR	Catalytic Subunit of DNA Polymerase	POLA1
Dyschromatoses			
Dyschromatosis Symmetrica Hereditaria	AD	Adenosine deaminase, RNA-specific	ADAR
Dyschromatosis Universalis Hereditaria	AD	ATP-binding cassette B6	ABCB6
Multiple Lentigines			
Carney Complex (LAMB/NAME Syndrome)	AD	Protein kinase A regulatory subunit 1a	PRKAR1A
Familial Generalized Lentiginosis	AD	Unknown	Unknown
LEOPARD	AD	Protein tyrosine phosphatase, nonreceptor Type 11	PTPN11 (SHP2)
LEOPARD	AD	v-Raf-1 murine leukemia viral oncogene homologue	RAF1
Peutz-Jeghers Syndromes	AD	Serine-threonine kinase 11	STK11 (LKB1)

Table 18.12: Disorders of Metabolism

Disorder	Inheritance	Protein	Gene
Disorders Due to Enzyme Deficiencies			
Alkaptonuria	AR	Homogentisic acid oxidase deficiency	HGD
Biotinidase Deficiency	AR	Biotinidase	BTD
Holocarboxylase Synthetase Defic	AR	Holocarboxylase synthetase	HLCS
Fabry Disease	XR	Alpha galactosidase A	GLA
Fucosidosis	AR	Alpha L fucosidase	FUCA1
Farber Lipogranulomatosis	AR	Acid ceramidase	ASAH
Gaucher Disease Types I-III	AR	Acid beta glucosidase (glucocerebrosidase)	GBA
Hereditary Angioedema Type 1, II	AD	Serpin peptidase inhibitor (C1 inhibitor)	SERPING1
Hereditary Angioedema, Type III	AD	Factor XII (Hageman factor)	F12
Homocystinuria	AR	Cystathionine beta synthase	CBS
Niemann Pick Disease Type A	AR	Acid sphingomyelinase	SMPD1
Phenylketonuria	AR	Phenylalanine hydroxylase	PAH
Phenylketonuria	AR	Quinoid dihydropteridine reductase	QDPR
Phenylketonuria	AR	6-Pyruvoyltetrahydropterin synthase	PTS
Prolidase Deficiency	AR	Prolidase (peptidase D)	PEPD
Defective Transporters/Related Proteins			
Acrodermatitis Enteropathica	AR	Solute carrier family 39, member 4 (Zinc transporter)	SLC39A4
Hartnup Disease	AR	Solute carrier family 6, member 0 (Neutral amino acid transporter)	SLC6A19
Hemochromatosis	AR	Hemochromatosis	HFE
Hemochromatosis	AR	Transferrin receptor 2	TFR2
Hemochromatosis	AD	Solute carrier family 40, member 1 (Ferroportin)	SLC11A3
Hemochromatosis, Juvenile	AR	Hepcidin antimicrobial peptide	HAMP
Hemochromatosis, Juvenile	AR	Hemojuvelin	HFE2
Wilson Disease	AR	Cu2+ transporting P-type ATPase 7B	ATP7B
Hyperlipidemias			
Lipoprotein Lipase Deficiency (Type 1 Hyperlipoproteinemia)	AR	Lipoprotein lipase	LPL
Apolipoprotein CII Deficiency (Type 1 Hyperlipoproteinemia)	AR	Apolipoprotein C-II	APOC2
Familial Hypercholesterolemia (Type II Lipoproteinemia)	AD	LDL receptor	LDLR
Familial Hypercholesterolemia (Type II Lipoproteinemia)	AD	Apolipoprotein B-100, LDL receptor binding domain	APOB
Familial Hypercholesterolemia (Type II Lipoproteinemia)	AD	Proprotein convertase subtilisin /kexin Type 9	PCSK9
Dysbetalipoproteinemia (Type III Hyperlipoproteinemia)	AR	Apolipoprotein E	APOE

Table 18.12: Disorders of Metabolism

Disorder	Inheritance	Protein	Gene
Familial Hypertriglyceridemia (Type IV Hyperlipoproteinemia)	AD	Lipase member I	LIPI
	AD	Apolipoprotein A-V	APOA5
Cerebrotendinous Xanthomatosis	AR	Cytochrome P-450, subfamily 27A, polypeptide 1 (sterol 27 hydroxylase)	CYP27
Hypoalpha-Lipoproteinemia	AD	Apolipoprotein A-1	APOA1
Tangier Disease	AR	ATP-binding cassette 1, subfamily A, member 1 (cholesterol efflux regulatory protein)	ABCA1
Sitosterolemia	AR	ATP-binding cassette, sub fam G, member 5 (Sterolin 1)	ABCG5
	AR	ATP-binding cassette, sub fam G, member 8 (Sterolin 2)	ABCG8
Porphyrias			
Congenital Erythropoietic Porphyria (Gunther Disease)	AR	Uroporphyrinogen-III synthase	UROS
Hepatoerythropoietic Porphyria	AR	Uroporphyrinogen –III decarboxylase	UROD
Porphyria Cutanea Tarda	AD	Uroporphyrinogen-III decarboxylase	UROD
Hereditary Coproporphyria	AD	Coproporphyrinogen oxidase	CPOX
Variegate Porphyria	AD	Protoporphyrinogen oxidase	PPOX
Erythropoietic Protoporphyria	AD	Ferrochelatase	FECH

Table 18.13: Disorders with Vascular Anomalies

Disorder	Inheritance	Protein	Gene
Capillary Malformations			
Port Wine Stain	NI		GNAQ
Sturge-Weber	NI	Gaq	GNAQ
Hereditary Hemorrhagic Telangiectasia (HHT, Rendu-Osler-Weber Syndrome) –Type 1	AD	Endoglin (component of endothelial cell TGF-b receptor)	ENG
HHT, Type 2	AD	Activin A receptor Type II-like 1 (component of endothelial cell TGF-B receptor)	ACVRL1 (ALK1)
HHT, Type 3	AD		Unknown
HHT, Type 4	AD	SMAD family member 4 (transmits signals from TGF-B receptor)	SMAD4
Hereditary Hemorrhagic Telangiectasia with Juvenile Polyposis	AD	SMAD family member 4 (transmits signals from TGF-B receptor)	SMAD4
CMTC	NI	Unknown	unknown
Capillary Malformation-AVM	AD	RAS p21 protein activator 1 (GTPase activating protein)	RASA1
Beckwith-Weidemann	AD	p57	CDKN1C
Von-Hippel Lindau	AD	VHL gene (many protein products)	VHL
Lymphatic Malformations			
Milroy Syndrome	AD	VEGF receptor 3	FLT4 / VEGFR3
Primary Hereditary Lymphedema	AD	Gap Junction C2 (Connexin 47)	GJC2
	AD	Vascular Endothelial Growth Factor C	VEGFC
Lymphedema with Distichiasis	AD	Forkhead box C2	FOXC2
Yellow Nail Syndrome	AD	Forkhead box C2	FOXC2
Primary Lymphedema with Myelodysplasia	AD	Gata-Binding Protein 2	GATA2
Hennekam Lymphangiectasia-Lymphedema Syndrome (Primary Generalized Lymphatic Anomaly)	AR	Collagen And Calcium-Binding EGF Domain	CCBE1
Lymphedema-Choanal Atresia	AR	Protein-Tyrosine Phosphatase, Nonreceptor-type, 14	PTPN14
Lymphedema Praecox (Meige Lymphedema)	AD	Forkhead box C2	FOXC2
Hypotrichosis-Lymphedema-Telangiectasia Syndrome	AD, AR	Sex determining region Y (SRY)-box 18	SOX18

Table 18.13: Disorders with Vascular Anomalies

Disorder	Inheritance	Protein	Gene
Lymphedema, Hereditary Early Onset-type (Milroy Disease)	AD	FMA-related tyrosine kinase 4 (vascular endothelial growth factor receptor 3)	FLT4
Venous Malformations			
Glomuvenous Malformations (Glomangiomatosis)	AD	Glomulin	GLMN
Blue Rubber Bleb Nevus Syndrome	Sporadic	Unknown	Unknown
Familial Cutaneous and Mucosal Venous Malformation	AD	Tyrosine Kinase, Endothelial	TEK (TIE2)
Maffucci's Syndrome (Multiple Enchondromatosis)	Somatic	Isocitrate Dehydrogenase 1 and 2	IDH1 and 2
Familial Glomangiomatosis (Glomuvenous Malformations)	AD	Glomulin	GLMN
Vascular Malformations with Other Anomalies			
Parkes Weber Syndrome	Sporadic > AD	p120-RasGAP	RASA1
Sturge-Weber Syndrome	Somatic	Gaq	GNAQ
Klippel-Trenaunay Syndrome	Sporadic	Phosphatidylinositol 3-kinase (p110a subunit)	PIK3CA
Maffucci Syndrome	Somatic	Isocitrate dehydrogenase 1 and 2	IDH1 and 2
Macrocephaly-CM (M-CM or MCAP)	Sporadic	Phosphatidylinositol 3-kinase (p110a subunit)	PIK3CA
Microcephaly-CM (MICCAP)	AR	STAM Binding Protein	STAMBP
CLOVES Syndrome	Somatic	Phosphatidylinositol 3-kinase (p110a subunit)	PIK3CA
Proteus Syndrome	Sporadic	AKT1 Kinase	AKT1
Bannayan-Riley-Ruvalcaba	AD	Phosphatase and tensin homolog	PTEN
Disorders with AVMs			
Cerebral Capillary Malformations, Familial (Associated with Hyperkeratotic Cutaneous Capillary-Venous Malformations)	AD	Krev interaction trapped-1	KRIT1
Other Vascular Disorders			
Ataxia-Telangiectasia	AR	phosphatidylinositol 3-kinase	ATM
Primary Erythromelalgia	AD	Sodium channel, voltage-gated, Type IX, alpha-subunit	SCN9A

Table 18.14: Other Inherited Skin Disorders

Disorder	Inheritance	Protein	Gene
Craniosynostosis / Skeletal Dysplasia Syndromes			
Apert Syndrome	AD	Fibroblast growth factor receptor 2	FGFR2
Beare-Stevenson Cutis Gyrata Syndrome	AD	Fibroblast growth factor receptor 2	FGFR2
Crouzon Syndrome with Acanthosis Nigricans; SADDAN; Thanatophoric Dysplasia	AD	Fibroblast growth factor receptor 3	FGFR3
Oral Facial Digital Syndrome	XD	Oral Facial Digital Syndrome	OFD1
Prominent Neuro Abnormalities			
Cockayne Syndrome CSA	AR	ERCC8 (transcription-coupled repair protein)	ERCC8
Cockayne Syndrome CSB	AR	ERCC6 (transcription coupled repair protein)	ERCC6
Cold-induced Sweating Syndrome	AR	Cytokine receptor-like factor 1	CRLF1
	AR	Cardiotrophin-like cytokine factor 1	CLCF1
Familial Dysautonomia (Riley-Day Syndrome)	AR	Inhibitor of k light polypeptide gene enhancer in B cells, kinase complex-assoc protein	IKBKAP
Insensitivity to Pain with Anhidrosis	AR	Neurotrophic tyrosine kinase receptor Type 1	NTRK1
Defects in Coagulation or Platelet Plugging			
Activated Protein C Resistance (Factor V Leiden)	AD	Factor V	F5
Protein C Deficiency	AD	Protein C	PROC
Protein S Deficiency	AD	Protein S	PROS1
Antithrombin III Deficiency	AD	Serpin peptidase inhibitor C1 (antithrombin III)	SERPINC1
Hypoprothrombinemia	AD	Prothrombin, G20210A polymorphism	F2
Thrombotic Dhrombocytopenic Purpura, Familial	AR	ADAM metallopeptidase with thrombospondin Type 1 motif, 13 (VWF cleaving protease)	ADAMTS13
Premature Aging Syndromes			
Progeria (Hutchinson-Gilford)	AD>>AR	Lamin A/C	LMNA
Mandibuloacral Dysplasia	AR	Lamin A/C	LMNA
Atypical Werner Syndrome	AD	Lamin A/C	LMNA
	AR	Zinc metallopeptidase (STE24 homologue)	ZMPSTE24
Werner Syndrome	AR	RecQ protein-like 2 (DNA helicase)	WRN (REC-QL2)

J. Finch & M. Payette

Table 18.14: Other Inherited Skin Disorders

Disorder	Inheritance	Protein	Gene
Lipodystrophy Syndromes			
Leprechaunism (Rabson-Mendenhall Syndrome)	AR	Insulin receptor	INSR
Lipodystrophy, Congenital Generalized (Berardinelli Seip)	AR	Seipen	BSCL2
Lipodystrophy, Familial Partial	AD	Lamin A/A	LMNA
	AD	Peroxisome proliferators activated receptor g	PPARG
Lipodystrophy, Acquired Partial (Barraquer Simons Syndrome)	AD	LMNB2	Lamin B2
Cutaneous Calcification			
Albright's Hereditary Osteodystrophy	AD	Stimulatory G protein, alpha subunit	GNAS
Progressive Osseous Heteroplasia	AD	Stimulatory G protein, alpha subunit	GNAS
Fibrodysplasia Ossificans Progresiva	AD	Activin A receptor, Type I	ACVR1
Hyperphosphatemic Familial Tumoral Calcinosis	AR	UDP-N-acetyl aD galactosamine polypeptide	GALNT3
	AR	Fibroblast growth factor 23	FGF23
	AR	Klotho	KL
Normophophatemic Familial Tumoral Calcinosis	AR	Sterile alpha motif domain-containing 9	SAMD9

Table 18.15: Autoinflammatory Syndromes

Disorder	Inheritance	Protein	Gene
Blau Syndrome	AD	Nucleotide-binding oligomerization domain containing 2	NOD2 (CARD15)
CINCA/NOMID (Chronic Infantile Neurologic Cutaneous and Articular Syndrome)	AD	NLR family, pyrin domain containing 3 (cryopyrin)	NLRP3 (CIAS1)
Cyclic neutropenia	AD	Neutrophil elastase	ELA2
DIRA (Deficiency in IL-1 Receptor Antagonist)	AR	IL-1 Receptor antagonist	IL1RN
Familial chilblain lupus	AD	3' repair TREX1 endonuclease 1	TREX1
Familial Cold Autoinflammatory Syndrome	AD	NLR family, pyrin domain containing 3 (cryopyrin)	NLRP3 (CIAS1)
Familial Hibernian Fever (TRAPS)	AD	TNF receptor superfamily, member 1A	TNFRSF1A
Familial Mediterranean Fever	AR	Pyrin (marenostrin)	MEFV
Hyperimmunoglobulin-emia D Syndrome	AR	Mevalonate kinase	MVK
Majeed Syndrome	AR	Lipin 2	LPIN2
Muckle-Wells Syndrome	AD	NLR family, pyrin domain containing 3 (cryopyrin)	NLRP3 (CIAS1)
PAPA (Pyogenic Arthritis, Pyoderma Gangrenosum, Acne Syndrome)	AD	Protein serine threonine phosphatase interacting protein 1	PSTPIP1
PFAPA Syndrome		Binds pyrin	PSTPIP1

Table 18.16: Immunodeficiency Syndromes

Disorder	Inheritance	Protein	Gene
Autoimmune Polyendocrinopathy (APECED, Candidiasis-Ectodermal Dystrophy)	AR	Autoimmune regulator	AIRE
Candidiasis, Familial Chronic Mucocutaneous	AD	Caspase recruitment domain-containing protein 9; Interleukin-17 receptor C; Signal transducer and activator of transcription 1	CARD9, IL17RC, STAT1
Chronic Granulomatous Disease	XR	Cytochrome b beta-polypeptide (p91-phox)	CYBB
	AR	Cytochrome b alpha-polypeptide (p22-phox)	CYBA
	AR	Neutrophil cytosolic factor 1 (p47 phox component of NADPH oxidase)	NCF1
	AR	Neutrophil cytosolic factor 2 (p67 phox component of NADPH oxidase)	NCF2
Hyperimmunoglobulinemia E (Job) AD Syndrome	AD	Signal transducer and activator of transcription 3	STAT3
	AR	Tyrosine kinase 2	TYK2
IPEX (Immune Dysregulation Polyendocrinopathy, Enteropathy X-linked Syndrome)	XR	Forkhead box P3	FOXP3
Leukocyte Adhesion Deficiency Type 1	AR	Beta2-integrin	ITGB2
Leukocyte adhesion Deficiency Type 2	AR	Solute carrier family 35, member C1 (GDP-fucose transporter 1)	SLC35G1
Leukocyte Adhesion Deficiency Type 3	AR	RAS guanyl releasing protein 2	RASGRP2
Omenn Syndrome	AR	Recombination activating gene 1	RAG1
	AR	Recombination activating gene 2	RAG2
	AR	DNA cross-link repair 1C (artemis)	DCLRE1C
WHIM (Warts, Hypogammaglobulinemia, Infections, and Myelokathexis Syndrome	AD	Chemokine (C-X-C motif) receptor 4	CXCR4
Wiskot Aldrich Syndrome	XR	WAS protein	WAS

Table 18.17: Non-EB Skin Fragility Syndromes

Disorder	Inheritance	Protein	Gene
Ectodermal Dysplasia/ Skin Fragility Syndrome	AR	Plakophilin 1	PKP1
Kindler Syndrome	AR	Kindlin 1	KIND1 (C20orf42)
Laryngo-onycho-Cutaneous (Shabbir) Syndrome	AR	Laminin-5 (332) polypeptide Subunit a3	LAMA3
Lethal acantholytic Epidermolysis Bullosa	AR	Desmoplakin	DSP
Skin Fragility/Woolly Hair Syndrome	AR	Desmoplakin	DSP
Mendes da Costa Syndrome (Macular-type Hereditary Bullous Dystrophy)	XR	Unknown	Unknown
Nephropathy with Pretibial Epidermolysis Bullosa and Deafness	AR	Platelet-endothelial cell tetraspanin Antigen 3 (CD151)	CD151

J. Finch & M. Payette

Disorder	Inheritance	Gene	Protein
Acral Peeling Skin Syndrome	AR	TGM5	Transglutaminase 5
Acro-Dermato-Ungual-Lacrimal Tooth (ADULT) Syndrome	AD	TP63	p63
Acrodermatitis Enteropathica	AR	SLC39A4	Solute carrier family 39, member 4 (zinc transporter)
Acrokeratosis Verruciformis of Hopf	AD	ATP2A2	Sarcoplasmic/endoplasmic reticulum Ca2+ ATPase 2 (SERCA2)
Activated protein C resistance (Factor V Leiden)	AD	F5	Factor V
Acute Megakaryocyte Leukemia	Somatic	GATA1	Mutation seen in 20% of transient myeloproliferation d/o of Down Syndrome
ADA2 Deficiency	AR	ADA2	Adenosine deaminase
Adams-Oliver Syndrome 1	AD	ARHGAP31	Rho-GTPase-Activating Protein 31
Adams-Oliver Syndrome 2	AR	DOCK6	Dedicator of cytokinesis 6
Alagille-Watson Syndrome	AD	JAG1	Jagged 1
Albinism Deafness Syndrome (Woolf Syndrome, Ziprkowski-Margolis Syndrome)	XLR	ADFN	Unknown
Albinism, Black lock, Cell migration Disorder of the Neurocytes of the Gut and Deafness (ABCD)	AR	EDNRB	Endothelin Receptor, Type B
Albinism, Ocular Type 1 (Nettleship-Falls)	XLR	GPR143	G protein coupled receptor 143
Albright's Hereditary Osteodystrophy	AD	GNAS	G protein, α subunit
Alkaptonuria (Ochronosis)	AR	HGD	Homogentisic acid oxidase
Angelman Syndrome	NI	UBE3A	Ubiquitin-Protein Ligase E3A; genomic imprinting caused by deletion or inactivation of genes on the maternally inherited chromosome 15
Anhidrotic Ectodermal Dysplasia (Hypohidrotic Ectodermal Dysplasia)	XLR	EDA	Ectodysplasin A

Disorder	Inheritance	Gene	Protein
Ankyloblepharon-Ectodermal Dysplasia-Cleft Lip/Palate (AEC) Syndrome (Hay-Wells Syndrome, Rapp-Hodgkin Syndrome)	AD	TP63	p63
Anonychia Congenita	AR	RSPO4	R-spondin family, member 4
Antithrombin III Deficiency	AD	SERPINC1	Serpin peptidase inhibitor C1 (antithrombin III)
Apert Syndrome	AD	FGFR2	Fibroblast growth factor receptor 2
Apolipoprotein CII Deficiency (Type I Hyperlipoproteinemia)	AR	APOC2	Apolipoprotein C-II
Aquagenic Wrinkling of the Palms	AR	CFTR	Cystic Fibrosis Transmembrane Conductance Regulator
Argininosuccinic Aciduria	AR	ASL	Argininosuccinate lysase
Arrhythmogenic Right Ventricular Dysplasia/Cardiomyopathy (ARVD/C)	AD	DSG2	Desmoglein 2
Arterial Tortuosity Syndrome	AR	SLC2A10	Solute carrier family 2, member 10 (facilitated glucose transporter)
Arthrogryposis–Renal Dysfunction–Cholestasis (ARC) Syndrome	AR	VPS33B	Vacuolar protein sorting 33 homolog B
Ataxia-Telangiectasia	AR	ATM	Ataxia-telangiectasia mutated (phosphatidy-linositol 3-kinase like serine/threonine protein kinase)
Athabascan-type Severe Combined Immunodeficiency (SCIDA)	AR	DCLRE1C	Protein artemis (Endonuclease involved in V(D)J recombination and DNA repair)
Atrichia with Papules	AR	HR	Hairless (zinc finger transcription factor)
Autoimmune Polyendocrinopathy (APECED, Candidiasis-Ectodermal Dystrophy)	AR>AD	AIRE	Autoimmune regulator
Azathioprine Myelosuppression	NI	---	Thiopurine methyltransferase (TPMT)

Disorder	Inheritance	Gene	Protein
Bannayan-Riley-Ruvalcaba Syndrome	AD	PTEN	Phosphatase and tensin homolog (tyrosine kinase)
Bart-Pumphrey Syndrome	AD	GJB2	Gap junction protein β2 (connexin 26)
Bart's Syndrome	AD	COL7A1	α1 chain of Type VII collagen
Basal Cell Carcinoma, Sporadic	Sporadic	PTCH1, PTCH2, SUFU	Sonic hedgehog pathway mutations
Basal Cell Carcinoma, Sporadic	Sporadic	SMO	Smoothened (G protein-coupled receptor-like receptor)
Basal Cell Carcinoma, sporadic	Sporadic	TP53	p53
Basal Cell Nevus Syndrome (Gorlin Syndrome)	AD	PTCH1	Patched homolog 1
Bazex-Dupré-Christol Syndrome (Bazex Syndrome, Follicular Atrophoderma and Basal Cell Carcinomas)	XLD	UBE2A*	Protein involved in repair of UV-damaged DNA
Beare-Stevenson Cutis Gyrata Syndrome	AD	FGFR2	Fibroblast growth factor receptor 2
Beckwith-Wiedemann	AD	IGF2, (also H19, p57 (KIP2), CDKN1C, NSD1, and LIT1)	Insulin-like growth factor 2
Berardinelli-Seip Syndrome Type 1 (Congenital Generalized Lipodystrophy Type 1)	AR	AGPAT2	1-Acylglycerol-3-phosphate O-acyltransferase 2
Biotinidase Deficiency	AR	BTD	Biotinidase
Birt-Hogg-Dubé Syndrome	AD	FLCN	Folliculin
Björnstad Syndrome	AR	BCS1L	ATPase needed for mitochondrial assembly
Blau Syndrome (Familial Granulomatous Arthritis, Dermatitis and Uveitis)	AD	NOD2 (CARD 15)	Nucleotide-binding oligomerization domain containing 2
Bloom Syndrome	AR	RECQL3	RecQ protein like 3 (DNA helicase)
Brooke-Spiegler Syndrome	AD	CYLD	Deubiquitinating enzyme (removes lys63-linked ubiquitin chains)
Burkitt's Lymphoma	NI	MYC	V-MYC Avian Myelocytomatosis Viral Oncogene Homolog

Disorder	Inheritance	Gene	Protein
Buschke-Ollendorff Syndrome	AD	LEMD3 (MAN1)	LEM domain containing 3 (Man 1, an inner nuclear membrane protein)
CADASIL (Cerebral Autosomal-Dominant Arteriopathy with Subcortical Infarcts and Leukoencephalopathy)	AD	NOTCH-3	Notch Drosophila Homolog, 3
Candidiasis, Familial Chronic Mucocutaneous Type 1	AD	Unknown	Unknown
Candidiasis, Familial Chronic Mucocutaneous Type 2	AR	CARD9	Caspase recruitment domain-containing protein 9
Candidiasis, Familial Chronic Mucocutaneous Type 3	AD	Unknown	Unknown
Candidiasis, Familial Chronic Mucocutaneous Type 4	AR	CLEC7A	Dectin-1 (pattern recognition receptor)
Candidiasis, Familial Chronic Mucocutaneous Type 5	Unknown	IL17RA	Interleukin-17 Receptor A
Candidiasis, Familial Chronic Mucocutaneous Type 6	Unknown	IL17F	Interleukin-17
CANDLE (Chronic Atypical Neutrophilic Dermatosis with Lipodystrophy and Elevated Temperature) Syndrome	AD	PSMB8	Proteasome subunit, β-type, 8
CAP (Craniosynostosis, Anal Anomalies and Porokeratoses) Syndrome	AR	FGFR1, FGFR2, FGFR3	Fibroblast growth factor receptor 1, 2, 3
Capillary Malformation-Arteriovenous Malformation	AD	RASA1	RAS p21 protein activator 1 (GTPase activating protein)
Cardio-Facio-Cutaneous Syndrome	AD	BRAF	V-RAF murine sarcoma viral oncogene homolog
Cardio-Facio-Cutaneous Syndrome	AD	KRAS	V-KI-RAS2 Kirsten rat sarcoma viral oncogene homolog
Cardio-Facio-Cutaneous Syndrome	AD	MAP2K1 (MEK1)	Mitogen-activated protein kinase 1
Cardio-Facio-Cutaneous Syndrome	AD	MAP2K2 (MEK2)	Mitogen-activated protein kinase 2
Carney Complex (LAMB/NAME Syndrome)	AD	PRKAR1A	Protein kinase A regulatory subunit 1a

Disorder	Inheritance	Gene	Protein
Cartilage-Hair Hypoplasia Syndrome	AR	RMRP	RNA component of mitochondrial RNA-processing endoribonuclease
Carvajal Syndrome	AR	DSP	Desmoplakin
CEDNIK (Cerebral Dysgenesis, Neuropathy, Ichthyosis and Keratoderma) Syndrome	AR	SNAP29	Synaptosomal-associated protein, 29 kDa
Cerebral Capillary Malformations, Familial (associated with hyperkeratotic cutaneous capillary-venous malformations)	AD	KRIT1 (CCM1)	Krev interaction trapped-1
Cerebrotendinous Xanthomatosis	AR	CYP27A1	Cytochrome P450, subfamily 27A1 (sterol 27 hydroxylase)
Chédiak-Higashi Syndrome	AR	LYST	Lysosomal trafficking regulator
CHILD Syndrome (Congenital Hemidysplasia with Ichthyosiform Erythroderma and Limb Defects)	XLD	NSDHL	3ß-hydroxysteroid dehydrogenase
Childhood Cancer Syndrome (CNS, Hematologic and GI malignancies) with NF 1 Phenotype (Formerly Lynch Syndrome)	AR	PMS2	Postmeiotic segregation increased
Chronic Granulomatous Disease	AR	CYBA	α subunit of cytochrome b(-245)
Chronic Granulomatous Disease	XLR	CYBB	α subunit of cytochrome b(-245)
Chronic Granulomatous Disease	AR	NCF1, NCF2, NCF4	Neutrophil cytosolic factor 1, 2, or 4
CINCA Syndrome (NOMID)	AD	CIAS1 (NLRP3)	NLR family, pyrin domain containing 3 (cryopyrin)
Citrullinemia	AR	ASS1	Argininosuccinate synthetase 1
CLOVE (Congenital, Lipomatous, Overgrowth, Vascular Malformations, Epidermal Nevi and Spinal/Skeletal Anomalies and/or Scoliosis) Syndrome	Somatic	PIK3CA	Phosphatidy-linositol 3-kinase, catalytic, α
Cockayne Syndrome A	AR	ERCC8	DNA helicase, excision repair cross-complementing, group 6

Disorder	Inheritance	Gene	Protein
Cockayne Syndrome B	AR	ERCC6	DNA helicase, excision repair cross-complementing, group 6
Cold-Induced Sweating Syndrome Type 1	AR	CRLF1	Cytokine receptor-like factor 1
Cold-Induced Sweating Syndrome Type 2	AR	CLCF1	Cardiotrophin-like cytokine factor 1
Common Variable Immunodeficiency	AR	CD19	CD19 B-lymphocyte antigen
Common Variable Immunodeficiency	AR	CD20 (MS4A1)	Membrane-spanning 4 Domains, Subfamily A, Member 1
Common Variable Immunodeficiency	AR	CD81	CD81 antigen
Common Variable Immunodeficiency	AR	ICOS	Inducible T-cell costimulator
Common Variable Immunodeficiency	Sporadic > AR > AD	TNFRSF13B	Transmembrane activator & CAML interactor (TACI)
Congenital Contractural Arachnodactyly	AD	FBN2	Fibrillin 2
Congenital Corneal Dystrophy	AD	DCN	Decorin
Congenital Insensitivity to Pain	AR	SCN9A	Voltage-gated sodium channel
Conradi-Hünermann-Happle Syndrome	XLD	EBP	D8-D7 sterol isomerase (emoparmil binding protein)
Conradi-Hünermann-Happle Syndrome	AR	PEX7	Peroxin 7
Cornea Plana Congenita	AR	KERA	Keratocan
Costello Syndrome	AD	HRAS	V-HA-RAS Harvey rat sarcoma viral oncogene homolog
Costello Syndrome	AD	KRAS	V-KI-RAS2 Kirsten rat sarcoma viral oncogene homolog
Cowden Syndrome	AD	PTEN	Phosphatase and tensin homolog (tyrosine kinase)
Cowden-like Polyposis Syndrome	AD	BMPR1A	Bone morphogenetic protein receptor Type IA
Crouzon Syndrome with Acanthosis Nigricans (SADDAN Syndrome, Thanatophoric Dysplasia)	AD	FGFR3	Fibroblast growth factor receptor 3
Cutis Laxa, AD	AD	ELN	Elastin

Disorder	Inheritance	Gene	Protein
Cutis Laxa, Neonatal Marfanoid-type	AD	LAMB1	Laminin polypeptide, β1 subunit
Cutis Laxa, Type IA	AR	FBLN5	Fibulin 5
Cutis Laxa, Type IB	AR	EFEMP2 (FBLN4)	EGF-containing fibulin-like extracellular matrix protein 2 (fibulin-4)
Cutis Laxa, Type IIA	AR	ATP6V0A2	ATPase, H+ transporting, lysosomal, V0 Subunit A2
Cutis Laxa, Type IIB	AR	PYCR1	Pyrroline-5-carboxylate reductase 1
Cutis Laxa, X-linked	XLR	ATP7A	ATPase, Cu2+-transporting, α-polypeptide
Cyclic Neutropenia	AD	ELA2	Neutrophil elastase
Cylindroma, sporadic tumor	sporadic	CYLD	Deubiquitinating enzyme (removes lys63-linked ubiquitin chains)
Darier's Disease (Keratosis Follicularis)	AD	ATP2A2	Sarcoplasmic/endoplasmic reticulum Ca2+ ATPase 2 (SERCA2)
De Barsy Syndrome (AR Cutis Laxa IIIa)	AR	ALDH18A1	Aldehyde dehydrogenase family 18, member A1 (Glutamate γ-semialdehyde synthetase)
De Sanctis-Cacchione Syndrome	AR	ERCC6	DNA helicase, excision repair cross-complementing, group 6
Dermatofibrosarcoma Protuberans (DFSP)	sporadic	PDGFB/COL1A1	t(17;22) chromosome translocation; fusion of COL1A1 and PDGFB genes
Dermatopathia Pigmentosa Reticularis	AD	K14	Keratin 14
Diffuse Neonatal Hemangiomatosis	NI	---	---
DiGeorge Syndrome (CATCH-22, Thymic Hypoplasia)	AD	TBX1	T-box 1
Dimethylglycine Dehydrogenase Deficiency	AR	DMGDH	Dimethylglycine dehydrogenase
DIRA (Deficiency of the Interleukin-1 Receptor Antagonist) Syndrome	AR	IL1RN	Interleukin 1 receptor antagonist

Disorder	Inheritance	Gene	Protein
Disseminated Superficial Porokeratosis	AD	SART3	Squamous Cell Carcinoma Antigen Recognized by T cells 3
Dolichol Kinase Deficiency	AR	DOLK	Dolichol kinase
Dowling-Meara Epidermolysis Bullosa	AD	K14	Keratin 14
Dowling-Meara Epidermolysis Bullosa	AD	K5	Keratin 5
Dowling–Degos Disease (Reticulate Pigment Anomaly of Flexures)	AD	K5	Keratin 5
Down Syndrome	Chromosome 21	Trisomy 21	N/A
Dysbetalipoproteinemia (Type III Hyperlipoproteinemia)	AR	APOE	Apolipoprotein E
Dyschromatosis Symmetrica Hereditaria	AD	ADAR	Adenosine deaminase, RNA-specific
Dyschromatosis Universalis Hereditaria	AD	Unknown	Unknown
Dyskeratosis Congenita (Zinsser-Engman-Cole Syndrome)	AD or AR	ACD	Telomere protein
Dyskeratosis Congenita (Zinsser-Engman-Cole Syndrome)	AR	CTC1, NHP2, NOP10, PARN, WRAP53	Telomerase complex components
Dyskeratosis Congenita (Zinsser-Engman-Cole Syndrome)	XLR	DKC1	Dyskerin
Dyskeratosis Congenita (Zinsser-Engman-Cole Syndrome)	AD or AR	RTEL1	Regulator of telomere elongation helicase 1
Dyskeratosis Congenita (Zinsser-Engman-Cole Syndrome)	AD	TERC, TINF2	Telomerase complex components
Dyskeratosis Congenita (Zinsser-Engman-Cole Syndrome)	AD or AR	TERT	Telomerase catalytic subunit
Dyskeratosis, Hereditary Benign Intraepithelial	AD	Unknown	Unknown
Ectodermal Dysplasia, Hypohidrotic, with Immune Deficiency	XLR	NEMO	NF-Kappa-B Essential Modulator
Ectodermal Dysplasia/Skin Fragility Syndrome	AR	PKP1	Plakophilin 1
Ectrodactyly Ectodermal Dysplasia Cleft Lip/Palate (EEC) Syndrome	AD	TP63	p63

Ludicrous 17-Page Genoderm Table (sorted by disease)

Disorder	Inheritance	Gene	Protein
Ectrodactyly Ectodermal Dysplasia Cleft Lip/Palate (EED) Syndrome	AR	CDH3	Cadherin 3 (P-cadherin)
Ehlers-Danlos Syndrome, Arthrochalasia-type	AD	COL1A1	α1 chain of Type I collagen
Ehlers-Danlos Syndrome, Arthrochalasia-type	AD	COL1A2	α2 chain of Type I collagen
Ehlers-Danlos Syndrome, Cardiac Valvular-type	AR	COL1A2	α2 chain of Type I collagen
Ehlers-Danlos Syndrome, Classic	AD	COL5A1	α1 chain of Type V collagen
Ehlers-Danlos Syndrome, Classic	AD	COL5A2	α2 chain of Type V collagen
Ehlers-Danlos Syndrome, Classic	AR	TNXB	Tenascin X, a glycoprotein of the extracellular matrix
Ehlers-Danlos Syndrome, Cleft Lip/Palate-type	AR	PVRL1	Nectin-1 poliovirus receptor related 1
Ehlers-Danlos Syndrome, Dermatosparaxis-type	AR	ADAMTS-2	A disintegrin-like and metalloproteinase with thrombospondin Type 1 motif, 2 (Procollagen I N-peptidase)
Ehlers-Danlos Syndrome, Hypermobility-type	AD	TNXB	Tenascin X, a glycoprotein of the extracellular matrix
Ehlers-Danlos Syndrome, Kyphoscoliosis-type	AR	PLOD1	Lysyl hydroxylase
Ehlers-Danlos Syndrome, Progeroid-type	AR	B4GALT7	Xylosylprotein b-galactosyl transferase, polypeptide 7
Ehlers-Danlos Syndrome, Vascular-type	AD	COL3A1	α1 chain of Type III collagen
Ehlers-Danlos Syndrome, with Periventricular Nodular Heterotopia	XLD	FLNA	Filamin A (actin-binding protein 280)
Ellis-van Creveld (EVC)	AR	EVC	EVC (single-pass Type I transmembrane protein)
Epidermal Nevus	somatic	NRAS	Neuroblastoma Ras viral oncogene homolog

Ludicrous 17-Page Genoderm Table (sorted by disease)

Disorder	Inheritance	Gene	Protein
Epidermal Nevus	somatic	PIK3CA	Phosphatidy-linositol 3-kinase, catalytic, α
Epidermal Nevus	somatic	FGFR3	Fibroblast growth factor receptor 3
Epidermal Nevus	somatic	HRAS	V-HA-RAS Harvey rat sarcoma viral oncogene homolog
Epidermodysplasia Verruciformis	AR	TMC6 (EVER1)	Transmembrane channel-like 6
Epidermodysplasia Verruciformis	AR	TMC8 (EVER2)	Transmembrane channel-like 8
Epidermolysis Bullosa Simplex (EBS)	AD	K14	Keratin 14
Epidermolysis Bullosa Simplex (EBS)	AD	K5	Keratin 5
Epidermolysis Bullosa Simplex (EBS) Ogna-type	AD	PLEC1	Plectin
Epidermolysis Bullosa Simplex (EBS) Weber-Cockayne	AD	K14	Keratin 14
Epidermolysis Bullosa Simplex (EBS) Weber-Cockayne	AD	K5	Keratin 5
Epidermolysis Bullosa Simplex (EBS) with Muscular Dystrophy	AR	PLEC1	Plectin
Epidermolysis Bullosa, Dominant Dystrophic	AD	COL7A1	α1 chain of Type VII collagen
Epidermolysis Bullosa, Junctional	AR	LAMB3	Laminin polypeptide β3 subunit (component of laminin 332)
Epidermolysis Bullosa, Junctional with Pyloric Atresia	AR	ITGB4	β4 integrin
Epidermolysis Bullosa, Junctional, Generalized Atrophic Benign-type	AR	LAMA3	Laminin polypeptide α3 subunit (component of laminin 332)
Epidermolysis Bullosa, Junctional, Herlitz-type	AR	LAMA3	Laminin polypeptide α3 subunit (component of laminin 332)
Epidermolysis Bullosa, Junctional, Herlitz-type	AR	LAMB3	Laminin polypeptide β3 subunit (component of laminin 332)

Disorder	Inheritance	Gene	Protein
Epidermolysis Bullosa, Junctional, Herlitz-type	AR	LAMC2	Laminin polypeptide γ2 subunit (component of laminin 332)
Epidermolysis Bullosa, Junctional, Non-Herlitz-type	AR	LAMA3, LAMB3, LAMC2, COL17A1, ITGB4	Laminin polypeptide α3, β3, or γ2 subunit (components of laminin 332)
Epidermolysis Bullosa, Recessive Dystrophic	AR	COL7A1	α1 chain of Type VII collagen
Erythrokeratodermia Variabilis (Mendes da Costa)	AD	GJB3	Gap junction protein β3 (connexin 31)
Erythrokeratodermia Variabilis (Mendes da Costa)	AD	GJB4	Gap junction protein β4 (connexin 30.3)
Erythromelalgia, primary	AD	SCN9A	Voltage-gated sodium channel
Erythropoietic Protoporphyria	AD	FECH	Ferrochelatase
Fabry Disease	XLR	GLA	α galactosidase A, (↑ in glycosphingolipid trihexidosyl ceramide)
Familial Adenomatous Polyposis	AD	APC	Adenomatous polyposis coli
Familial Atypical Mole-malignant Melanoma (FAMMM) Syndrome	AD	CDK4	Cyclin-dependent kinase 4
Familial Atypical Mole-Malignant Melanoma (FAMMM) Syndrome	AD	CDKN2A	Cyclin-dependent kinase inhibitor 2A (p16 (INK) and p14 (ARF)
Familial Chilblain Lupus	AD	TREX1	3' repair TREX1 endonuclease 1
Familial Cold Autoinflammatory/ Urticaria Syndrome (FCAS)	AD	CIAS1 (NLRP3)	NLR family, pyrin domain containing 3 (cryopyrin)
Familial Cylindromatosis	AD	CYLD	Deubiquitinating enzyme (removes lys63-linked ubiquitin chains)
Familial Dysautonomia (Riley-Day Syndrome)	AR	IKBKAP	Inhibitor of κ light polypeptide gene enhancer in B cells, kinase complex-associated protein; component of Elongator, a transcription elongation factor complex that has histone acetyltransferase activity

Disorder	Inheritance	Gene	Protein
Familial Generalized Lentiginosis	AD	Unknown	Unknown
Familial Hibernian Fever (Tumor Necrosis Factor Receptor Associated Periodic Syndrome; TRAPS)	AD	TNFRSF1A	Tumor necrosis factor receptor superfamily, member 1A
Familial Hypercholesterolemia (Type II Lipoproteinemia)	AR	APOB	Apolipoprotein B-100, LDL receptor binding domain
Familial Hypercholesterolemia (Type II Lipoproteinemia)	AD	LDLR	LDL receptor
Familial Hypercholesterolemia (Type II Lipoproteinemia)	AD	PCSK9	Proprotein convertase subtilisin /kexin Type 9
Familial Hypertriglyceridemia (Type IV Hyperlipoproteinemia)	AD	APOA5	Apolipoprotein A-V
Familial Hypertriglyceridemia (Type IV Hyperlipoproteinemia)	AD	LIPI	Lipase member I
Familial Mastocytosis	AD	KIT	KIT proto-oncogene (stem cell factor receptor)
Familial Mediterranean Fever	AR, AD	MEFV	Pyrin (marenostrin)
Familial Tooth Agenesis (Witkop Syndrome)	AD	MSX1	Muscle segment homeobox 1
Farber Lipogranulomatosis	AR	ASAH	Acid ceramidase
Ferguson-Smith Syndrome (Multiple self-healing Squamous Epitheliomas)	AD	TGFβR1	TGF-β receptor 1
Fibrodysplasia Ossificans Progressiva	AD	ACVR1	Activin A receptor, Type I
Focal Dermal Hypoplasia (Goltz Syndrome)	XLD	PORCN	Porcupine homolog
Fraser Syndrome	AR	FREM2	Fras1-related extracellular matrix protein 2
Fraser Syndrome	AR	FRAS1	Extracellular matrix protein
Fucosidosis	AR	FUCA1	α L fucosidase
Gardner Syndrome	AD	APC	Adenomatous polyposis coli
Gaucher Disease Types I-III	AR	GBA	Acid-β-glucosidase, ↓ glucocere-brosidase (in histiocytes)

Disorder	Inheritance	Gene	Protein
Giant Axonal Neuropathy with Curly Hair	AR	GAN1	Gigatoxin
Glomuvenous Malformations (Familial Glomangiomatosis)	AD	GLMN	Glomulin
Goeminne (Torticollis, Keloids, Cryptorchidism, Renal Dysplasia) Syndrome	XLD	TKCR	Unknown
Gorham-Stout Syndrome	NI	Unknown	Unknown
Griscelli Syndrome, Type 1 (Elejalde Syndrome)	AR	MYO5A	Myosin 5A
Griscelli Syndrome, Type 2	AR	RAB27A	Ras-associated protein
Griscelli Syndrome, Type 3	AR	MLPH	Melanophilin
Grzybowski Syndrome	NI	---	---
H Syndrome	AR	SLC29A3	Solute carrier family 29, member 3 (nucleoside transporter)
Hailey-Hailey	AD	ATP2C1	Human secretory pathway Ca2+ ATPase 1 (hSPCA1)
Haim-Munk Syndrome	AR	CTSC	Cathepsin C
HAIR-AN (HyperAndrogenism, Insulin Resistance, Acanthosis Nigricans) Syndrome	NI	Unknown	Unknown
Hallermann-Streiff Syndrome (Oculomandibulofacial Syndrome)	Somatic	GJA1	Gap junction protein α1 (connexin 43)
Harlequin Ichthyosis	AR	ABCA12	ATP-binding cassette, subfamily A, member 12
Hartnup Disease	AR	SLC6A19	Solute carrier family 6, member 19 (BOAT1 neutral amino acid transporter)
Hemochromatosis	AR	HFE	Hemochromatosis, ↑ iron absorption and deposition
Hemochromatosis	AD	SLC11A3	Solute carrier family 40, member 1 (ferroportin)
Hemochromatosis	AR	TFR2	Transferrin receptor 2
Hemochromatosis, Juvenile	AR	HAMP	Hepcidin antimicrobial peptide
Hemochromatosis, Juvenile	AR	HFE2	Hemojuvelin

Disorder	Inheritance	Gene	Protein
Hennekam Lymphangiectasia-Lymphedema Syndrome, Type 1	AR	CCBE1	Collagen and calcium-binding EGF domain-containing protein 1
Hepatoerythropoietic Porphyria	AR	UROD	Uroporphyrinogen-III decarboxylase
Hereditary Angioedema, Type 1	AD	C1INH (SERPING1)	C1 inhibitor protein
Hereditary Angioedema, Type 2	AD	C1INH (SERPING1)	C1 inhibitor protein
Hereditary Angioedema, Type 3	AD	F12	Factor XII (Hageman factor)
Hereditary Coproporphyria	AD	CPOX	Copropor-phyrinogen oxidase
Hereditary Gelsolin Amyloidosis	AD	GSN	Gelsolin
Hereditary Hemorrhagic Telangiectasia, Type 1	AD	ENG	Endoglin (component of endothelial cell TGF-β receptor)
Hereditary Hemorrhagic Telangiectasia, Type 2	AD	ACVRL1 (ALK1)	Activin A receptor, Type II-like 1
Hereditary Hemorrhagic Telangiectasia, Type 3	Unknown	Unknown	Unknown
Hereditary Hemorrhagic Telangiectasia, Type 4	AD	Unknown	Unknown
Hereditary Hemorrhagic Telangiectasia, with Juvenile Polyposis	AD	SMAD4	SMAD family member 4 (transmits signals from TGF-β receptor)
Hereditary Hypotrichosis Simplex	AD	APCDD1	APC Down-Regulated-1 gene encodes a membrane-bound glycoprotein expressed in human hair follicles
Hereditary Leiomyomatosis and Renal Cell Cancer	AD	FH	Fumarate hydratase
Heredofamilial Systemic Amyloidosis (Familial Amyloid Polyneuropathy)	AD	APOA1	Apolipoprotein A-I
Heredofamilial Systemic Amyloidosis (Familial Amyloid Polyneuropathy)	AD	TTR	Transthyretin
Hermansky-Pudlak (Type 1)	AR	HPS1	HPS1 (BLOC-3 component)
Hermansky-Pudlak (Type 2)	AR	AP3B1	Adaptor protein 3, β1 subunit
Hermansky-Pudlak (Type 3)	AR	HPS3	HPS3 (BLOC-2 component)
Hermansky-Pudlak (Type 4)	AR	HPS4	HPS4 (BLOC-3 component)

Disorder	Inheritance	Gene	Protein
Hermansky-Pudlak (Type 5)	AR	HPS5	α-integrin-binding protein (BLOC-2 component)
Hermansky-Pudlak (Type 6)	AR	HPS6	BLOC-2 component
Hermansky-Pudlak (Type 7)	AR	DTNBP1	Dysbindin (dystrobrevin-binding protein 1)
Hermansky-Pudlak (Type 8)	AR	BLOC1S3	Biogenesis of lysosome-related organelles complex 1, subunit 3 (BLOC1 component)
Hidrotic Ectodermal Dysplasia (Clouston Syndrome)	AD	GJB6	Gap junction protein β6 (connexin 30)
Holocarboxylase Synthetase Deficiency	AR	HLCS	Holocarboxylase synthetase
Homocystinuria	AR	CBS	Cystathione β-synthase (methionine metabolism defect)
Howel-Evans Syndrome (Tylosis-Esophageal CA)	AD	TOC (RHBDF2)	Inhibitory rhomboid-like (rhomboid 5) pseudoproteases, inhibit EGFR signaling
Hyper IgE Syndrome (Job Syndrome)	AR	DOCK8	Dedicator of cytokinesis 8
Hyper IgE Syndrome (Job Syndrome)	AR	PGM3	Phosphoglu-comutase-3
Hyper IgE Syndrome (Job Syndrome)	AD	STAT3	Signal transducer and activator of transcription 3
Hyper IgE Syndrome (Job Syndrome)	AR	TYK2	Tyrosine kinase 2
Hyper IgM Syndrome	AR	AICDA	Activation-induced cytidine deaminase
Hyper IgM Syndrome	AR	CD40	Costimulatory protein found on antigen presenting cells
Hyper IgM Syndrome	XLR	CD40LG	Costimulatory protein found on activated T cells
Hyper IgM Syndrome	AR	UNG	Uracil-DNA glycosylase
Hyper-IgD with Periodic Fever Syndrome	AR	MVK	Mevalonate kinase
Hyperphosphatemic Familial Tumoral Calcinosis	AR	FGF23	Fibroblast growth factor 23
Hyperphosphatemic Familial Tumoral Calcinosis	AR	GALNT3	UDP-N-acetyl-α-D-galactosa-mine, polypeptide N-acetylgalactosa-minyltransferase 3

Disorder	Inheritance	Gene	Protein
Hyperphosphatemic Familial Tumoral Calcinosis	AR	KL	Klotho
Hypertrichosis Universalis Congenita (Ambras Syndrome)	AD	HTC1	Function unknown
Hypertrichosis, Generalized, X-Linked	XLD	HTC2	Palindrome-mediated interchromosomal insertion at chromosome Xq27.1
Hypertrophic Osteoarthropathy Pachydermoperiostosis, Touraine-Solente-Golé Syndrome)	AR	HPGD	15-Hydroxyprosta-glandin Dehydrogenase-
Hypertrophic Osteoarthropathy (Pachydermoperio-stosis, Touraine-Solente-Golé Syndrome)	AR	SLCO2A1	Solute carrier family 21, member 2 (prostaglandin transporter)
Hypoalphalipo-proteinemia	AD	APOA1	Apolipoprotein A-I
Hypohidrotic Ectodermal Dysplasia	XLR	EDA	Ectodysplasin A
Hypohidrotic Ectodermal Dysplasia	AD	EDAR	Ectodysplasin A receptor
Hypohidrotic Ectodermal Dysplasia	AD	EDARADD	EDAR-associated death domain
Hypohidrotic Ectodermal Dysplasia, with Immunodeficiency	XLR	IKBKG (NEMO)	Inhibitor of κ light polypeptide gene enhancer in B cells kinase γ (nuclear factor-κB essential modulator)
Hypoprothrombinemia	AD	F2	Prothrombin, G20210A polymorphism
Hypotrichosis Simplex of the Scalp	AD	CDSN	Corneodesmosin
Hypotrichosis with Juvenile Macular Dystrophy	AR	CDH3	Cadherin 3 (P-cadherin)
Hypotrichosis-Lymphedema-Telangiectasia Syndrome	AD, AR	SOX18	Sex determining region Y (SRY)-box 18
Hypotrichosis, Mari-type	AR	LIPH	Lipase H
Hystrix-like Ichthyosis–Deafness (HID) Syndrome	AD	GJB2	Gap junction protein β2 (connexin 26)
Ichthyosis Vulgaris	AD	FLG	Filaggrin
Ichthyosis, Bullosa of Siemens	AD	K2e	Keratin 2e
Ichthyosis, Congenital AR-type	AR	NIPAL4	Ichthyin, NIPA-like domain-containing 4
Ichthyosis, Congenital with Hypotrichosis	AR	ST14	Matriptase (serine protease)

Disorder	Inheritance	Gene	Protein
Ichthyosis, Epidermolytic (Bullous CIE)	AD	K1	Keratin 1
Ichthyosis, Epidermolytic (Bullous CIE)	AD	K10	Keratin 10
Ichthyosis, Hypotrichosis-Sclerosing Cholangitis (IHSC)	AR	CLDN1	Claudin 1
Ichthyosis, Hystrix Curth–Macklin	AD	K1	Keratin 1
Ichthyosis, Prematurity Syndrome	AR	SLC27A4	Solute carrier family 27, member 4 (fatty acid transporter)
Ichthyosis, X-linked Recessive	XLR	STS	Steroid sulfatase (arylsulfatase c)
IFAP (Ichthyosis-Follicularis-Atrichia-Photophobia) Syndrome	XLR	MBTPS2	Membrane-embedded zinc metalloprotease
IgA Deficiency Type I	Unknown	MSH5	Inability to produce IgA
IgA Deficiency Type II	Unknown	TNFRSF13B	Transmembrane activator & CAML interactor (TACI)
IL 12/23 Deficiency	AR	IL12β, IL12Rβ	p40 subunit of IL-12 & IL-23 or its receptor
Incontinentia Pigmenti	XLD	IKBKG (NEMO)	Inhibitor of κ light polypeptide gene enhancer in B cells, kinase γ (nuclear factor-κB essential modulator)
Infantile Hemangiomas, Hereditary	AD	ANTXR1	Anthrax toxin receptor 1
Infantile Systemic Hyalinosis	AR	ANTXR2 (CMG2)	Anthrax toxin receptor 2 (capillary morphogenesis Protein 2)
Insensitivity to Pain with Anhidrosis	AR	NTRK1	Neurotrophic tyrosine kinase receptor Type 1
IPEX (Immune dysregulation, Polyendocrinopathy, Enteropathy, X-linked) Syndrome	XLR	FOXP3	Forkhead box P3
Isolated Congenital Nail Dysplasia	AD	Unknown	Unknown
Isolated Toenail Dystrophy	AD	COL7A1	α1 chain of Type VII collagen
Isovaleric Acidemia	AR	IVD	Isovaleryl-coA dehydrogenase
Johanson-Blizzard Syndrome	AR	UBR1	Ubiquitin-protein ligase E3 component N-recognin 1

Disorder	Inheritance	Gene	Protein
Juvenile Hyaline Fibromatosis (Murray-Puretic-Drescher Syndrome)	AR	ANTXR2 (CMG2)	Anthrax toxin receptor 2 (capillary morphogenesis Protein 2)
Kallmann Syndrome Type 1	XLR	ANOS1	Anosmin 1
Kallmann Syndrome Type 2	AD/AR	FGFR1	Fibroblast growth factor receptor 1
Kallmann Syndrome Type 3	AD/AR	PROKR2	Prokineticin receptor 2 (a G-protein coupled receptor)
Kallmann Syndrome Type 4	AD/AR	PROK2	Prokineticin
Keratolytic Winter Erythema (Oudtshoorn Skin Disease)	AD	Unknown	Unknown
Keratosis Follicularis Spinulosa Decalvans	XLR	MBTPS2	Membrane-embedded zinc metalloprotease
Keratosis Follicularis Spinulosa Decalvans	XLR > AD	SAT1	Spermidine/spermine N(1)-acetyltransferase
Keratosis Pilaris Atrophicans Faciei (Ulerythema Ophryogenes)	AD	Unknown	Unknown
KID (Keratitis–Ichthyosis–Deafness) Syndrome	AD>AR	GJB2	Gap junction protein β2 (connexin 26)
Kindler Syndrome	AR	KIND1 (C20orf42)	Kindlin 1
Klinefelter Syndrome	NI	XXY	N/A
Klippel-Trenaunay Syndrome	NI		
Lamellar Ichthyosis	AR	ABCA12	ATP-binding cassette, subfamily A, member 12
Lamellar Ichthyosis	AR	CYP4F22	Cytochrome P450, family 4, subfamily F22
Lamellar Ichthyosis	AR	TGM1	Transglutaminase 1
Laron Syndrome (Pituitary Dwarfism II)	AR	GHR	Growth hormone receptor
Laryngo-Onycho-Cutaneous (Shabbir) Syndrome	AR	LAMA3	Laminin polypeptide α3 subunit (component of laminin 332)
Laugier-Hunziker Syndrome	NI	Unknown	May be simply acquired pigmentation, not a genetic syndrome

Disorder	Inheritance	Gene	Protein
Legius Syndrome	AD	SPRED1	Sprouty-Related EVH1 Domain-containing Protein 1; regulate growth factor-induced activation of the MAP kinase cascade
Leigh Syndrome	Mt	>12 genes	Various components of mitochondrial respiratory chain complexes
Leigh Syndrome	AR	SURF1	Surfeit 1
Leiner's Disease	Unknown	C5	C5 deficiency
Leprechaunism (Rabson-Mendenhall Syndrome, Donohue Syndrome)	AR	INSR	Insulin receptor
Lesch-Nyhan	XLR	HGPT	Hypoxanthine guanine sphoribosyl-transferase, ↑ uric acid
Lethal Acantholytic Epidermolysis Bullosa	AR	DSP	Desmoplakin
Leukocyte Adhesion Deficiency Type I	AR	ITGB2	β2 integrin
Leukocyte Adhesion Deficiency Type II (Congenital Disorder of Glycosylation Type IIc)	AR	SLC35C1	Solute carrier family 35, member c1 (neutrophil sialyl-LewisX)
Leukocyte Adhesion Deficiency Type III	AR	FERMT3, KIND3	Intracellular protein that interacts with β-integrins in hematopoietic cells
Leukocyte Adhesion Deficiency Type III	AR	KIND3	Fermitin Family Homolog 3
Li-Fraumeni Syndrome	AD	TP53	p53
Limb-Mammary Syndrome	AD	TP63	p63
Lipodystrophy, Acquired Partial (Barraquer Simons Syndrome)	AD	LMNB2	Lamin B2
Lipodystrophy, Congenital Generalized (Berardinelli-Seip Type 2)	AR	BSCL2	Seipen
Lipodystrophy, Familial Partial	AD	LMNA	Lamin A/C
Lipodystrophy, Familial Partial	AD	PPARG	Peroxisome proliferators activated receptor γ
Lipoid Proteinosis	AR	ECM1	Extracellular matrix Protein 1

Disorder	Inheritance	Gene	Protein
Lipomatosis, Benign Symmetric (Madelung Disease)	Most Unknown. Some Mt	MT-TK	Mitochondrial lysine tRNA
Lipomatosis, Familial Multiple	AD	Unknown	Unknown
Lipoprotein Lipase Deficiency (Type 1 Hyperlipoproteinemia)	AR	LPL	Lipoprotein lipase
Localized Autosomal Recessive Hypotrichosis	AR	DSG4	Desmoglein 4
Loeys-Dietz Syndrome Type I	AD	TGFβR1	TGF-β receptor 1
Loeys-Dietz Syndrome Type II	AD	TGFβR2	TGF-β receptor 2
LUMBAR Syndrome (SACRAL Syndrome, PELVIS Syndrome)	NI	---	---
Lymphangioleio-myomatosis	Somatic	TSC2	Tuberin / GTPase activating protein of rap1 GAP family
Lymphangiomatosis	Unknown	Unknown	Unknown
Lymphedema Praecox (Meige Lymphedema)	AD	FOXC2	Forkhead box C2
Lymphedema-Distichiasis	AD	FOXC2	Forkhead box C2
Lymphedema, Hereditary early onset-type (Milroy Disease)	AD	FLT4	FMA-related tyrosine kinase 4 (vascular endothelial growth factor receptor 3)
Macrocephaly-Capillary Malformation Syndrome	Somatic	PIK3CA	Phosphati-dylinositol 3-kinase, catalytic, α
Macular-type Hereditary Bullous Dystrophy (Mendes da Costa Syndrome)	XLR	Unknown	Unknown
Maffucci Syndrome (Multiple Enchondromatosis)	AD	IDH1/IDH2	Isocitrate dehydrogenase 1 or 2
Majeed Syndrome (Recurrent Sweet's + Osteomyelitis)	AR	LPIN2	Lipin 2
Mal de Meleda	AR	SLURP1	Secreted LY6/Plaur Domain-containing protein 1
Mammalian Sterile 20-like Kinase 1 Deficiency	AR	MST1 (STK4)	Serine-threonine kinase
Mandibuloacral Dysplasia Syndrome	AR	LMNA	Lamin A/C
Mandibuloacral Dysplasia Syndrome	AR	ZMPSTE24	Zinc metallopeptidase (STE24 homolog)

Disorder	Inheritance	Gene	Protein
Maple Syrup Urine Disease	AR	BCKDHA	E1-α subunit of the branched-chain α-keto acid (BCAA) dehydrogenase complex
Maple Syrup Urine Disease	AR	CKDHB	E1-β subunit of the branched-chain α-keto acid (BCAA) dehydrogenase complex
Maple Syrup Urine Disease	AR	DBT	Lipoamide acyltransferase component of branched-chain α-keto acid dehydrogenase complex
Maple Syrup Urine Disease	AR	DLD	Dihydrolipoamide dehydrogenase
Marfan Syndrome Type 1	AD	FBN1	Fibrillin 1
Marfan Syndrome Type 2	AD	TGFβR2	TGF-β receptor 2
Marie-Unna Hypotrichosis	AR	HR	Hairless (zinc finger transcription factor)
Mastocytosis, adult-onset	Somatic	KIT	KIT proto-oncogene (stem cell factor receptor)
McCune–Albright Syndrome	AD	GNAS	G protein, α subunit
MEDNIK Syndrome	AR	AP1S1	Adaptor-related protein complex 1, sigma-1 subunit
Meesmann Corneal Dystrophy	AD	K12	Keratin 12
Meesmann Corneal Dystrophy	AD	K3	Keratin 3
Melorheostosis	Somatic	LEMD3 (MAN1)	LEM domain containing 3 (Man 1, an inner nuclear membrane protein)
Menkes Kinky Hair	XLR	ATP7A	ATPase, Cu2+-transporting, α-polypeptide
Methionine Adenosyltransferase Deficiency	AD/AR	MAT1A	Methionine adenosyl-transferase I, α
Microcephaly-Capillary Malformation Syndrome	AR	STAMBP	Stam-binding protein
MIDAS (Microphthalmia, Dermal Aplasia, and Sclerocornea) Syndrome	XLD	HCCS	Holocytochrome C Synthase

Disorder	Inheritance	Gene	Protein
Milroy Disease (Hereditary Lymphedema)	AD	FLT4	FMA-related tyrosine kinase 4 (vascular endothelial growth factor receptor 3)
Milroy's Disease (Hereditary Lymphedema)	AD	FOXC2, SOX18, GATA2, CCBE1, PTPN14, KIF11, VEGFC	Multiple proteins
Milroy's Disease (Hereditary Lymphedema)	AD	GJC2	Gap junction protein γ2 (connexin 47)
Monilethrix	AR	DSG4	Desmoglein 4
Monilethrix	AD	K81, K83, K86	Hair cortex keratins
Monocytopenia and Mycobacterial Infection (MonoMAC) Syndrome	AD	GATA2	Zinc finger transcription factor
Muckle–Wells Syndrome	AD	CIAS1 (NLRP3)	NLR family, pyrin domain containing 3 (cryopyrin)
Mucopolysaccharidosis Type I (Hurler Syndrome)	AR	IDUA	α-L-iduronidase; dermatan, heparan sulfate
Mucopolysaccharidosis Type II (Hunter Syndrome)	XLR	IDS	Iduronate-2-sulfatase; dermatan, heparan sulfate
Muir-Torre Syndrome	AD	MLH1	MutL homolog 1 (mismatch repair enzyme)
Muir-Torre Syndrome	AD	MSH2	MutS homolog 2
Muir-Torre Syndrome	AD	MSH6	MutS homolog 6
Multiple Carboxylase Deficiency	AR	BTD	Biotinidase
Multiple Carboxylase Deficiency	AR	HLCS	Holocarboxylase synthetase
Multiple Endocrine Neoplasia (MEN) Syndrome Type 1 (Wermer)	AD	MEN1	Menin, nuclear scaffold protein
Multiple Endocrine Neoplasia (MEN) Syndrome Type 2A (Sipple)	AD	RET	Ret-proto-oncogene (cysteine-rich extracellular domain)
Multiple Endocrine Neoplasia (MEN) Syndrome Type 4	AD	CDKN1B	Cyclin-dependent kinase inhibitor 1B (p27, Kip1)
Multiple Pterygium Syndrome	AR	CHRNG	Cholinergic receptor, nicotinic, γ polypeptide
Multiple Sulfatase Deficiency	AR	SUMF1	Sulfatase-modifying factor 1

Disorder	Inheritance	Gene	Protein
Naegeli–Franceschetti–Jadassohn Syndrome	AD	K14	Keratin 14
Nail-Patella Syndrome (Hereditary Osteo-Onychodysplasia)	AD	LMX1B	LIM homeodomain protein (involved in dorsal-ventral limb patterning)
Naxos Syndrome	AR	JUP	Junction Plakoglobin
Nephropathy with Pretibial Epidermolysis Bullosa and Deafness	AR	CD151	Platelet-endothelial cell tetraspanin antigen 3 (CD151)
Netherton Syndrome	AR	SPINK5	Serine protease inhibitor, Kazal Type 5 (lymphoepithelial Kazal-type-related inhibitor, LEKTI)
Neurofibromatosis-1	AD	NF1	Neurofibromin 1 (GTPase activating protein)
Neurofibromatosis-2	AD	NF2	Neurofibromin 2 (merlin)
Neutral Lipid Storage Disease (Chanarin–Dorfman Syndrome)	AR	ABHD5 (CGI-58)	Abhydrolase domain-containing 5 (comparative gene identification 58, esterase-lipase-thioesterase subfamily)
Nezelof Syndrome (Thymic Dysplasia with Normal Immunoglobulins)	AR	Unknown	Purine nucleoside phosphorylase (PNP) deficiency
Nicolau-Balus Syndrome	Unknown	Unknown	Unknown
Niemann-Pick Disease Type A	AR	SMPD1	Sphingomyelin Sphingo-myelinphospho-diesterase 1
Nodulosis, Arthropathy, Osteolysis (NAO) Syndrome	AR	MMP2	Matrix metalloproteinase 2
Non-bullous Congenital Ichthyosiform Erythroderma	AR	ALOX12B	12R-Lipoxygenase
Non-bullous Congenital Ichthyosiform Erythroderma	AR	ALOXE3	Epidermal lipoxygenase 3
Non-bullous Congenital Ichthyosiform Erythroderma	AR	NIPAL4	Ichthyin
Non-bullous Congenital Ichthyosiform Erythroderma	AR	TGM1	Transglutaminase 1
Noonan Syndrome Type 1	AD	PTPN11	Protein tyrosine phosphatase, nonreceptor Type 11

Disorder	Inheritance	Gene	Protein
Noonan Syndrome Type 10	AD	LZTR1	Leucine zipper-like transcriptional regulator 1
Noonan Syndrome Type 2	AR	Unknown	Unknown
Noonan Syndrome Type 3	Unknown	KRAS	V-KI-RAS2 Kirsten rat sarcoma viral oncogene homolog
Noonan Syndrome Type 4	AD	SOS1	Son of sevenless homolog 1 (guanine nucleotide exchange factor)
Noonan Syndrome Type 5	AD	RAF1	V-Raf-1 murine leukemia viral oncogene homolog
Noonan Syndrome Type 6	AD	NRAS	Neuroblastoma Ras viral oncogene homolog
Noonan Syndrome Type 7	Unknown	BRAF	V-RAF murine sarcoma viral oncogene homolog
Noonan Syndrome Type 8	AD	RIT1	RIC-like protein without CAAX motif 1 (RAS-like protein)
Noonan Syndrome Type 9	AD	SOS2	Son of sevenless homolog 2 (guanine nucleotide exchange factor)
Noonan Syndrome with Multiple Lentigines (formerly LEOPARD Syndrome)	AD	PTPN11 > RAF1 > BRAF, MAP2K1	Protein tyrosine phosphatase, nonreceptor Type 11
Noonan-Like Syndrome with Loose Anagen Hair	AD	SHOC2	Suppressor of Clear, C. elegans
Normophosphatemic Familial Tumoral Calcinosis	AR	SAMD9	Sterile α motif domain-containing 9
Oasthouse Urine Syndrome (Methionine Malabsorption Syndrome)	AR	Unknown	Unknown
Oculocutaneous Albinism Type 2 (OCA2)	AR	OCA2	P protein (pink eye dilution homolog)
Oculocutaneous Albinism Type 3 (OCA3)	AR	TYRP1	Tyrosinase-related protein 1
Oculocutaneous Albinism Type 4 (OCA4)	AR	SLC45A2 (MATP)	Solute carrier family 45, member 2
Oculocutaneous Albinism Types 1A, 1B (OCA1A, 1B)	AR	TYR	Tyrosinase (absent-OCA1; or decreased OCA1B activity)

J. Finch & M. Payette

Disorder	Inheritance	Gene	Protein
Oculodentodigital Dysplasia	AD/AR	GJA1	Gap junction protein α1 (connexin 43)
Odonto-Onycho-Dermal Dysplasia	AR	WNT10A	Wingless-type MMTV integration site family, member 10A
Olmsted Syndrome	AD	TRPV3	Transient receptor potential cation channel, subfamily V, member 3
Omenn Syndrome (SCID)	AR	DCLRE1C	Protein artemis (Endonuclease involved in V(D)J recombination and DNA repair)
Oral-Facial-Digital Syndrome	XLD	OFD1	Centriole and centriolar satellite protein
Osteogenesis Imperfecta	AD	COL1A1	α1 chain of Type I collagen
Osteogenesis Imperfecta	AD	COL1A2	α2 chain of Type I collagen
P14 Deficiency, Immunodeficiency Syndrome	AR	TP14	p14 (MAPBP-interacting protein)
Pachyonychia Congenita Type I (Jadassohn-Lewandowsky)	AD	K16	Keratin 16
Pachyonychia Congenita Type I (Jadassohn-Lewandowsky)	AD	K6a	Keratin 6a
Pachyonychia Congenita Type II (Jackson-Lawler)	AD	K17	Keratin 17
Pachyonychia Congenita Type II (Jackson-Lawler)	AD	K6b	Keratin 6b
Palmoplantar Keratoderma (PPK) with cutaneous SCC and sex reversal	AR	RSPO1	R-spondin family, member 1
Palmoplantar Keratoderma (PPK) with Deafness	AD	GJB2	Gap junction protein β2 (connexin 26)
Palmoplantar Keratoderma (PPK) with Deafness	Mt	MT-TS1	Mitochondrial serine tRNA
PAPA (Pyogenic Arthritis, Pyoderma Gangrenosum, Acne) Syndrome	AD	PSTPIP1 (CD2BP1)	Protein serine threonine phosphatase interacting protein 1
Papillon-Lefèvre Syndrome	AR	CTSC	Cathepsin C
Parkes Weber Syndrome	NI	RASA1	p120-Ras GTPase-activating protein
Peutz-Jeghers Syndrome	AD	STK11 (LKB1)	Serine-threonine kinase 11

Disorder	Inheritance	Gene	Protein
PFAPA (Periodic Fever, Aphthous Stomatitis, Pharyngitis, Adenitis) Syndrome	Unknown	SPAG7*	Functionally linked to antiviral and inflammatory responses
PHACES Syndrome	NI	---	---
Phenylketonuria	AR	PAH	Phenylalanine hydroxylase
Phenylketonuria	AR	PTS	6-Pyruvoyl-tetrahydropterin synthase
Phenylketonuria	AR	QDPR	Quinoid dihydropteridine reductase
Piebaldism	AD	KIT	KIT proto-oncogene (stem cell factor receptor)
Piebaldism	AD	SNAI2	Snail homolog 2
Pili Annulati (Ringed Hair)	AD	Unknown	Unknown
Pili Torti (Twisted Hair)	Unknown	Unknown	Unknown
Pilomatricoma	Somatic	CTNNB1	β-Catenin
Plate-Like Osteoma Cutis	AD	GNAS	G protein, α subunit
Poland Syndrome	Sporadic	Unknown	Unknown
Polycythemia Vera, Essential Thrombocythemia	Somatic	JAK2	Janus Kinase 2
Popliteal Pterygium Syndrome	AD	IRF6	Interferon regulatory factor 6
Porokeratosis, Disseminated Superficial Actinic	AD	MVK	Mevalonate kinase
Porphyria, Acute Intermittent	AD	HMBS	Hydroxy-methylbilane synthase; also known as porphobilinogen deaminase (PBGD)
Porphyria, ALA Dehydratase Deficiency	AR	ALAD	Delta-aminolevulinate (ALA) dehydratase
Porphyria, Congenital Erythropoietic (Gunther Disease)	AR	UROS	Uroporphyrinogen-III synthase
Porphyria, Cutanea Tarda (PCT)	AD	UROD	Uroporphyrinogen-III decarboxylase
Porphyria, Variegate	AD	PPOX	Protoporphy-rinogen oxidase
Prader-Willi	NI	NDN, SNRPN	Genomic imprinting caused by deletion or inactivation of genes on the paternally inherited chromosome 15

Disorder	Inheritance	Gene	Protein
Primary Localized Cutaneous Amyloidosis 1	AD	OSMR	Oncostatin M receptor
Progeria (Hutchinson-Gilford)	AD>>AR	LMNA	Lamin A/C
Progressive Osseous Heteroplasia	AD	GNAS	G protein, α subunit
Progressive Symmetric Erythrokeratoderma	AD	LOR	Loricrin
Prolidase Deficiency	AR	PEPD	Prolidase (peptidase D)
Properdin Deficiency (Complement Factor Properdin Deficiency)	XLR	PFC	Properdin P Factor, Complement
Protein C Deficiency	AD	PROC	Protein C
Protein S Deficiency	AD	PROS1	Protein S
Proteus Syndrome	Somatic	AKT1	V-AKT Murine Thymoma Viral Oncogene Homolog 1
Proteus-like Syndrome (Cohen-Hayden Syndrome)	AD	PTEN	Phosphatase and tensin homolog (tyrosine kinase)
Pseudoxanthoma Elasticum	AR	ABCC6	ATP-binding cassette, subfamily C, member 6 (Multidrug resistance-associated protein 6)
Pseudoxanthoma Elasticum-like Disorder with Multiple Coagulation Factor Deficiency	AR	GGCX	γ-glutamyl carboxylase
Pure Hair-Nail-Type Ectodermal Dysplasia	AR	K85	Keratin 85
Rasmussen Syndrome	Unknown	Unknown	Unknown
Refsum Syndrome (Hereditary Motor & Sensory Neuropathy Type 4, Phytanic Acid Storage Disease)	AR	PHYH	Phytanoyl-CoA 2-hydroxylase
Refsum Syndrome (Hereditary Motor & Sensory Neuropathy Type 4)	AR	PEX7	Peroxin 7
Restrictive Dermopathy	AD	LMNA	Lamin A/C
Restrictive Dermopathy	AR	ZMPSTE24	Zinc metallopeptidase (STE24 homolog)
Reticulate Acropigmentation of Dohi	AD	DSRAD	Adenosine deaminase, RNA-specific
Reticulate Acropigmentation of Kitamura	AD	ADAM10	A disintegrin and metalloproteinase domain 10

Disorder	Inheritance	Gene	Protein
Retinoblastoma	Somatic > AD	RB1, MYCN	Rb
Rhizomelic Chondrodysplasia Punctata	AR	PEX7	Peroxin 7
Richner-Hanhart Syndrome	AR	TAT	Tyrosine aminotransferase
Rombo Syndrome	AD	Unknown	Unknown
Rothmund-Thomson Syndrome	AR	RECQL4	RecQ protein like 1 (DNA helicase)
Rubinstein-Taybi Syndrome Type 1 (Thumb-Hallux Syndrome)	AD	CREBBP	CREB-binding protein
Rubinstein-Taybi Syndrome Type 2	Sporadic	EP300	E1A-binding protein
Russell-Silver Syndrome	Sporadic	Unknown	Unknown
Schimmelpenning-Feuerstein-Mims Syndrome (Linear Sebaceous Nevus Syndrome)	Somatic	HRAS	V-HA-RAS Harvey rat sarcoma viral oncogene homolog
Schimmelpenning-Feuerstein-Mims Syndrome (Linear Sebaceous Nevus Syndrome)	Somatic	KRAS	V-KI-RAS2 Kirsten rat sarcoma viral oncogene homolog
Schimmelpenning-Feuerstein-Mims Syndrome (Linear Sebaceous Nevus Syndrome)	Somatic	NRAS	Neuroblastoma Ras viral oncogene homolog
Schöpf-Schulz-Passarge Syndrome	AR	WNT10A	Wingless-type MMTV integration site family, member 10A
Schwartz-Jampel Syndrome	AR	HSPG2	Heparan sulfate proteoglycan of basement membrane
Sclerotylosis (Huriez Syndrome)	AD	TYS	Unknown
Seborrhea-like Dermatitis with Psoriasiform Elements	AD	ZNF750	Zinc finger protein 750
Selective Tooth Agenesis	XLD	EDA	Ectodysplasin A
Senter Syndrome (Desmons' Syndrome)	Unknown	Unknown	Unknown
Setleis Syndrome	AR	TWIST2	Twist, Drosophila, Homolog of, 2
Severe Combined Immunodeficiency Syndrome (SCID) (B-NK-)	AR	ADA	"Adenosine Deaminase"
Severe Combined Immunodeficiency Syndrome (SCID) (B-NK+)	AR	Artemis gene (DCLRE1C)	DNA cross-link repair protein 1C (artemis)

J. Finch & M. Payette

Disorder	Inheritance	Gene	Protein
Severe Combined Immunodeficiency Syndrome (SCID) (B-NK+) (Omenn Syndrome)	AR	RAG1	Recombination activating gene 1
Severe Combined Immunodeficiency Syndrome (SCID) (B-NK+) (Omenn Syndrome)	AR	RAG2	Recombination activating gene 2
Severe Combined Immunodeficiency Syndrome (SCID) (B+ NK-)	XLR	IL2RG	γ chain of IL-2 receptor
Severe Combined Immunodeficiency Syndrome (SCID) (B+ NK-)	AR	JAK3	Janus Kinase 3, TAP1, TAP2, defective MHCl, defective CD8
Severe Combined Immunodeficiency Syndrome (SCID) (B+ NK+)	AR	CD3D	OKT3 δ-chain (T-cell antigen receptor)
Severe Combined Immunodeficiency Syndrome (SCID) (B+ NK+)	AR	CD45 (PTPRC)	Leukocyte Common Antigen (LCA) (Protein-Tyrosine Phosphatase, Receptor-type, C)
Severe Combined Immunodeficiency Syndrome (SCID) (B+ NK+)	AR	IL7R	IL-7 receptor
SHORT (Short Stature, Hyperextensibility, Ocular Depression (Deeply set eyes), Rieger Anomaly, and Teething Delay) Syndrome	AD	PIK3R1	Phosphatidy-linositol 3-kinase, regulatory subunit 1
Sialidosis	AR	NEU1	Neuramidase (skin fragility)
Sitosterolemia	AR	ABCG5	ATP-binding cassette, subfamily G, member 5 (Sterolin 1)
Sitosterolemia	AR	ABCG8	ATP-binding cassette, subfamily G, member 8 (Sterolin 2)
Sjögren–Larsson Syndrome	AR	ALDH3A2 (FALDH)	Aldehyde dehydrogenase family 3, member A2 (fatty aldehyde dehydrogenase)
Skin Fragility/ Woolly Hair Syndrome	AR	DSP	Desmoplakin
Slow Acetylator Phenotype	AR	NAT1	N-Acetyl Transferase

Disorder	Inheritance	Gene	Protein
Smith-Lemli-Opitz Syndrome	AR	DHCR7	Delta-7-sterol reductase
Squamous Cell Carcinoma, sporadic cutaneous	Sporadic	RAS / tp53	
Squamous Cell Carcinoma, sporadic cutaneous	Sporadic	TP53	p53
Steatocystoma Multiplex	AD	K17	Keratin 17
Stiff Skin Syndrome	AD	FBN1	Fibrillin 1
Striate Palmoplantar Keratoderma (PPK)	AD	DSG1	Desmoglein 1
Striate Palmoplantar Keratoderma (PPK)	AD	DSP	Desmoplakin
Striate Palmoplantar Keratoderma (PPK)	AD	K1	Keratin 1
Sturge-Weber Syndrome	Somatic	GNAQ	Guanine Nucleotide-binding protein, Q polypeptide
Systemic Mastocytosis	Somatic	FIPL1/ PDGFRA fusion	FIPL1/PDGFRA fusion protein
T-cell Immunodeficiency and Congenital Alopecia	AR	FOXN1	Forkhead box N1 (winged helix nude)
Tangier Disease	AR	ABCA1	ATP-binding cassette, subfamily A, member 1 (cholesterol efflux regulatory protein)
Thrombotic Thrombocytopenic Purpura (TTP)	AR	ADAMTS-13	A disintegrin-like and metalloprotease with thrombospondin Type 1 motif, 13 (von Willebrand factor-cleaving protease)
Thymic Hypoplasia (DiGeorge Syndrome)	AD	TBX1	T-box 1
Tietz Syndrome	AD	MITF	Microphthalmia-associated transcription factor
Tricho-Dento-Osseous Syndrome	AD	DLX3	Distal-less homeobox 3
Trichoepitheliomas, Multiple Familial	AD	CYLD	Deubiquitinating enzyme (removes lys63-linked ubiquitin chains)
Trichorhinophalangeal Syndrome Type I	AD	TRPS1	Zinc finger transcription factor

Disorder	Inheritance	Gene	Protein
Trichorhinophalangeal Syndrome Type II (Langer-Giedion Syndrome)	AR	TRPS1, EXT1	Contiguous gene deletion, zinc finger transcription factor/Exostosin glycosyltrans-ferase 1
Trichorhinophalangeal Syndrome Type III	AR	TRPS1	Zinc finger transcription factor
Trichorrhexis Invaginata (Netherton Syndrome)	AR	SPINK5	Serine protease inhibitor, Kazal Type 5 (lymphoepithelial Kazal-type-related inhibitor, LEKTI)
Trichothiodystrophy	AR	ERCC2 (XPD)	DNA helicase (5' to 3' DNA helicase in nucleotide excision repair)
Trichothiodystrophy	AR	ERCC3 (XPB)	DNA helicase (3' to 5' DNA helicase in nucleotide excision repair)
Trichothiodystrophy	AR	GTF2H5 (TTDA)	Transcription/repair factor TFIIH
Trichothiodystrophy without photosensitivity or ichthyosis	AR	MPLKIP	M-phase-specific PLK1-interacting protein
Trimethylaminuria	AR	FMO3	Flavin-containing monooxygenase 3
Tuberous Sclerosis-1	AD	TSC1	Hamartin / GTPase activating protein of rap1 GAP family
Tuberous Sclerosis-2	AD	TSC2	Tuberin / GTPase activating protein of rap1 GAP family
Tuberous Sclerosis-associated Polycystic Kidney Disease	AD	PKD1	Polycystin 1
Turner Syndrome	XO	XO	Single X chromosome
Tyrosinemia Type I	AR	FAH	Fumarylacetoacetate hydrolase
Tyrosinemia Type II (Richner-Hanhart Syndrome)	AR	TAT	Tyrosine aminotransferase
Ullrich Scleroatonic Muscular Dystrophy	AR	COL6A1	α1 chain of type VI collagen
Ullrich Scleroatonic Muscular Dystrophy	AR	COL6A2	α2 chain of type VI collagen
Ullrich Scleroatonic Muscular Dystrophy	AR	COL6A3	α3 chain of type VI collagen
Uncombable Hair Syndrome (Spun Glass Hair, Pili Trianguli et Canaliculi)	AD	Unknown	Unknown
Unna-Thost PPK (Non-Epidermolytic PPK)	AD	K1	Keratin 1

Disorder	Inheritance	Gene	Protein
UV Apoptosis	NI	BCL2	Protein phosphatase 1, regulatory subunit 50
Van der Woude Syndrome	AD	IRF6	Interferon regulatory factor 6
Venous Malformations, Multiple Cutaneous and Mucosal	AD	TEK (TIE2)	Endothelial-specific tyrosine kinase receptor
Vitamin D-dependent Rickets with Alopecia	AR	VDR	Vitamin D receptor
Vohwinkel Syndrome	AD	GJB2	Gap junction protein β2 (connexin 26)
Vohwinkel Syndrome, Variant	AD	LOR	Loricrin
Von Hippel-Lindau Syndrome	AD	VHL	VHL tumor suppressor
Vörner PPK (Epidermolytic PPK)	AD	K1	Keratin 1 (feet)
Vörner PPK (Epidermolytic PPK)	AD	K9	Keratin 9 (hands)
Waardenburg Syndrome Type 1	AD	PAX3	Paired box gene 3
Waardenburg Syndrome Type 2	AD	MITF	Microphthalmia-associated transcription factor
Waardenburg Syndrome Type 2	AR	SLUG	Snail homolog 2
Waardenburg Syndrome Type 3	AD	PAX3	Paired box gene 3
Waardenburg Syndrome Type 4	AD	SOX10	SRY-related HMG-box gene 10
Waardenburg Syndrome Type 4A	AD, AR	EDNRB	Endothelin Receptor, type B
Waardenburg Syndrome Type 4B	AD, AR	EDN3	Endothelin 3
Waardenburg-Shah Syndrome	AD/AR	EDNRB	Endothelin Receptor, type B
Wagner Syndrome	AD	VCAN	Versican
Watson Syndrome; Neurofibromatosis	AD	NF1	Neurofibromin 1 (GTPase activating protein)
Werner Syndrome (Adult Progeria)	AR	RECQL2	RecQ protein-like 2 (DNA helicase)
Werner Syndrome, Atypical	AD	LMNA	Lamin A/C
Werner Syndrome, Atypical	AR	ZMPSTE24	Zinc metallopeptidase (STE24 homolog)
WHIM (Warts, Hypogammaglobu-linemia, Infections, and Myelokathexis) Syndrome	AD	CXCR4	Chemokine (C-X-C motif) receptor 4

J. Finch & M. Payette

Disorder	Inheritance	Gene	Protein
White Sponge Nevus	AD	K13	Keratin 13
White Sponge Nevus	AD	K4	Keratin 4
Williams Syndrome	AD	CLIP2, ELN, GTF2I, GTF2IRD1, LIMK1	Deletion of genetic material from a specific region of chromosome 7
Wilms Tumor	Somatic > AD	WT-1, BRCA2, GPC3	Wilms tumor 1. Tumor suppressor gene
Wilson's Disease	AR	ATP7B	ATPase, Cu2+-transporting, β-polypeptide
Winchester Syndrome	AR	MMP2	Matrix metalloproteinase 2
Wiskott-Aldrich Syndrome	XLR	WAS	WAS Protein, regulates transduction of Cdc42 protein which regulates cytoskeleton in T-cells
Woolly Hair (without other associated anomalies)	AD	K74	Keratin 74
Wrinkly Skin Syndrome	AR	ATP6V0A2	ATPase, H+ transporting, lysosomal, V0 Subunit A2
X-Linked Agammaglobulinemia (Bruton)	XLR	BTK	B cell tyrosine kinase
X-Linked Recessive Chondrodysplasia punctata	XLR	ARSE	Arylsulfatase E, Contiguous with X-linked Ichthyosis
X-linked Reticulate Pigmentary Disorder	XLR	POLA1	Catalytic subunit of DNA polymerase-α
X-linked Reticulate Pigmentary Disorder, Partington-type	XLR	Unknown	Unknown
Xeroderma Pigmentosum A (XPA)	AR	DDB1	DNA damage binding protein
Xeroderma Pigmentosum B (XPB)	AR	ERCC3 (XPB)	DNA helicase (3' to 5' DNA helicase in nucleotide excision repair)
Xeroderma Pigmentosum C (XPC)	AR	XPC	DNA damage-binding protein in nucleotide excision repair
Xeroderma Pigmentosum D (XPD)	AR	ERCC2 (XPD)	DNA helicase (5' to 3' DNA helicase in nucleotide excision repair)
Xeroderma Pigmentosum E (XPE)	AR	DDB2	DNA damage binding protein

Disorder	Inheritance	Gene	Protein
Xeroderma Pigmentosum F (XPF)	AR	ERCC4	5' endonuclease
Xeroderma Pigmentosum G (XPG)	AR	ERCC5	3' endonuclease
Xeroderma Pigmentosum, Variant (XP Variant)	AR	POLH	DNA Polymerase η (intact nucleotide excision repair)
Yellow Nail Syndrome	AD	FOXC2	Forkhead box C2
Yemenite Deaf-Blind Hypopigmentation	AD	SOX10	SRY-related HMG box gene 10
Zimmerman-Lanband Syndrome	AD	KCNH1	Voltage-gated potassium channel, Subfamily H, Member 1

Disorder	Inheritance	Gene	Protein
Grzybowski Syndrome	NI		
Azathioprine Myelosuppression	NI		Thiopurine methyltransferase (TPMT)
Diffuse Neonatal Hemangiomatosis	NI		
Klippel-Trenaunay Syndrome	NI		
LUMBAR Syndrome (SACRAL Syndrome, PELVIS Syndrome)	NI		
PHACES Syndrome	NI		
Leigh Syndrome	Mt	>12 genes	Various components of mitochondrial respiratory chain complexes
Tangier Disease	AR	ABCA1	ATP-binding cassette, subfamily A, member 1 (cholesterol efflux regulatory protein)
Harlequin Ichthyosis	AR	ABCA12	ATP-binding cassette, subfamily A, member 12
Lamellar Ichthyosis	AR	ABCA12	ATP-binding cassette, subfamily A, member 12
Pseudoxanthoma Elasticum	AR	ABCC6	ATP-binding cassette, subfamily C, member 6 (Multidrug resistance-associated protein 6)
Sitosterolemia	AR	ABCG5	ATP-binding cassette, subfamily G, member 5 (Sterolin 1)
Sitosterolemia	AR	ABCG8	ATP-binding cassette, subfamily G, member 8 (Sterolin 2)
Neutral Lipid Storage Disease (Chanarin–Dorfman Syndrome)	AR	ABHD5 (CGI-58)	Abhydrolase domain-containing 5 (comparative gene identification 58, esterase-lipase-thioesterase subfamily)
Dyskeratosis Congenita (Zinsser-Engman-Cole Syndrome)	AD or AR	ACD	Telomere protein
Fibrodysplasia Ossificans Progressiva	AD	ACVR1	Activin A receptor, Type I
Hereditary Hemorrhagic Telangiectasia, Type 2	AD	ACVRL1 (ALK1)	Activin A receptor, Type II-like 1
Severe Combined Immunodeficiency Syndrome (SCID) (B-NK-)	AR	ADA	"Adenosine Deaminase"
ADA2 Deficiency	AR	ADA2	Adenosine deaminase

Disorder	Inheritance	Gene	Protein
Reticulate Acropigmentation of Kitamura	AD	ADAM10	A disintegrin and metalloproteinase domain 10
Thrombotic Thrombocytopenic Purpura (TTP)	AR	ADAMTS-13	A disintegrin-like and metalloprotease with thrombospondin Type 1 motif, 13 (von Willebrand factor-cleaving protease)
Ehlers-Danlos Syndrome, Dermatosparaxis-type	AR	ADAMTS-2	A disintegrin-like and metalloproteinase with thrombospondin Type 1 motif, 2 (Procollagen I N-peptidase)
Dyschromatosis Symmetrica Hereditaria	AD	ADAR	Adenosine deaminase, RNA-specific
Albinism Deafness Syndrome (Woolf Syndrome, Ziprkowski-Margolis Syndrome)	XLR	ADFN	Unknown
Berardinelli-Seip Syndrome Type 1 (Congenital generalized lipodystrophy Type 1)	AR	AGPAT2	1-Acylglycerol-3-phosphate O-acyltransferase 2
Hyper IgM Syndrome	AR	AICDA	Activation-induced cytidine deaminase
Autoimmune Polyendocrinopathy (APECED, Candidiasis-Ectodermal Dystrophy)	AR>AD	AIRE	Autoimmune regulator
Proteus Syndrome	Somatic	AKT1	V-AKT Murine Thymoma Viral Oncogene Homolog 1
Porphyria, ALA Dehydratase Deficiency	AR	ALAD	Delta-aminolevulinate (ALA) dehydratase
De Barsy Syndrome (AR Cutis Laxa IIIa)	AR	ALDH18A1	Aldehyde dehydrogenase family 18, member A1 (Glutamate γ-semialdehyde synthetase)
Sjögren–Larsson Syndrome	AR	ALDH3A2 (FALDH)	Aldehyde dehydrogenase family 3, member A2 (fatty aldehyde dehydrogenase)
Non-bullous Congenital Ichthyosiform Erythroderma	AR	ALOX12B	12R-Lipoxygenase
Non-bullous Congenital Ichthyosiform Erythroderma	AR	ALOXE3	Epidermal lipoxygenase 3

J. Finch & M. Payette

Disorder	Inheritance	Gene	Protein
Kallmann Syndrome Type 1	XLR	ANOS1	Anosmin 1
Infantile Hemangiomas, Hereditary	AD	ANTXR1	Anthrax toxin receptor 1
Infantile Systemic Hyalinosis	AR	ANTXR2 (CMG2)	Anthrax toxin receptor 2 (capillary morphogenesis protein 2)
Juvenile Hyaline Fibromatosis (Murray-Puretic-Drescher Syndrome)	AR	ANTXR2 (CMG2)	Anthrax toxin receptor 2 (capillary morphogenesis Protein 2)
MEDNIK Syndrome	AR	AP1S1	Adaptor-related protein complex 1, sigma-1 subunit
Hermansky-Pudlak (Type 2)	AR	AP3B1	Adaptor protein 3, β1 subunit
Gardner Syndrome	AD	APC	Adenomatous polyposis coli
Familial Adenomatous Polyposis	AD	APC	Adenomatous polyposis coli
Hereditary Hypotrichosis Simplex	AD	APCDD1	APC Down-Regulated-1 gene encodes a membrane-bound glycoprotein expressed in human hair follicles
Heredofamilial Systemic Amyloidosis (Familial Amyloid Polyneuropathy)	AD	APOA1	Apolipoprotein A-I
Hypoalphalipo-proteinemia	AD	APOA1	Apolipoprotein A-I
Familial Hypertriglyceridemia (Type IV Hyperlipoproteinemia)	AD	APOA5	Apolipoprotein A-V
Familial Hypercholesterolemia (Type II Lipoproteinemia)	AR	APOB	Apolipoprotein B-100, LDL receptor binding domain
Apolipoprotein CII Deficiency (Type I Hyperlipoproteinemia)	AR	APOC2	Apolipoprotein C-II
Dysbetalipo-proteinemia (Type III Hyperlipo-proteinemia)	AR	APOE	Apolipoprotein E
Adams-Oliver Syndrome 1	AD	ARHGAP31	Rho-GTPase-Activating Protein 31
X-Linked Recessive Chondrodysplasia Punctata	XLR	ARSE	Arylsulfatase E, Contiguous with X-linked Ichthyosis
Severe Combined Immunodeficiency Syndrome (SCID) (B-NK+)	AR	Artemis gene (DCLRE1C)	DNA cross-link repair protein 1C (artemis)

Disorder	Inheritance	Gene	Protein
Farber Lipogranulomatosis	AR	ASAH	Acid ceramidase
Argininosuccinic Aciduria	AR	ASL	Argininosuccinate lysase
Citrullinemia	AR	ASS1	Argininosuccinate synthetase 1
Ataxia-Telangiectasia	AR	ATM	Ataxia-telangiectasia mutated (phosphatidylinositol 3-kinase like serine/threonine protein kinase)
Acrokeratosis Verruciformis of Hopf	AD	ATP2A2	Sarcoplasmic/endoplasmic reticulum Ca2+ ATPase 2 (SERCA2)
Darier's Disease (Keratosis Follicularis)	AD	ATP2A2	Sarcoplasmic/endoplasmic reticulum Ca2+ ATPase 2 (SERCA2)
Hailey-Hailey	AD	ATP2C1	Human secretory pathway Ca2+ ATPase 1 (hSPCA1)
Cutis Laxa, Type IIA	AR	ATP6V0A2	ATPase, H+ transporting, lysosomal, V0 Subunit A2
Wrinkly Skin Syndrome	AR	ATP6V0A2	ATPase, H+ transporting, lysosomal, V0 subunit A2
Cutis Laxa, X-linked	XLR	ATP7A	ATPase, Cu2+-transporting, α-polypeptide
Menkes Kinky Hair	XLR	ATP7A	ATPase, Cu2+-transporting, α-polypeptide
Wilson's Disease	AR	ATP7B	ATPase, Cu2+-transporting, β-polypeptide
Ehlers-Danlos Syndrome, Progeroid-type	AR	B4GALT7	Xylosylprotein 4b-galactosyl-transferase, polypeptide 7
Maple Syrup Urine Disease	AR	BCKDHA	E1-α subunit of the branched-chain α-keto acid (BCAA) dehydrogenase complex
UV Apoptosis	NI	BCL2	Protein phosphatase 1, regulatory subunit 50
Björnstad Syndrome	AR	BCSIL	ATPase needed for mitochondrial assembly
Hermansky-Pudlak (Type 8)	AR	BLOC1S3	Biogenesis of lysosome-related organelles complex 1, subunit 3 (BLOC1 component)

Disorder	Inheritance	Gene	Protein
Cowden-like Polyposis Syndrome	AD	BMPR1A	Bone morphogenetic protein receptor Type IA
Cardio-facio-cutaneous Syndrome	AD	BRAF	V-RAF murine sarcoma viral oncogene homolog
Noonan Syndrome Type 7	Unknown	BRAF	V-RAF murine sarcoma viral oncogene homolog
Lipodystrophy, Congenital Generalized (Berardinelli-Seip Type 2)	AR	BSCL2	Seipen
Biotinidase Deficiency	AR	BTD	Biotinidase
Multiple Carboxylase Deficiency	AR	BTD	Biotinidase
X-Linked Agammaglobulinemia (Bruton)	XLR	BTK	B cell tyrosine kinase
Hereditary Angioedema, Type 1	AD	C1INH (SERPING1)	C1 inhibitor protein
Hereditary Angioedema, Type 2	AD	C1INH (SERPING1)	C1 inhibitor protein
Leiner's Disease	Unknown	C5	C5 deficiency
Candidiasis, Familial Chronic Mucocutaneous Type 2	AR	CARD9	Caspase recruitment domain-containing protein 9
Homocystinuria	AR	CBS	Cystathione β-synthase (methionine metabolism defect)
Hennekam Lymphangiectasia-Lymphedema Syndrome, Type 1	AR	CCBE1	Collagen and calcium-binding EGF domain-containing protein 1
Nephropathy with Pretibial Epidermolysis Bullosa and Deafness	AR	CD151	Platelet-endothelial cell tetraspanin antigen 3 (CD151)
Common Variable Immunodeficiency	AR	CD19	CD19 B-lymphocyte antigen
Common Variable Immunodeficiency	AR	CD20 (MS4A1)	Membrane-spanning 4 Domains, Subfamily A, Member 1
Severe Combined Immunodeficiency Syndrome (SCID) (B+ NK+)	AR	CD3D	OKT3 δ-chain (T-cell antigen receptor)
Hyper IgM Syndrome	AR	CD40	Costimulatory protein found on antigen presenting cells
Hyper IgM Syndrome	XLR	CD40LG	Costimulatory protein found on activated T cells
Severe Combined Immunodeficiency Syndrome (SCID) (B+ NK+)	AR	CD45 (PTPRC)	Leukocyte Common Antigen (LCA) (Protein-Tyrosine Phosphatase, receptor-type, C)

Disorder	Inheritance	Gene	Protein
Common Variable Immunodeficiency	AR	CD81	CD81 antigen
Ectrodactyly Ectodermal Dysplasia Cleft Lip/Palate (EED) Syndrome	AR	CDH3	Cadherin 3 (P-cadherin)
Hypotrichosis with Juvenile Macular Dystrophy	AR	CDH3	Cadherin 3 (P-cadherin)
Familial Atypical Mole-malignant Melanoma (FAMMM) Syndrome	AD	CDK4	Cyclin-dependent kinase 4
Multiple Endocrine Neoplasia (MEN) Syndrome Type 4	AD	CDKN1B	Cyclin-dependent kinase inhibitor 1B (p27, Kip1)
Familial Atypical Mole-malignant Melanoma (FAMMM) Syndrome	AD	CDKN2A	Cyclin-dependent kinase inhibitor 2A (p16 (INK) and p14 (ARF)
Hypotrichosis Simplex of the Scalp	AD	CDSN	Corneodesmosin
Aquagenic Wrinkling of the Palms	AR	CFTR	Cystic Fibrosis Transmembrane Conductance Regulator
Multiple Pterygium Syndrome	AR	CHRNG	Cholinergic receptor, nicotinic, γ polypeptide
CINCA Syndrome (NOMID)	AD	CIAS1 (NLRP3)	NLR family, pyrin domain containing 3 (cryopyrin)
Familial Cold Autoinflammatory/ Urticaria Syndrome (FCAS)	AD	CIAS1 (NLRP3)	NLR family, pyrin domain containing 3 (cryopyrin)
Muckle–Wells Syndrome	AD	CIAS1 (NLRP3)	NLR family, pyrin domain containing 3 (cryopyrin)
Maple Syrup Urine Disease	AR	CKDHB	E1-β subunit of the branched-chain α-keto acid (BCAA) dehydrogenase complex
Cold-Induced Sweating Syndrome Type 2	AR	CLCF1	Cardiotrophin-like cytokine factor 1
Ichthyosis, Hypotrichosis-Sclerosing Cholangitis (IHSC)	AR	CLDN1	Claudin 1
Candidiasis, Familial Chronic Mucocutaneous Type 4	AR	CLEC7A	Dectin-1 (pattern recognition receptor)
Williams Syndrome	AD	CLIP2, ELN, GTF2I, GTF2IRD1, LIMK1	Deletion of genetic material from a specific region of chromosome 7

J. Finch & M. Payette

Disorder	Inheritance	Gene	Protein
Ehlers-Danlos Syndrome, Arthrochalasia-type	AD	COL1A1	α1 chain of Type I collagen
Osteogenesis Imperfecta	AD	COL1A1	α1 chain of Type I collagen
Ehlers-Danlos Syndrome, Arthrochalasia-type	AD	COL1A2	α2 chain of Type I collagen
Ehlers-Danlos Syndrome, Cardiac Valvular-type	AR	COL1A2	α2 chain of Type I collagen
Osteogenesis Imperfecta	AD	COL1A2	α2 chain of Type I collagen
Ehlers-Danlos Syndrome, Vascular-type	AD	COL3A1	α1 chain of Type III collagen
Ehlers-Danlos Syndrome, Classic	AD	COL5A1	α1 chain of Type V collagen
Ehlers-Danlos Syndrome, Classic	AD	COL5A2	α2 chain of Type V collagen
Ullrich Scleroatonic Muscular Dystrophy	AR	COL6A1	α1 chain of Type VI collagen
Ullrich Scleroatonic Muscular Dystrophy	AR	COL6A2	α2 chain of Type VI collagen
Ullrich Scleroatonic Muscular Dystrophy	AR	COL6A3	α3 chain of Type VI collagen
Bart's Syndrome	AD	COL7A1	α1 chain of Type VII collagen
Epidermolysis Bullosa, Dominant Dystrophic	AD	COL7A1	α1 chain of Type VII collagen
Epidermolysis Bullosa, Recessive Dystrophic	AR	COL7A1	α1 chain of Type VII collagen
Isolated Toenail Dystrophy	AD	COL7A1	α1 chain of Type VII collagen
Hereditary Coproporphyria	AD	CPOX	Coproporphyrinogen oxidase
Rubinstein-Taybi Syndrome Type 1 (Thumb-Hallux Syndrome)	AD	CREBBP	CREB-binding protein
Cold-Induced Sweating Syndrome Type 1	AR	CRLF1	Cytokine receptor-like factor 1
Dyskeratosis Congenita (Zinsser-Engman-Cole Syndrome)	AR	CTC1, NHP2, NOP10, PARN, WRAP53	Telomerase complex components
Pilomatricoma	Somatic	CTNNB1	β-Catenin
Haim-Munk Syndrome	AR	CTSC	Cathepsin C
Papillon-Lefèvre Syndrome	AR	CTSC	Cathepsin C

Disorder	Inheritance	Gene	Protein
WHIM (Warts, Hypogammaglobulinemia, Infections, and Myelokathexis) Syndrome	AD	CXCR4	Chemokine (C-X-C motif) receptor 4
Chronic Granulomatous Disease	AR	CYBA	α subunit of cytochrome b(-245)
Chronic Granulomatous Disease	XLR	CYBB	α subunit of cytochrome b(-245)
Brooke-Spiegler Syndrome	AD	CYLD	Deubiquitinating enzyme (removes lys63-linked ubiquitin chains)
Cylindroma, Sporadic Tumor	sporadic	CYLD	Deubiquitinating enzyme (removes lys63-linked ubiquitin chains)
Familial Cylindromatosis	AD	CYLD	Deubiquitinating enzyme (removes lys63-linked ubiquitin chains)
Trichoepitheliomas, Multiple Familial	AD	CYLD	Deubiquitinating enzyme (removes lys63-linked ubiquitin chains)
Cerebrotendinous Xanthomatosis	AR	CYP27A1	Cytochrome P450, subfamily 27A1 (sterol 27 hydroxylase)
Lamellar Ichthyosis	AR	CYP4F22	Cytochrome P450, family 4, subfamily F22
Maple Syrup Urine Disease	AR	DBT	Lipoamide acyltransferase component of branched-chain α-keto acid dehydrogenase complex
Athabascan-type Severe Combined Immunodeficiency (SCIDA)	AR	DCLRE1C	Protein artemis (Endonuclease involved in V(D)J recombination and DNA repair)
Omenn Syndrome (SCID)	AR	DCLRE1C	Protein artemis (Endonuclease involved in V(D)J recombination and DNA repair)
Congenital Corneal Dystrophy	AD	DCN	Decorin
Xeroderma Pigmentosum A (XPA)	AR	DDB1	DNA damage binding protein
Xeroderma Pigmentosum E (XPE)	AR	DDB2	DNA damage binding protein
Smith-Lemli-Opitz Syndrome	AR	DHCR7	Delta-7-sterol reductase

Disorder	Inheritance	Gene	Protein
Dyskeratosis Congenita (Zinsser-Engman-Cole Syndrome)	XLR	DKC1	Dyskerin
Maple Syrup Urine Disease	AR	DLD	Dihydrolipoamide dehydrogenase
Tricho-Dento-Osseous Syndrome	AD	DLX3	Distal-less homeobox 3
Dimethylglycine Dehydrogenase Deficiency	AR	DMGDH	Dimethylglycine dehydrogenase
Adams-Oliver Syndrome 2	AR	DOCK6	Dedicator of cytokinesis 6
Hyper IgE Syndrome (Job Syndrome)	AR	DOCK8	Dedicator of cytokinesis 8
Dolichol Kinase Deficiency	AR	DOLK	Dolichol kinase
Striate Palmoplantar Keratoderma (PPK)	AD	DSG1	Desmoglein 1
Arrhythmogenic Right Ventricular Dysplasia/Cardiomyopathy (ARVD/C)	AD	DSG2	Desmoglein 2
Localized Autosomal Recessive Hypotrichosis	AR	DSG4	Desmoglein 4
Monilethrix	AR	DSG4	Desmoglein 4
Carvajal Syndrome	AR	DSP	Desmoplakin
Lethal Acantholytic Epidermolysis Bullosa	AR	DSP	Desmoplakin
Skin Fragility/Woolly Hair Syndrome	AR	DSP	Desmoplakin
Striate Palmoplantar Keratoderma (PPK)	AD	DSP	Desmoplakin
Reticulate Acropigmentation of Dohi	AD	DSRAD	Adenosine deaminase, RNA-specific
Hermansky-Pudlak (Type 7)	AR	DTNBP1	Dysbindin (dystrobrevin-binding protein 1)
Conradi-Hünermann-Happle Syndrome	XLD	EBP	D8-D7 sterol isomerase (emopamil binding protein)
Lipoid Proteinosis	AR	ECM1	Extracellular matrix Protein 1
Anhidrotic Ectodermal Dysplasia (Hypohidrotic Ectodermal Dysplasia)	XLR	EDA	Ectodysplasin A
Hypohidrotic Ectodermal Dysplasia	XLR	EDA	Ectodysplasin A

Disorder	Inheritance	Gene	Protein
Selective Tooth Agenesis	XLD	EDA	Ectodysplasin A
Hypohidrotic Ectodermal Dysplasia	AD	EDAR	Ectodysplasin A receptor
Hypohidrotic Ectodermal Dysplasia	AD	EDARADD	EDAR-associated death domain
Waardenburg Syndrome Type 4B	AD, AR	EDN3	Endothelin 3
Albinism, Black lock, Cell migration Disorder of the Neurocytes of the Gut and Deafness (ABCD)	AR	EDNRB	Endothelin Receptor, Type B
Waardenburg Syndrome Type 4A	AD, AR	EDNRB	Endothelin Receptor, Type B
Waardenburg-Shah Syndrome	AD/AR	EDNRB	Endothelin Receptor, Type B
Cutis Laxa, Type IB	AR	EFEMP2 (FBLN4)	EGF-containing fibulin-like extracellular matrix protein 2 (fibulin-4)
Cyclic Neutropenia	AD	ELA2	Neutrophil elastase
Cutis Laxa, AD	AD	ELN	Elastin
Hereditary Hemorrhagic Telangiectasia, Type 1	AD	ENG	Endoglin (component of endothelial cell TGF-β receptor)
Rubinstein-Taybi Syndrome Type 2	Sporadic	EP300	E1A-binding protein
Trichothiodystrophy	AR	ERCC2 (XPD)	DNA helicase (5' to 3' DNA helicase in nucleotide excision repair)
Xeroderma Pigmentosum D (XPD)	AR	ERCC2 (XPD)	DNA helicase (5' to 3' DNA helicase in nucleotide excision repair)
Trichothiodystrophy	AR	ERCC3 (XPB)	DNA helicase (3' to 5' DNA helicase in nucleotide excision repair)
Xeroderma Pigmentosum B (XPB)	AR	ERCC3 (XPB)	DNA helicase (3' to 5' DNA helicase in nucleotide excision repair)
Xeroderma Pigmentosum F (XPF)	AR	ERCC4	5' endonuclease
Xeroderma Pigmentosum G (XPG)	AR	ERCC5	3' endonuclease
Cockayne Syndrome B	AR	ERCC6	DNA helicase, excision repair cross-complementing, group 6

Disorder	Inheritance	Gene	Protein
De Sanctis-Cacchione Syndrome	AR	ERCC6	DNA helicase, excision repair cross-complementing, group 6
Cockayne Syndrome A	AR	ERCC8	DNA helicase, excision repair cross-complementing, group 6
Ellis-van Creveld (EVC)	AR	EVC	EVC (single-pass Type I transmembrane protein)
Hereditary Angioedema, Type 3	AD	F12	Factor XII (Hageman factor)
Hypoprothrombinemia	AD	F2	Prothrombin, G20210A polymorphism
Activated Protein C Resistance (Factor V Leiden)	AD	F5	Factor V
Tyrosinemia Type I	AR	FAH	Fumarylacetoacetate hydrolase
Cutis Laxa, Type IA	AR	FBLN5	Fibulin 5
Marfan Syndrome Type 1	AD	FBN1	Fibrillin 1
Stiff Skin Syndrome	AD	FBN1	Fibrillin 1
Congenital Contractural Arachnodactyly	AD	FBN2	Fibrillin 2
Erythropoietic Protoporphyria	AD	FECH	Ferrochelatase
Leukocyte Adhesion Deficiency Type III	AR	FERMT3, KIND3	Intracellular protein that interacts with β-integrins in hematopoietic cells
Hyperphosphatemic Familial Tumoral Calcinosis	AR	FGF23	Fibroblast growth factor 23
Kallmann Syndrome Type 2	AD/AR	FGFR1	Fibroblast growth factor receptor 1
CAP (Craniosynostosis, Anal Anomalies and Porokeratoses) Syndrome	AR	FGFR1, FGFR2, FGFR3	Fibroblast growth factor receptor 1, 2, 3
Apert Syndrome	AD	FGFR2	Fibroblast growth factor receptor 2
Beare-Stevenson Cutis Gyrata Syndrome	AD	FGFR2	Fibroblast growth factor receptor 2
Crouzon Syndrome with Acanthosis Nigricans (SADDAN Syndrome, Thanatophoric Dysplasia)	AD	FGFR3	Fibroblast growth factor receptor 3

Disorder	Inheritance	Gene	Protein
Epidermal Nevus	somatic	FGFR3	Fibroblast growth factor receptor 3
Hereditary Leiomyomatosis and Renal Cell Cancer	AD	FH	Fumarate hydratase
Systemic Mastocytosis	Somatic	FIPL1/ PDGFRA fusion	FIPL1/PDGFRA fusion protein
Birt-Hogg-Dubé Syndrome	AD	FLCN	Folliculin
Ichthyosis Vulgaris	AD	FLG	Filaggrin
Ehlers-Danlos Syndrome, with Periventricular Nodular Heterotopia	XLD	FLNA	Filamin A (actin-binding protein 280)
Lymphedema, Hereditary early onset-type (Milroy Disease)	AD	FLT4	FMA-related tyrosine kinase 4 (vascular endothelial growth factor receptor 3)
Milroy Disease (Hereditary Lymphedema)	AD	FLT4	FMA-related tyrosine kinase 4 (vascular endothelial growth factor receptor 3)
Trimethylaminuria	AR	FMO3	Flavin-containing monooxygenase 3
Lymphedema Praecox (Meige Lymphedema)	AD	FOXC2	Forkhead box C2
Lymphedema-Distichiasis	AD	FOXC2	Forkhead box C2
Yellow Nail Syndrome	AD	FOXC2	Forkhead box C2
Milroy's Disease (Hereditary Lymphedema)	AD	FOXC2, SOX18, GATA2, CCBE1, PTPN14, KIF11, VEGFC	Multiple proteins
T-cell Immunodeficiency and Congenital Alopecia	AR	FOXN1	Forkhead box N1 (winged helix nude)
IPEX (Immune dysregulation, Polyendocrinopathy, Enteropathy, X-linked) Syndrome	XLR	FOXP3	Forkhead box P3
Fraser Syndrome	AR	FRAS1	Extracellular matrix protein
Fraser Syndrome	AR	FREM2	Fras1-related extracellular matrix protein 2
Fucosidosis	AR	FUCA1	α L fucosidase
Hyperphosphatemic Familial Tumoral Calcinosis	AR	GALNT3	UDP-N-acetyl-α-D-galactosamine, polypeptide N-acetylgalactosaminyl-transferase 3

Disorder	Inheritance	Gene	Protein
Giant Axonal Neuropathy with Curly Hair	AR	GAN1	Gigatoxin
Acute Megakaryocyte Leukemia	Somatic	GATA1	Mutation seen in 20% of transient myeloproliferation d/o a/w Down Syndrome
Monocytopenia and Mycobacterial Infection (MonoMAC) Syndrome	AD	GATA2	Zinc finger transcription factor
Gaucher Disease Types I-III	AR	GBA	Acid-β-glucosidase, ↓ glucocerebrosidase (in histiocytes)
Pseudoxanthoma Elasticum-like Disorder with Multiple Coagulation Factor Deficiency	AR	GGCX	γ-glutamyl carboxylase
Laron Syndrome (Pituitary Dwarfism II)	AR	GHR	Growth hormone receptor
Hallermann-Streiff Syndrome (Oculomandibulofacial Syndrome)	Somatic	GJA1	Gap junction protein α1 (connexin 43)
Oculodentodigital Dysplasia	AD/AR	GJA1	Gap junction protein α1 (connexin 43)
Bart-Pumphrey Syndrome	AD	GJB2	Gap junction protein β2 (connexin 26)
Hystrix-like Ichthyosis–Deafness (HID) Syndrome	AD	GJB2	Gap junction protein β2 (connexin 26)
KID (Keratitis–Ichthyosis–Deafness) Syndrome	AD>AR	GJB2	Gap junction protein β2 (connexin 26)
Palmoplantar Keratoderma (PPK) with Deafness	AD	GJB2	Gap junction protein β2 (connexin 26)
Vohwinkel Syndrome	AD	GJB2	Gap junction protein β2 (connexin 26)
Erythrokeratodermia Variabilis (Mendes da Costa)	AD	GJB3	Gap junction protein β3 (connexin 31)
Erythrokeratodermia Variabilis (Mendes da Costa)	AD	GJB4	Gap junction protein β4 (connexin 30.3)
Hidrotic Ectodermal Dysplasia (Clouston Syndrome)	AD	GJB6	Gap junction protein β6 (connexin 30)
Milroy's Disease (Hereditary Lymphedema)	AD	GJC2	Gap junction protein γ2 (connexin 47)
Fabry Disease	XLR	GLA	α galactosidase A , (↑ in glycosphingolipid trihexidosyl ceramide)

Disorder	Inheritance	Gene	Protein
Glomuvenous Malformations (Familial Glomangiomatosis)	AD	GLMN	Glomulin
Sturge-Weber Syndrome	Somatic	GNAQ	Guanine Nucleotide-binding protein, Q polypeptide
Albright's Hereditary Osteodystrophy	AD	GNAS	G protein, α subunit
McCune–Albright Syndrome	AD	GNAS	G protein, α subunit
Plate-Like Osteoma Cutis	AD	GNAS	G protein, α subunit
Progressive Osseous Heteroplasia	AD	GNAS	G protein, α subunit
Albinism, Ocular Type 1 (Nettleship-Falls)	XLR	GPR143	G protein coupled receptor 143
Hereditary Gelsolin Amyloidosis	AD	GSN	Gelsolin
Trichothiodystrophy	AR	GTF2H5 (TTDA)	Transcription/repair factor TFIIH
Hemochromatosis, Juvenile	AR	HAMP	Hepcidin antimicrobial peptide
MIDAS (Microphthalmia, Dermal Aplasia, and Sclerocornea) Syndrome	XLD	HCCS	Holocytochrome C Synthase
Hemochromatosis	AR	HFE	Hemochromatosis, ↑ iron absorption and deposition
Hemochromatosis, Juvenile	AR	HFE2	Hemojuvelin
Alkaptonuria (Ochronosis)	AR	HGD	Homogentisic acid oxidase
Lesch-Nyhan	XLR	HGPT	Hypoxanthine guanine phosphoribosyl-transferase, ↑ uric acid
Holocarboxylase Synthetase Deficiency	AR	HLCS	Holocarboxylase synthetase
Multiple Carboxylase Deficiency	AR	HLCS	Holocarboxylase synthetase
Porphyria, Acute Intermittent	AD	HMBS	Hydroxymethylbilane synthase; also known as porphobilinogen deaminase (PBGD)
Hypertrophic Osteoarthropathy (Pachydermo-periostosis, Touraine-Solente-Golé Syndrome)	AR	HPGD	15-Hydroxyprostag-landin Dehydrogenase
Hermansky-Pudlak (Type 1)	AR	HPS1	HPS1 (BLOC-3 component)
Hermansky-Pudlak (Type 3)	AR	HPS3	HPS3 (BLOC-2 component)

J. Finch & M. Payette

Disorder	Inheritance	Gene	Protein
Hermansky-Pudlak (Type 4)	AR	HPS4	HPS4 (BLOC-3 component)
Hermansky-Pudlak (Type 5)	AR	HPS5	α-integrin-binding protein (BLOC-2 component)
Hermansky-Pudlak (Type 6)	AR	HPS6	BLOC-2 component
Atrichia with Papules	AR	HR	Hairless (zinc finger transcription factor)
Marie-Unna Hypotrichosis	AR	HR	Hairless (zinc finger transcription factor)
Costello Syndrome	AD	HRAS	V-HA-RAS Harvey rat sarcoma viral oncogene homolog
Epidermal Nevus	somatic	HRAS	V-HA-RAS Harvey rat sarcoma viral oncogene homolog
Schimmelpenning-Feuerstein-Mims Syndrome (Linear Sebaceous Nevus Syndrome)	Somatic	HRAS	V-HA-RAS Harvey rat sarcoma viral oncogene homolog
Schwartz-Jampel Syndrome	AR	HSPG2	Heparan sulfate proteoglycan of basement membrane
Hypertrichosis Universalis Congenita (Ambras Syndrome)	AD	HTC1	Function unknown
Hypertrichosis, Generalized, X-Linked	XLD	HTC2	Palindrome-mediated interchromosomal insertion at chromosome Xq27.1
Common Variable Immunodeficiency	AR	ICOS	Inducible T-cell costimulator
Maffucci Syndrome (Multiple Enchondromatosis)	AD	IDH1/IDH2	Isocitrate dehydrogenase 1 or 2
Mucopolysaccharidosis Type II (Hunter Syndrome)	XLR	IDS	Iduronate-2-sulfatase; dermatan, heparan sulfate
Mucopolysaccharidosis Type I (Hurler Syndrome)	AR	IDUA	α-L-iduronidase; dermatan, heparan sulfate
Beckwith-Wiedemann	AD	IGF2, (also H19, p57 (KIP2), CDKN1C, NSD1, and LIT1)	Insulin-like growth factor 2

Disorder	Inheritance	Gene	Protein
Familial Dysautonomia (Riley-Day Syndrome)	AR	IKBKAP	Inhibitor of κ light polypeptide gene enhancer in B cells, kinase complex-associated protein; component of Elongator, a transcription elongation factor complex that has histone acetyltransferase activity
Hypohidrotic Ectodermal Dysplasia, with Immunodeficiency	XLR	IKBKG (NEMO)	Inhibitor of κ light polypeptide gene enhancer in B cells kinase γ (nuclear factor-κB essential modulator)
Incontinentia Pigmenti	XLD	IKBKG (NEMO)	Inhibitor of κ light polypeptide gene enhancer in B cells, kinase γ (nuclear factor-κB essential modulator)
IL 12/23 Deficiency	AR	IL12β, IL12Rβ	p40 subunit of IL-12 & IL-23 or its receptor
Candidiasis, Familial Chronic Mucocutaneous Type 6	Unknown	IL17F	Interleukin-17
Candidiasis, Familial Chronic Mucocutaneous Type 5	Unknown	IL17RA	Interleukin-17 Receptor A
DIRA (Deficiency of the Interleukin-1 Receptor Antagonist) Syndrome	AR	IL1RN	Interleukin 1 receptor antagonist
Severe Combined Immunodeficiency Syndrome (SCID) (B+ NK-)	XLR	IL2RG	γ chain of IL-2 receptor
Severe Combined Immunodeficiency Syndrome (SCID) (B+ NK+)	AR	IL7R	IL-7 receptor
Leprechaunism (Rabson-Mendenhall Syndrome, Donohue Syndrome)	AR	INSR	Insulin receptor
Popliteal Pterygium Syndrome	AD	IRF6	Interferon regulatory factor 6
Van der Woude Syndrome	AD	IRF6	Interferon regulatory factor 6
Leukocyte Adhesion Deficiency Type I	AR	ITGB2	β2 integrin
Epidermolysis Bullosa, Junctional with Pyloric Atresia	AR	ITGB4	β4 integrin

Disorder	Inheritance	Gene	Protein
Isovaleric Acidemia	AR	IVD	Isovaleryl-coA dehydrogenase
Alagille-Watson Syndrome	AD	JAG1	Jagged 1
Polycythemia Vera, Essential Thrombocythemia	Somatic	JAK2	Janus Kinase 2
Severe Combined Immunodeficiency Syndrome (SCID) (B+ NK-)	AR	JAK3	Janus Kinase 3, TAP1, TAP2, defective MHCI, defective CD8
Naxos Syndrome	AR	JUP	Junction Plakoglobin
Ichthyosis, Epidermolytic (Bullous CIE)	AD	K1	Keratin 1
Ichthyosis, Hystrix Curth–Macklin	AD	K1	Keratin 1
Striate Palmoplantar Keratoderma (PPK)	AD	K1	Keratin 1
Unna-Thost PPK (Non-Epidermolytic PPK)	AD	K1	Keratin 1
Vörner PPK (Epidermolytic PPK)	AD	K1	Keratin 1 (feet)
Ichthyosis, Epidermolytic (Bullous CIE)	AD	K10	Keratin 10
Meesmann Corneal Dystrophy	AD	K12	Keratin 12
White Sponge Nevus	AD	K13	Keratin 13
Dermatopathia Pigmentosa Reticularis	AD	K14	Keratin 14
Dowling-Meara Epidermolysis Bullosa	AD	K14	Keratin 14
Epidermolysis Bullosa Simplex (EBS)	AD	K14	Keratin 14
Epidermolysis Bullosa Simplex (EBS) Weber-Cockayne	AD	K14	Keratin 14
Naegeli–Franceschetti–Jadassohn Syndrome	AD	K14	Keratin 14
Pachyonychia Congenita Type I (Jadassohn-Lewandowsky)	AD	K16	Keratin 16
Pachyonychia Congenita Type II (Jackson-Lawler)	AD	K17	Keratin 17
Steatocystoma Multiplex	AD	K17	Keratin 17
Ichthyosis, Bullosa of Siemens	AD	K2e	Keratin 2e

Disorder	Inheritance	Gene	Protein
Meesmann Corneal Dystrophy	AD	K3	Keratin 3
White Sponge Nevus	AD	K4	Keratin 4
Dowling-Meara Epidermolysis Bullosa	AD	K5	Keratin 5
Dowling–Degos Disease (Reticulate Pigment Anomaly of Flexures)	AD	K5	Keratin 5
Epidermolysis Bullosa Simplex (EBS)	AD	K5	Keratin 5
Epidermolysis Bullosa Simplex (EBS) Weber-Cockayne	AD	K5	Keratin 5
Pachyonychia Congenita Type I (Jadassohn-Lewandowsky)	AD	K6a	Keratin 6a
Pachyonychia Congenita Type II (Jackson-Lawler)	AD	K6b	Keratin 6b
Woolly Hair (without other associated anomalies)	AD	K74	Keratin 74
Monilethrix	AD	K81, K83, K86	Hair cortex keratins
Pure Hair-Nail-type Ectodermal Dysplasia	AR	K85	Keratin 85
Vörner PPK (Epidermolytic PPK)	AD	K9	Keratin 9 (hands)
Zimmerman-Lanband Syndrome	AD	KCNH1	Voltage-gated potassium channel, Subfamily H, Member 1
Cornea Plana Congenita	AR	KERA	Keratocan
Kindler Syndrome	AR	KIND1 (C20orf42)	Kindlin 1
Leukocyte Adhesion Deficiency Type III	AR	KIND3	Fermitin Family Homolog 3
Familial Mastocytosis	AD	KIT	KIT proto-oncogene (stem cell factor receptor)
Mastocytosis, adult-onset	Somatic	KIT	KIT proto-oncogene (stem cell factor receptor)
Piebaldism	AD	KIT	KIT proto-oncogene (stem cell factor receptor)
Hyperphosphatemic Familial Tumoral Calcinosis	AR	KL	Klotho
Cardio-Facio-Cutaneous Syndrome	AD	KRAS	V-KI-RAS2 Kirsten rat sarcoma viral oncogene homolog

J. Finch & M. Payette

Disorder	Inheritance	Gene	Protein
Costello Syndrome	AD	KRAS	V-KI-RAS2 Kirsten rat sarcoma viral oncogene homolog
Noonan Syndrome Type 3	Unknown	KRAS	V-KI-RAS2 Kirsten rat sarcoma viral oncogene homolog
Schimmelpenning-Feuerstein-Mims Syndrome (Linear Sebaceous Nevus Syndrome)	Somatic	KRAS	V-KI-RAS2 Kirsten rat sarcoma viral oncogene homolog
Cerebral Capillary Malformations, Familial (Associated with Hyperkeratotic Cutaneous Capillary-Venous Malformations)	AD	KRIT1 (CCM1)	Krev interaction trapped-1
Epidermolysis Bullosa, Junctional, Generalized Atrophic Benign-type	AR	LAMA3	Laminin polypeptide α3 subunit (component of laminin 332)
Epidermolysis Bullosa, Junctional, Herlitz-type	AR	LAMA3	Laminin polypeptide α3 subunit (component of laminin 332)
Laryngo-Onycho-Cutaneous (Shabbir) Syndrome	AR	LAMA3	Laminin polypeptide α3 subunit (component of laminin 332)
Epidermolysis Bullosa, Junctional, Non-Herlitz-type	AR	LAMA3, LAMB3, LAMC2, COL17A1, ITGB4	Laminin polypeptide α3, β3, or γ2 subunit (components of laminin 332)
Cutis Laxa, Neonatal Marfanoid-type	AD	LAMB1	Laminin polypeptide, β1 subunit
Epidermolysis Bullosa, Junctional	AR	LAMB3	Laminin polypeptide β3 subunit (component of laminin 332)
Epidermolysis Bullosa, Junctional, Herlitz-type	AR	LAMB3	Laminin polypeptide β3 subunit (component of laminin 332)
Epidermolysis Bullosa, Junctional, Herlitz-type	AR	LAMC2	Laminin polypeptide γ2 subunit (component of laminin 332)
Familial Hypercholesterolemia (Type II Lipoproteinemia)	AD	LDLR	LDL receptor
Buschke-Ollendorff Syndrome	AD	LEMD3 (MAN1)	LEM domain containing 3 (Man 1, an inner nuclear membrane protein)
Melorheostosis	Somatic	LEMD3 (MAN1)	LEM domain containing 3 (Man 1, an inner nuclear membrane protein)
Hypotrichosis, Mari-type	AR	LIPH	Lipase H

Disorder	Inheritance	Gene	Protein
Familial Hypertriglyceridemia (Type IV Hyperlipoproteinemia)	AD	LIPI	Lipase member I
Lipodystrophy, Familial Partial	AD	LMNA	Lamin A/C
Mandibuloacral Dysplasia Syndrome	AR	LMNA	Lamin A/C
Progeria (Hutchinson-Gilford)	AD>>AR	LMNA	Lamin A/C
Restrictive Dermopathy	AD	LMNA	Lamin A/C
Werner Syndrome, Atypical	AD	LMNA	Lamin A/C
Lipodystrophy, Acquired Partial (Barraquer Simons Syndrome)	AD	LMNB2	Lamin B2
Nail-Patella Syndrome (Hereditary Osteo-Onychodysplasia)	AD	LMX1B	LIM homeodomain protein (involved in dorsal-ventral limb patterning)
Progressive Symmetric Erythrokeratoderma	AD	LOR	Loricrin
Vohwinkel Syndrome, Variant	AD	LOR	Loricrin
Majeed Syndrome (Recurrent Sweet's + Osteomyelitis)	AR	LPIN2	Lipin 2
Lipoprotein Lipase Deficiency (Type 1 Hyperlipoproteinemia)	AR	LPL	Lipoprotein lipase
Chédiak-Higashi Syndrome	AR	LYST	Lysosomal trafficking regulator
Noonan Syndrome Type 10	AD	LZTR1	Leucine zipper-like transcriptional regulator 1
Cardio-Facio-Cutaneous Syndrome	AD	MAP2K1 (MEK1)	Mitogen-activated protein kinase 1
Cardio-Facio-Cutaneous Syndrome	AD	MAP2K2 (MEK2)	Mitogen-activated protein kinase 2
Methionine Adenosyltransferase Deficiency	AD/AR	MAT1A	Methionine adenosyltransferase I, α
IFAP (Ichthyosis-Follicularis-Atrichia-Photophobia) Syndrome	XLR	MBTPS2	Membrane-embedded zinc metalloprotease
Keratosis Follicularis Spinulosa Decalvans	XLR	MBTPS2	Membrane-embedded zinc metalloprotease
Familial Mediterranean Fever	AR, AD	MEFV	Pyrin (marenostrin)

Disorder	Inheritance	Gene	Protein
Multiple Endocrine Neoplasia (MEN) Syndrome Type 1 (Wermer)	AD	MEN1	Menin, nuclear scaffold protein
Tietz Syndrome	AD	MITF	Microphthalmia-associated transcription factor
Waardenburg Syndrome Type 2	AD	MITF	Microphthalmia-associated transcription factor
Muir-Torre Syndrome	AD	MLH1	MutL homolog 1 (mismatch repair enzyme)
Griscelli Syndrome, Type 3	AR	MLPH	Melanophilin
Nodulosis, Arthropathy, Osteolysis (NAO) Syndrome	AR	MMP2	Matrix metalloproteinase 2
Winchester Syndrome	AR	MMP2	Matrix metalloproteinase 2
Trichothiodystrophy without Photosensitivity or Ichthyosis	AR	MPLKIP	M-phase-specific PLK1-interacting protein
Muir-Torre Syndrome	AD	MSH2	MutS homolog 2
IgA Deficiency Type I	Unknown	MSH5	Inability to produce IgA
Muir-Torre Syndrome	AD	MSH6	MutS homolog 6
Mammalian Sterile 20-like Kinase 1 Deficiency	AR	MST1 (STK4)	Serine-threonine kinase
Familial Tooth Agenesis (Witkop Syndrome)	AD	MSX1	Muscle segment homeobox 1
Lipomatosis, Benign Symmetric (Madelung Disease)	Most Unknown. Some Mt	MT-TK	Mitochondrial lysine tRNA
Palmoplantar Keratoderma (PPK) with Deafness	Mt	MT-TS1	Mitochondrial serine tRNA
Hyper-IgD with Periodic Fever Syndrome	AR	MVK	Mevalonate kinase
Porokeratosis, Disseminated Superficial Actinic	AD	MVK	Mevalonate kinase
Burkitt's Lymphoma	NI	MYC	V-MYC Avian Myelocytomatosis Viral Oncogene Homolog
Griscelli Syndrome, Type 1 (Elejalde Syndrome)	AR	MYO5A	Myosin 5A
Slow Acetylator Phenotype	AR	NAT1	N-Acetyl Transferase
Chronic Granulomatous Disease	AR	NCF1, NCF2, NCF4	Neutrophil cytosolic factor 1, 2, or 4

Disorder	Inheritance	Gene	Protein
Prader-Willi	NI	NDN, SNRPN	Genomic imprinting caused by deletion or inactivation of genes on the paternally inherited chromosome 15
Ectodermal Dysplasia, Hypohidrotic, with Immune Deficiency	XLR	NEMO	NF-Kappa-B Essential Modulator
Sialidosis	AR	NEU1	Neuramidase (skin fragility)
Neurofibromatosis-1	AD	NF1	Neurofibromin 1 (GTPase activating protein)
Watson Syndrome; Neurofibromatosis	AD	NF1	Neurofibromin 1 (GTPase activating protein)
Neurofibromatosis-2	AD	NF2	Neurofibromin 2 (merlin)
Ichthyosis, Congenital AR-type	AR	NIPAL4	Ichthyin, NIPA-like domain-containing 4
Non-bullous Congenital Ichthyosiform Erythroderma	AR	NIPAL4	Ichthyin
Blau Syndrome (Familial Granulomatous Arthritis, Dermatitis and Uveitis)	AD	NOD2 (CARD 15)	Nucleotide-binding oligomerization domain containing 2
CADASIL (Cerebral Autosomal-Dominant Arteriopathy with Subcortical Infarcts and Leukoencephalopathy)	AD	NOTCH-3	Notch Drosophila Homolog, 3
Epidermal Nevus	somatic	NRAS	Neuroblastoma Ras viral oncogene homolog
Noonan Syndrome Type 6	AD	NRAS	Neuroblastoma Ras viral oncogene homolog
Schimmelpenning-Feuerstein-Mims Syndrome (Linear Sebaceous Nevus Syndrome)	Somatic	NRAS	Neuroblastoma Ras viral oncogene homolog
CHILD Syndrome (Congenital Hemidysplasia with Ichthyosiform Erythroderma and Limb Defects)	XLD	NSDHL	3ß-hydroxysteroid dehydrogenase
Insensitivity to Pain with Anhidrosis	AR	NTRK1	Neurotrophic tyrosine kinase receptor Type 1
Oculocutaneous Albinism Type 2 (OCA2)	AR	OCA2	P protein (pink eye dilution homolog)
Oral-Facial-Digital Syndrome	XLD	OFD1	Centriole and centriolar satellite protein

Disorder	Inheritance	Gene	Protein
Primary Localized Cutaneous Amyloidosis 1	AD	OSMR	Oncostatin M receptor
Phenylketonuria	AR	PAH	Phenylalanine hydroxylase
Waardenburg Syndrome Type 1	AD	PAX3	Paired box gene 3
Waardenburg Syndrome Type 3	AD	PAX3	Paired box gene 3
Familial Hypercholesterolemia (Type II Lipoproteinemia)	AD	PCSK9	Proprotein convertase subtilisin /kexin Type 9
Dermatofibrosarcoma Protuberans (DFSP)	sporadic	PDGFB/ COL1A1	t(17;22) chromosome translocation; fusion of COL1A1 and PDGFB genes
Prolidase Deficiency	AR	PEPD	Prolidase (peptidase D)
Conradi-Hünermann-Happle Syndrome	AR	PEX7	Peroxin 7
Refsum Syndrome (Hereditary Motor & Sensory Neuropathy Type 4)	AR	PEX7	Peroxin 7
Rhizomelic Chondrodysplasia Punctata	AR	PEX7	Peroxin 7
Properdin Deficiency (Complement Factor Properdin Deficiency)	XLR	PFC	Properdin P Factor, Complement
Hyper IgE Syndrome (Job Syndrome)	AR	PGM3	Phosphoglucomutase-3
Refsum Syndrome (Hereditary Motor & Sensory Neuropathy Type 4, Phytanic Acid Storage Disease)	AR	PHYH	Phytanoyl-CoA 2-hydroxylase
CLOVE (Congenital, Lipomatous, Overgrowth, Vascular Malformations, Epidermal Nevi and Spinal/Skeletal Anomalies and/or Scoliosis) Syndrome	Somatic	PIK3CA	Phosphatidylinositol 3-kinase, catalytic, α
Epidermal Nevus	somatic	PIK3CA	Phosphatidylinositol 3-kinase, catalytic, α
Macrocephaly-Capillary Malformation Syndrome	Somatic	PIK3CA	Phosphatidylinositol 3-kinase, catalytic, α
SHORT (Short Stature, Hyperextensibility, Ocular Depression (Deeply Set Eyes), Rieger Anomaly, and Teething delay) Syndrome	AD	PIK3R1	Phosphatidylinositol 3-kinase, regulatory subunit 1

Disorder	Inheritance	Gene	Protein
Tuberous Sclerosis-associated Polycystic Kidney Disease	AD	PKD1	Polycystin 1
Ectodermal Dysplasia/ Skin Fragility Syndrome	AR	PKP1	Plakophilin 1
Epidermolysis Bullosa Simplex (EBS) Ogna-type	AD	PLEC1	Plectin
Epidermolysis Bullosa Simplex (EBS) with Muscular Dystrophy	AR	PLEC1	Plectin
Ehlers-Danlos Syndrome, Kyphoscoliosis-type	AR	PLOD1	Lysyl hydroxylase
Childhood Cancer Syndrome (CNS, Hematologic and GI Malignancies) with NF 1 Phenotype (formerly Lynch Syndrome)	AR	PMS2	Postmeiotic segregation increased
X-linked Reticulate Pigmentary Disorder	XLR	POLA1	Catalytic subunit of DNA polymerase-α
Xeroderma Pigmentosum, Variant (XP Variant)	AR	POLH	DNA Polymerase η (intact nucleotide excision repair)
Focal Dermal Hypoplasia (Goltz Syndrome)	XLD	PORCN	Porcupine homolog
Lipodystrophy, Familial Partial	AD	PPARG	Peroxisome proliferators activated receptor γ
Porphyria, Variegate	AD	PPOX	Protoporphyrinogen oxidase
Carney Complex (LAMB/NAME Syndrome)	AD	PRKAR1A	Protein kinase A regulatory subunit 1a
Protein C Deficiency	AD	PROC	Protein C
Kallmann Syndrome Type 4	AD/AR	PROK2	Prokineticin
Kallmann Syndrome Type 3	AD/AR	PROKR2	Prokineticin receptor 2 (a G-protein coupled receptor)
Protein S Deficiency	AD	PROS1	Protein S
CANDLE (Chronic Atypical Neutrophilic Dermatosis with Lipodystrophy and Elevated Temperature) Syndrome	AD	PSMB8	Proteasome subunit, β-type, 8
PAPA (Pyogenic Arthritis, Pyoderma Gangrenosum, Acne) Syndrome	AD	PSTPIP1 (CD2BP1)	Protein serine threonine phosphatase interacting protein 1

Disorder	Inheritance	Gene	Protein
Basal Cell Nevus Syndrome (Gorlin Syndrome)	AD	PTCH1	Patched homolog 1
Basal Cell Carcinoma, Sporadic	Sporadic	PTCH1, PTCH2, SUFU	Sonic hedgehog pathway mutations
Bannayan-Riley-Ruvalcaba Syndrome	AD	PTEN	Phosphatase and tensin homolog (tyrosine kinase)
Cowden Syndrome	AD	PTEN	Phosphatase and tensin homolog (tyrosine kinase)
Proteus-like Syndrome (Cohen-Hayden Syndrome)	AD	PTEN	Phosphatase and tensin homolog (tyrosine kinase)
Noonan Syndrome Type 1	AD	PTPN11	Protein tyrosine phosphatase, nonreceptor Type 11
Noonan Syndrome with Multiple Lentigines (formerly LEOPARD Syndrome)	AD	PTPN11 > RAF1 > BRAF, MAP2K1	Protein tyrosine phosphatase, nonreceptor Type 11
Phenylketonuria	AR	PTS	6-Pyruvoyl-tetrahydropterin synthase
Ehlers-Danlos Syndrome, Cleft Lip/Palate-type	AR	PVRL1	Nectin-1 poliovirus receptor related 1
Cutis Laxa, Type IIB	AR	PYCR1	Pyrroline-5-carboxylate reductase 1
Phenylketonuria	AR	QDPR	Quinoid dihydropteridine reductase
Griscelli Syndrome, Type 2	AR	RAB27A	Ras-associated protein
Noonan Syndrome Type 5	AD	RAF1	V-Raf-1 murine leukemia viral oncogene homolog
Severe Combined Immunodeficiency Syndrome (SCID) (B-NK+) (Omenn Syndrome)	AR	RAG1	Recombination activating gene 1
Severe Combined Immunodeficiency Syndrome (SCID) (B-NK+) (Omenn Syndrome)	AR	RAG2	Recombination activating gene 2
Squamous Cell Carcinoma, sporadic cutaneous	Sporadic	RAS / tp53	
Capillary Malformation-Arteriovenous Malformation	AD	RASA1	RAS p21 protein activator 1 (GTPase activating protein)
Parkes Weber Syndrome	NI	RASA1	p120-Ras GTPase-activating protein

Disorder	Inheritance	Gene	Protein
Retinoblastoma	Somatic > AD	RB1, MYCN	Rb
Werner Syndrome (Adult Progeria)	AR	RECQL2	RecQ protein-like 2 (DNA helicase)
Bloom Syndrome	AR	RECQL3	RecQ protein like 3 (DNA helicase)
Rothmund-Thomson Syndrome	AR	RECQL4	RecQ protein like 1 (DNA helicase)
Multiple Endocrine Neoplasia (MEN) Syndrome Type 2A (Sipple)	AD	RET	Ret-proto-oncogene (cysteine-rich extracellular domain)
Noonan Syndrome Type 8	AD	RIT1	RIC-like protein without CAAX motif 1 (RAS-like protein)
Cartilage-Hair Hypoplasia Syndrome	AR	RMRP	RNA component of mitochondrial RNA-processing endoribonuclease
Palmoplantar Keratoderma (PPK) with cutaneous SCC and sex reversal	AR	RSPO1	R-spondin family, member 1
Anonychia Congenita	AR	RSPO4	R-spondin family, member 4
Dyskeratosis Congenita (Zinsser-Engman-Cole Syndrome)	AD or AR	RTEL1	Regulator of telomere elongation helicase 1
Normophosphatemic Familial Tumoral Calcinosis	AR	SAMD9	Sterile α motif domain-containing 9
Disseminated Superficial Porokeratosis	AD	SART3	Squamous Cell Carcinoma Antigen Recognized by T cells 3
Keratosis Follicularis Spinulosa Decalvans	XLR > AD	SAT1	Spermidine/spermine N(1)-acetyltransferase
Congenital Insensitivity to Pain	AR	SCN9A	Voltage-gated sodium channel
Erythromelalgia, Primary	AD	SCN9A	Voltage-gated sodium channel
Antithrombin III Deficiency	AD	SERPINC1	Serpin peptidase inhibitor C1 (antithrombin III)
Noonan-Like Syndrome with Loose Anagen Hair	AD	SHOC2	Suppressor of Clear, C. elegans
Hemochromatosis	AD	SLC11A3	Solute carrier family 40, member 1 (ferroportin)
Ichthyosis, Prematurity Syndrome	AR	SLC27A4	Solute carrier family 27, member 4 (fatty acid transporter)
H Syndrome	AR	SLC29A3	Solute carrier family 29, member 3 (nucleoside transporter)

J. Finch & M. Payette

Disorder	Inheritance	Gene	Protein
Arterial Tortuosity Syndrome	AR	SLC2A10	Solute carrier family 2, member 10 (facilitated glucose transporter)
Leukocyte Adhesion Deficiency Type II (Congenital Disorder of Glycosylation Type IIc)	AR	SLC35C1	Solute carrier family 35, member c1 (neutrophil sialyl-LewisX)
Acrodermatitis Enteropathica	AR	SLC39A4	Solute carrier family 39, member 4 (zinc transporter)
Oculocutaneous Albinism Type 4 (OCA4)	AR	SLC45A2 (MATP)	Solute carrier family 45, member 2
Hartnup Disease	AR	SLC6A19	Solute carrier family 6, member 19 (BOAT1 neutral amino acid transporter)
Hypertrophic Osteoarthropathy (Pachydermo-periostosis, Touraine-Solente-Golé Syndrome)	AR	SLCO2A1	Solute carrier family 21, member 2 (prostaglandin transporter)
Waardenburg Syndrome Type 2	AR	SLUG	Snail homolog 2
Mal de Meleda	AR	SLURP1	Secreted LY6/Plaur Domain-containing protein 1
Hereditary Hemorrhagic Telangiectasia, with Juvenile Polyposis	AD	SMAD4	SMAD family member 4 (transmits signals from TGF-β receptor)
Basal Cell Carcinoma, Sporadic	Sporadic	SMO	Smoothened (G protein-coupled receptor-like receptor)
Niemann-Pick Disease Type A	AR	SMPD1	Sphingomyelin phosphodiesterase 1
Piebaldism	AD	SNAI2	Snail homolog 2
CEDNIK (Cerebral Dysgenesis, Neuropathy, Ichthyosis and Keratoderma) Syndrome	AR	SNAP29	Synaptosomal-associated protein, 29 kDa
Noonan Syndrome Type 4	AD	SOS1	Son of sevenless homolog 1 (guanine nucleotide exchange factor)
Noonan Syndrome Type 9	AD	SOS2	Son of sevenless homolog 2 (guanine nucleotide exchange factor)
Waardenburg Syndrome Type 4	AD	SOX10	SRY-related HMG-box gene 10
Yemenite Deaf-Blind Hypopigmentation	AD	SOX10	SRY-related HMG box gene 10

Disorder	Inheritance	Gene	Protein
Hypotrichosis-Lymphedema-Telangiectasia Syndrome	AD, AR	SOX18	Sex determining region Y (SRY)-box 18
PFAPA (Periodic Fever, Aphthous Stomatitis, Pharyngitis, Adenitis) Syndrome	Unknown	SPAG7*	Functionally linked to antiviral and inflammatory responses
Netherton Syndrome	AR	SPINK5	Serine protease inhibitor, Kazal Type 5 (lymphoepithelial Kazal-type-related inhibitor, LEKTI)
Trichorrhexis Invaginata (Netherton Syndrome)	AR	SPINK5	Serine protease inhibitor, Kazal Type 5 (lymphoepithelial Kazal-type-related inhibitor, LEKTI)
Legius Syndrome	AD	SPRED1	Sprouty-Related EVH1 Domain-containing Protein 1; regulate growth factor-induced activation of the MAP kinase cascade
Ichthyosis, Congenital with Hypotrichosis	AR	ST14	Matriptase (serine protease)
Microcephaly-Capillary Malformation Syndrome	AR	STAMBP	Stam-binding protein
Hyper IgE Syndrome (Job Syndrome)	AD	STAT3	Signal transducer and activator of transcription 3
Peutz-Jeghers Syndrome	AD	STK11 (LKB1)	Serine-threonine kinase 11
Ichthyosis, X-linked Recessive	XLR	STS	Steroid sulfatase (arylsulfatase c)
Multiple Sulfatase Deficiency	AR	SUMF1	Sulfatase-modifying factor 1
Leigh Syndrome	AR	SURF1	Surfeit 1
Richner-Hanhart Syndrome	AR	TAT	Tyrosine aminotransferase
Tyrosinemia Type II (Richner-Hanhart Syndrome)	AR	TAT	Tyrosine aminotransferase
DiGeorge Syndrome (CATCH-22, Thymic Hypoplasia)	AD	TBX1	T-box 1
Thymic Hypoplasia (DiGeorge Syndrome)	AD	TBX1	T-box 1
Venous Malformations, Multiple Cutaneous and Mucosal	AD	TEK (TIE2)	Endothelial-specific tyrosine kinase receptor
Dyskeratosis Congenita (Zinsser-Engman-Cole Syndrome)	AD	TERC, TINF2	Telomerase complex components

Disorder	Inheritance	Gene	Protein
Dyskeratosis Congenita (Zinsser-Engman-Cole Syndrome)	AD or AR	TERT	Telomerase catalytic subunit
Hemochromatosis	AR	TFR2	Transferrin receptor 2
Ferguson-Smith Syndrome (Multiple self-healing Squamous Epitheliomas)	AD	TGFβR1	TGF-β receptor 1
Loeys-Dietz Syndrome Type I	AD	TGFβR1	TGF-β receptor 1
Loeys-Dietz Syndrome Type II	AD	TGFβR2	TGF-β receptor 2
Marfan Syndrome Type 2	AD	TGFβR2	TGF-β receptor 2
Lamellar Ichthyosis	AR	TGM1	Transglutaminase 1
Non-bullous Congenital Ichthyosiform Erythroderma	AR	TGM1	Transglutaminase 1
Acral Peeling Skin Syndrome	AR	TGM5	Transglutaminase 5
Goeminne (Torticollis, Keloids, Cryptorchidism, Renal Dysplasia) Syndrome	XLD	TKCR	Unknown
Epidermodysplasia Verruciformis	AR	TMC6 (EVER1)	Transmembrane channel-like 6
Epidermodysplasia Verruciformis	AR	TMC8 (EVER2)	Transmembrane channel-like 8
Common Variable Immunodeficiency	Sporadic > AR > AD	TNFRSF13B	Transmembrane activator & CAML interactor (TACI)
IgA Deficiency Type II	Unknown	TNFRSF13B	Transmembrane activator & CAML interactor (TACI)
Familial Hibernian Fever (Tumor Necrosis Factor Receptor Associated Periodic Syndrome; TRAPS)	AD	TNFRSF1A	Tumor necrosis factor receptor superfamily, member 1A
Ehlers-Danlos Syndrome, Classic	AR	TNXB	Tenascin X, a glycoprotein of the extracellular matrix
Ehlers-Danlos Syndrome, Hypermobility-type	AD	TNXB	Tenascin X, a glycoprotein of the extracellular matrix
Howel-Evans Syndrome (Tylosis-Esophageal CA)	AD	TOC (RHBDF2)	Inhibitory rhomboid-like (rhomboid 5) pseudoproteases, inhibit EGFR signaling
P14 Deficiency, Immunodeficiency Syndrome	AR	TP14	p14 (MAPBP-interacting protein)

Disorder	Inheritance	Gene	Protein
Basal Cell Carcinoma, Sporadic	Sporadic	TP53	p53
Li-Fraumeni Syndrome	AD	TP53	p53
Squamous Cell Carcinoma, Sporadic Ccutaneous	Sporadic	TP53	p53
Acro-Dermato-Ungual-Lacrimal Tooth (ADULT) Syndrome	AD	TP63	p63
Ankyloblepharon-Ectodermal Dysplasia-Cleft Lip/Palate (AEC) Syndrome (Hay-Wells Syndrome, Rapp-Hodgkin Syndrome)	AD	TP63	p63
Ectrodactyly Ectodermal Dysplasia Cleft Lip/Palate (EEC) Syndrome	AD	TP63	p63
Limb-mammary Syndrome	AD	TP63	p63
Familial Chilblain Lupus	AD	TREX1	3' repair TREX1 endonuclease 1
Down Syndrome	Chromosome 21	Trisomy 21	N/A
Trichorhinophalangeal Syndrome Type I	AD	TRPS1	Zinc finger transcription factor
Trichorhinophalangeal Syndrome Type III	AR	TRPS1	Zinc finger transcription factor
Trichorhinophalangeal Syndrome Type II (Langer-Giedion Syndrome)	AR	TRPS1, EXT1	Contiguous gene deletion, zinc finger transcription factor/Exostosin glycosyltransferase 1
Olmsted Syndrome	AD	TRPV3	Transient receptor potential cation channel, subfamily V, member 3
Tuberous Sclerosis-1	AD	TSC1	Hamartin / GTPase activating protein of rap1 GAP family
Tuberous Sclerosis-2	AD	TSC2	Tuberin / GTPase activating protein of rap1 GAP family
Lymphangioleio-myomatosis	Somatic	TSC2	Tuberin / GTPase activating protein of rap1 GAP family
Heredofamilial Systemic Amyloidosis (Familial Amyloid Polyneuropathy)	AD	TTR	Transthyretin
Setleis Syndrome	AR	TWIST2	Twist, Drosophila, Homolog of, 2
Hyper IgE Syndrome (Job Syndrome)	AR	TYK2	Tyrosine kinase 2

J. Finch & M. Payette

Disorder	Inheritance	Gene	Protein
Oculocutaneous Albinism Types 1A, 1B (OCA1A, 1B)	AR	TYR	Tyrosinase (absent-OCA1; or decreased OCA1B activity)
Oculocutaneous Albinism Type 3 (OCA3)	AR	TYRP1	Tyrosinase-related protein 1
Sclerotylosis (Huriez Syndrome)	AD	TYS	Unknown
Bazex-Dupré-Christol Syndrome (Bazex Syndrome, Follicular Atrophoderma and Basal Cell Carcinomas)	XLD	UBE2A*	Protein involved in repair of UV-damaged DNA
Angelman Syndrome	NI	UBE3A	Ubiquitin-Protein Ligase E3A; genomic imprinting caused by deletion or inactivation of genes on the maternally inherited chromosome 15
Johanson-Blizzard Syndrome	AR	UBR1	Ubiquitin-protein ligase E3 component N-recognin 1
Hyper IgM Syndrome	AR	UNG	Uracil-DNA glycosylase
Candidiasis, Familial Chronic Mucocutaneous Type 1	AD	Unknown	Unknown
Candidiasis, Familial Chronic Mucocutaneous Type 3	AD	Unknown	Unknown
Dyschromatosis Universalis Hereditaria	AD	Unknown	Unknown
Dyskeratosis, Hereditary Benign Intraepithelial	AD	Unknown	Unknown
Familial Generalized Lentiginosis	AD	Unknown	Unknown
Gorham-Stout Syndrome	NI	Unknown	Unknown
HAIR-AN (HyperAndrogenism, Insulin Resistance, Acanthosis Nigricans) Syndrome	NI	Unknown	Unknown
Hereditary Hemorrhagic Telangiectasia, Type 3	Unknown	Unknown	Unknown
Hereditary Hemorrhagic Telangiectasia, Type 4	AD	Unknown	Unknown
Isolated Congenital Nail Dysplasia	AD	Unknown	Unknown

Disorder	Inheritance	Gene	Protein
Keratolytic Winter Erythema (Oudtshoorn Skin Disease)	AD	Unknown	Unknown
Keratosis Pilaris Atrophicans Faciei (Ulerythema Ophryogenes)	AD	Unknown	Unknown
Laugier-Hunziker Syndrome	NI	Unknown	May be simply acquired pigmentation, not a genetic syndrome
Lipomatosis, Familial Multiple	AD	Unknown	Unknown
Lymphangiomatosis	Unknown	Unknown	Unknown
Macular-type Hereditary Bullous Dystrophy (Mendes da Costa Syndrome)	XLR	Unknown	Unknown
Nezelof Syndrome (Thymic Dysplasia with Normal Immunoglobulins)	AR	Unknown	Purine nucleoside phosphorylase (PNP) deficiency
Nicolau-Balus Syndrome	Unknown	Unknown	Unknown
Noonan Syndrome Type 2	AR	Unknown	Unknown
Oasthouse Urine Syndrome (Methionine Malabsorption Syndrome)	AR	Unknown	Unknown
Pili Annulati (Ringed Hair)	AD	Unknown	Unknown
Pili Torti (Twisted Hair)	Unknown	Unknown	Unknown
Poland Syndrome	Sporadic	Unknown	Unknown
Rasmussen Syndrome	Unknown	Unknown	Unknown
Rombo Syndrome	AD	Unknown	Unknown
Russell-Silver Syndrome	Sporadic	Unknown	Unknown
Senter Syndrome (Desmons' Syndrome)	Unknown	Unknown	Unknown
Uncombable Hair Syndrome (Spun Glass Hair, Pili Trianguli et Canaliculi)	AD	Unknown	Unknown
X-linked Reticulate Pigmentary Disorder, Partington-type	XLR	Unknown	Unknown
Hepatoerythropoietic Porphyria	AR	UROD	Uroporphyrinogen-III decarboxylase
Porphyria, Cutanea Tarda (PCT)	AD	UROD	Uroporphyrinogen-III decarboxylase
Porphyria, Congenital Erythropoietic (Gunther Disease)	AR	UROS	Uroporphyrinogen-III synthase
Wagner Syndrome	AD	VCAN	Versican

Ludicrous 17-Page Genoderm Table (sorted by gene)

Disorder	Inheritance	Gene	Protein
Vitamin D-dependent Rickets with Alopecia	AR	VDR	Vitamin D receptor
Von Hippel-Lindau Syndrome	AD	VHL	VHL tumor suppressor
Arthrogryposis–Renal Dysfunction–Cholestasis (ARC) Syndrome	AR	VPS33B	Vacuolar protein sorting 33 homolog B
Wiskott-Aldrich Syndrome	XLR	WAS	WAS Protein, regulates transduction of Cdc42 protein, which regulates cytoskeleton in T-cells
Odonto-Onycho-Dermal Dysplasia	AR	WNT10A	Wingless-type MMTV integration site family, member 10A
Schöpf-Schulz-Passarge Syndrome	AR	WNT10A	Wingless-type MMTV integration site family, member 10A
Wilms Tumor	Somatic > AD	WT-1, BRCA2, GPC3	Wilms tumor 1. Tumor suppressor gene
Turner Syndrome	XO	XO	Single X chromosome
Xeroderma Pigmentosum C (XPC)	AR	XPC	DNA damage-binding protein in nucleotide excision repair
Klinefelter Syndrome	NI	XXY	N/A
Mandibuloacral Dysplasia Syndrome	AR	ZMPSTE24	Zinc metallopeptidase (STE24 homolog)
Restrictive Dermopathy	AR	ZMPSTE24	Zinc metallopeptidase (STE24 homolog)
Werner Syndrome, Atypical	AR	ZMPSTE24	Zinc metallopeptidase (STE24 homolog)
Seborrhea-like Dermatitis with Psoriasiform Elements	AD	ZNF750	Zinc finger protein 750

Index

Symbol

A

B

C

D

J. Finch & M. Payette

www.ingramcontent.com/pod-product-compliance
Lightning Source LLC
Chambersburg PA
CBHW041704210326
41598CB00007B/531